CULTURE OF EPITHELIAL CELLS

Second Edition

D0701721

Culture of Specialized Cells

Series Editor

R. Ian Freshney

CULTURE OF HEMATOPOIETIC CELLS
R. Ian Freshney, Ian B. Pragnell and Mary G. Freshney, Editors

CULTURE OF IMMORTALIZED CELLS
R. Ian Freshney and Mary G. Freshney, Editors

DNA TRANSFER TO CULTURED CELLS
Katya Ravid and R. Ian Freshney, Editors

CULTURE OF EPITHELIAL CELLS, SECOND EDITION
R. Ian Freshney and Mary Freshney, Editors

CULTURE OF EPITHELIAL CELLS

Second Edition

Editors

R. Ian Freshney and Mary G. Freshney
CRC Beatson Laboratories
Glasgow, Scotland

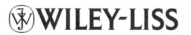

A JOHN WILEY & SONS, INC., PUBLICATION

Copyright © 2002 by Wiley-Liss, Inc., New York. All rights reserved.

Published simultaneously in Canada.

For ordering and customer service, call 1-800-CALL-WILEY.

Library of Congress Cataloging-in-Publication Data:

Culture of epithelial cells / editors, R. Ian Freshney and Mary G. Freshney. — 2nd ed.
    p. ; cm. — (Culture of specialized cells)
  Includes bibliographical references and index.
  ISBN 0-471-40121-8 (cloth : alk. paper)
    1. Epithelial cells. 2. Cell culture.. 3. Epithelium—Cultures and culture media.
I. Freshney, R. Ian. II. Freshney, Mary G. III. Series.
  [DNLM: 1. Epithelial Cells. 2. Cell Differentiation. 3. Cells, Cultured. 4. Cytological Techniques. QS 532.5.E7 C968 2002]
  QP88.4 .C85 2002
  611'.0187—dc21
                                       2001045535

Printed in the United States of America.

10 9 8 7 6 5 4 3 2 1

Contents

Contributors

(Email addresses are only provided for those who have been designated as corresponding authors)

Catherine Booth, EpiStem Ltd., Incubator Building, Grafton St., Manchester M13 9XX, UK. Email: *Cbooth@epistem.co.uk*.

Leland G. Dobbs, Suite 150, University of California Laurel Heights Campus, 3333 California Street, San Francisco, CA 94118, USA. Email: *dobbs@itsa.ucs.edu*.

R. Ian Freshney, CRC Department of Medical Oncology, CRC Beatson Laboratories, University of Glasgow, Garscube Estate, Bearsden, Glasgow G61 1BD, UK. Email: *I.Freshney@beatson.gla.ac.uk*.

Norbert E. Fusenig, Division of Carcinogenesis and Differentiation, German Cancer Research Center (Deutsches Krebsforschungszentrum), Im Neuenheimer Feld 280, D-69120 Heidelberg, Germany. Email: *n.fusenig@dkfz-heidelberg.de*.

Robert F. Gonzalez, Suite 150, University of California Laurel Heights Campus, 3333 California Street, San Francisco, CA 94118, USA.

Roland C. Grafström, Experimental Carcinogenesis, Inst. Environmental Medicine, Karolinska Institutet, S-171 77 Stockholm, Sweden. Email: *roland.grafstrom@imm.ki.se*.

Christiane Guguen-Guillouzo, INSERM U522, Régulations des Equilibres Fonctionnels du Foie Normal et Pathologique, Hôpital Pontchaillou, av. de la Bataille, F-35033 Rennes, France. Email: *christiane.guillouzo@rennes.inserm.fr*.

John F. Lechner, Bayer Diagnostics, Emeryville, CA 94608, USA. Email: *John.Lechner.B@bayer.com*.

Nicole Maas-Szabowski, Division of Carcinogenesis and Differentiation, German Cancer Research Center (Deutsches Krebsforschungszentrum), Im Neuenheimer Feld 280, D-69120 Heidelberg, Germany.

John R. W. Masters, Institute of Urology, University College, St. Paul's Hospital, 3rd Floor, 67 Riding House Street, London, UK.

Julie A. O'Shea, EpiStem Ltd., Incubator Building, Grafton St., Manchester M13 9XX, UK.

E. Kenneth Parkinson, The Beatson Institute for Cancer Research, Garscube Estate, Switchback Road, Bearsden, Glasgow G61 1BD, Scotland, UK. Email: *K.Parkinson@beatson.gla.ac.uk.*

Donna M. Peehl, Department of Urology, Stanford University School of Medicine, Stanford, CA 94305, USA. Email: *dpeehl@leland.stanford.edu.*

Jennifer Southgate, Jack Birch Unit of Molecular Carcinogenesis, Department of Biology University of York, York, UK. Email: *js35@york.ac.uk.*

Martha R. Stampfer, Lawrence Berkeley National Laboratory, Life Sciences Division, Bldg. 70A-1118, Berkeley, CA 94720, USA. Email: *mrstampfer@lbl.gov.*

Margaret A. Stanley, Department of Pathology, University of Cambridge, Tennis Court Road, Cambridge CB2 1QP, UK. Email: *mas@mole.bio.cam.ac.uk.*

Hans-Jürgen Stark, Division of Carcinogenesis and Differentiation, German Cancer Research Center (Deutsches Krebsforschungszentrum), Im Neuenheimer Feld 280, D-69120 Heidelberg, Germany.

Joyce Taylor-Papadimitriou, Guy's Hospital, 3rd Floor, Thomas Guy House, London SE1 9RT, UK.

Ludwik K. Trejdosiewicz, ICRF Cancer Medicine Research Unit, St. James's University Hospital, Leeds, UK.

John Wise, Yale University, School of Medicine, New Haven, CT 06520, USA.

Paul Yaswen, Lawrence Berkeley National Laboratory, Life Sciences Division, Bldg. 70A-1118, Berkeley, CA 94720, USA.

W. Andrew Yeudall, Molecular Carcinogenesis Group, Guy's King's & St. Thomas' Schools of Medicine & Dentistry, King's College London, London SE1 9RT, UK.

Preface

Culture of Epithelial Cells was first published in 1992, and, although many of the basic techniques described have not changed materially, there are a number of significant innovations that, together with a need to update references and suppliers, justify a second edition. In addition, several types of epithelia were not represented in the first edition and have been included here, either as new invited chapters or in the final chapter, where a number of different epithelia not covered in the invited chapters, are presented in review form with some additional protocols. It is hoped that this will give a more complete, as well as more up-to-date, guide to epithelial culture techniques and that, where protocols are not provided, for example, for some less widely used epithelia, the references provided will lead the reader into the relevant literature.

The layout is similar to other books in the "Culture of Specialized Cells" series, providing background, preparation of reagents, step-by-step protocols, applications, and alternative techniques, with the sources of the reagents and materials provided in an appendix to each chapter. The address of each supplier is provided at the end of the book. For the sake of consistency, tissue culture grade water is referred to ultra-pure water (UPW) regardless of the mode of preparation but assuming at least a triple stage purification, for example, distillation or reverse osmosis coupled to carbon filtration and deionization, usually with micropore filtration at the delivery point. Calcium- and magnesium-free phosphate-buffered saline is referred to as PBSA, the Ca^{2+} and Mg^{2+} supplement being referred to as PBSB, and the complete solution, PBS. Abbreviations are defined at the front of the book, after the Contents and Prefaces. Most abbreviations are standard, but some have been coined by individual authors and are explained when first introduced.

We are greatly indebted to the individual contributors for making their expertise available in these chapters and for their patience in responding to suggestions and queries during review. We hope that this compilation will provide a good starting point for those who wish to progress from routine culture of continuous cell lines into the realms of culture of specialized epithelia. It has not been possible to deal with every type of epithelium, and this was never the intention, but, hopefully, there is sufficient information at least to provide a rational approach to culturing the better-known epithelia and to provide a basis for approaching other epithelia not dealt with in detail here.

R. Ian Freshney and Mary G. Freshney

Preface to First Edition

It is now the age of the specialized cell in culture. Along with advances in biotechnology, which are gradually enabling specialized product formation in rather artificial host cells, there is an increasing need to understand the regulation of specialized functions in the very cells in which these functions are determined by ontogeny. This is the only way that the fundamental regulatory processes may be understood and that the aberrations that arise in disease can be defined and controlled. This volume, the first in a series of books on the culture and manipulation of specialized cells for experimentation in vitro, is devoted to epithelial cell culture.

The practice of tissue and cell culture is now firmly established as a standard research method in many laboratories. In the majority of cases, cultures are used as production substrates for cell products or as investigative tools for studying the control mechanisms of gene expression, cell proliferation, and transformation. Tissue culture has now progressed sufficiently, however, that investigators are prepared to ask questions about how specific cells express their specialized phenotypes and how regulatory processes fail in neoplasia and other forms of metabolic disease. While it might be sufficient in the study of molecular functions to have an all-purpose fibroblast or HeLa cell culture, if one wishes to study what makes a primitive stem cell mature into a keratinocyte or enterocyte, one must have the capacity to culture the specific lineage in question.

Much of the interest that has developed in recent years, both on the kinetics of stem cell regeneration and on the mechanisms of differentiation and neoplasia, has focused on epithelial cells. This is partly because these cells provide some of the best characterized models for cell proliferation, regeneration, and differentiation, but also because epithelial cells form the cellular environment where the majority of common solid tumors arise.

Culture of epithelium has, traditionally, been fraught with problems related to overgrowth of stromal cells for which the culture environment has seemed to be more suitable. Various physical separation methods and selective culture techniques have been developed over the years to reduce fibroblast contamination and suppress fibroblast overgrowth. A general consensus is emerging that the culture conditions have to be favorable and selective for epithelial survival in order for realistic studies to be performed in epithelial cell biology. Consequently, a common theme throughout much of this book is the definition of the correct selective environment to favor the survival of the particular cells of interest.

Authors have been chosen by virtue of the cell type in which their main research interest lies. They have also been chosen for their recognized expertise in the field, and the methods described will often have been documented previously in refereed publications. Our objective is not to present a procedure that is new and untried, but to provide an established technology on which the investigator can depend.

A fundamental ignorance of how cells work has previously permitted us to have been content to study any cell in culture. Now, although far from fully conversant with all aspects of fundamental cell biology, we need to move on to look at more complex systems—systems more complex in their regulation whereby the cell type may be highly specialized—and systems more complex that force us, when modeling three-dimensional tissue rather than simple cellular functions, to explore the regulatory information passing between different cell types as well as their specific responses to more general systemic signals. This book, and those planned to follow, will attempt to examine these complexities.

R. Ian Freshney
June 12, 1991

List of Abbreviations

2×AL-15	Leibowitz L-15 medium with double-strength antibiotics
ATCC	American Type Culture Collection
AUM	asymmetric unit membrane
BPE	bovine pituitary extract
BPH	benign prostatic hyperplasia
BrdU	bromodeoxyuridine
BSA	bovine serum albumin
CDK	cyclin-dependent kinase
CIN	cervical intraepithelial neoplasia
CFE	colony-forming efficiency
CG	clonal growth
CMRL	Connaught Medical Research Laboratory
CSFBS	charcoal-stripped fetal bovine serum
CT	cholera toxin
CYP	cytochrome P
DMEM	Dulbecco's modification of Eagle's medium
DMSO	dimethyl sulfoxide
DNase	deoxyribonuclease
DTT	dithiothreitol
EDTA	ethylene diaminetetraacetic acid
EHS	Engelbreth-Holm-Swarm
EGF	epidermal growth factor
EGTA	ethylene glycol-bis(β-aminoethyl ether) N,N,N',N'-tetraacetic acid
FBS	fetal bovine serum
FCS	fetal calf serum (used synonymously with FBS)
FGF	fibroblast growth factor
FN/V/BSA	fibronectin, Vitrogen 100, and bovine serum albumin
GI	growth inhibition
GM-CSF	granulocyte-macrophage colony-stimulating factor
GST	glutathione-S-transferase
HBS	HEPES-buffered salt solution
HBSS	Hanks' balanced salt solution

HCMF	Hanks' balanced salt solution without Ca^{2+} and Mg^{2+}
HEPES	4-(2-hydroxyethyl)-1-piperazine-ethanesulfonic acid
HGF	hepatocyte growth factor
HGSIL	high-grade squamous intraepithelial lesions
HLF	human lung fibroblasts
HMEC	human mammary epithelial cells
HMM	hepatocyte minimal medium
HPV	human papillomavirus
IGF	insulin-like growth factor
IgG	immuno-γ-globulin
IL-1,6,8	interleukin-1,6,8
i.p.	intraperitoneal
KGF	keratinocyte growth factor
KIU	kallikrein-inactivating units
KSFMc	complete keratinocyte serum-free medium
LGSIL	low-grade squamous intraepithelial lesions
LHC	Laboratory of Human Carcinogenesis
LTR	long terminal repeat
MCDB	Molecular, Cellular and Developmental Biology (U. Colorado, Boulder)
mRNA	messenger RNA
MM	low-serum-containing medium
MX	milk mix
NBS	newborn bovine serum
NGF	nerve growth factor
NHBE	normal human bronchial epithelium
NHU	normal human urothelial
PAP	prostatic acid phosphatase
PAS	periodic acid-Schiff reagent
PBS	Dulbecco's phosphate-buffered saline with 0.5 mM $MgCl_2$ and 0.9 mM $CaCl_2$
PBSA	Dulbecco's phosphate-buffered saline without Ca^{2+} and Mg^{2+}
PCNA	proliferating cell nuclear antigen
PD	population doublings
PD/D	population doublings per day
PDGF	platelet-derived growth factor
PEM	polymorphic epithelial mucin
PET	polyvinylpyrrolidone, EGTA, and trypsin
pH	hydrogen ion concentration
PSA	prostate-specific antigen
PVP	polyvinylpyrrolidone
RPMI	Rosewell Park Memorial Institute

R-point	restriction point
RPTC	renal proximal tubule cells
SBTI	soybean trypsin inhibitor
S-DMEM	DMEM containing sorbitol
SIL	squamous intraepithelial lesions
SV40T	simian virus 40 T antigen
T3	triiodothyronine
TCP	tissue culture plastic
TD	terminal differentiation (= squamous in Chapter 7)
TDLU	terminal ductal lobular units
TGF	transforming growth factor
TNF	tumor necrosis factor
TSD	terminal saturation density
UP	uroplakin protein
UPW	ultra-pure water

1

Introduction

R. Ian Freshney

CRC Department of Medical Oncology, CRC Beatson Laboratories,
University of Glasgow, Bearsden, Glasgow G61 1BD, United Kingdom.
I.Freshney@beatson.gla.ac.uk

"Epithelium" describes the various layers of cells that either coat surfaces on the exterior of the organism or line internal organs, ducts, or secretory acini. They may act as a total barrier, such as the epidermis, with minimum permeation of polar substances, or a regulated barrier, for example, in the intestine and the lung, where selected substances are able to cross the plasma membrane or the whole epithelium via specific transporters. Although other tissue cells assume transitory or permanent polarity along the long axis of the cell, basal to apical polarization is fundamental to the normal function of all epithelia. Epithelia are associated with the major functional role of many tissues, such as hepatocytes and liver metabolism, epidermal keratinocytes and the barrier properties of skin, pancreatic acinar cells and digestive enzyme secretion, and so on, and have been a focus of interest in the development of in vitro models for many years. Because most epithelia are renewable, they have proliferating precursor compartments and stem cells capable of self-renewal and hence form attractive models for studying the regulation of cell proliferation and differentiation.

Because of their regenerative nature, many epithelia are frequent sites for malignant transformation in vivo, and the most common solid tumors are the carcinomas of lung, breast, colon, prostate, and bladder, derived from the epithelial cells of these tissues. Epithelial cell systems have therefore been adopted as appropriate models for studies of carcinogenesis, and of differentiation, on the assumption that malignancy results, at least in part, from a failure to differentiate. This has produced many excellent models for differentiation and, owing to the geometry of tissues such as skin and intestine, some of the clearest examples of stem cell maturation, although without the supporting detail on stem cell identity that has exemplified progress in the hemopoietic system.

I. FUNCTIONS OF EPITHELIUM

Epithelium usually is found at the interface between the organism and the environment (epidermis, bronchial, or alveolar epithelium) or between an organ and a fluid space (enterocytes of the gut, tubular epithelium of the kidney, or hepatocytes and biliary epithelium of the liver). This location implies that the regulation of permeability, transport, endocytosis, and exocytosis is a major requirement. Furthermore, if permeability is to be regulated, then transcellular transport is likely to predominate and pericellular transport to be restricted. Characteristically, epithelium expresses active control of transcellular permeability and a passive, but stringent, blockade of pericellular permeability.

Epithelial cells transport fluid, ions, oxygen, and essential nutrients, and secrete products, in a polarized fashion; as we see below and in later chapters, shape and polarity are vital elements in the expression of the differentiated epithelial phenotype. Furthermore, epithelium is well suited to monolayer culture, as many epithelia are simple avascular monolayers or multilayers that are sufficiently thin to be still dependent on diffusion for nutrient supply.

2. HISTOLOGY

Epithelial cell layers are separated from other cellular compartments (e.g., connective tissue, capillaries) by a basement membrane made up of collagen, laminin, fibronectin, and proteoglycans, and the reconstitution of this basement membrane in vitro has been featured in many attempts to grow functional epithelium. The basement membrane is usually a joint product of the epithelium and the underlying stroma and, together with soluble factors from the stroma, serves to regulate the differentiated function of the epithelium (see below) as well as providing physical support and a barrier separating epithelial and stromal compartments.

Epithelial cells are closely associated in vivo, as implied by their regulated permeability and transport functions; to maintain this structural integrity, they are usually joined by desmosomes (Fig. 1.1a), the mechanical junctions connected to the intermediate filament cytoskeleton that hold epithelium together and are characteristic markers of epithelial identity [Moll et al., 1986]. Where barrier properties are particularly crucial (e.g., kidney ductal epithelium, or secretory acini), the desmosomes are accompanied by tight junctions forming a junctional complex that is quite specific to epithelium (Fig. 1.1b). The presence of these junctional complexes, together with cytokeratin intermediate filaments (see Chapter 5), provide very useful and specific markers for recognizing epithelial cells in vitro.

3. EMBRYOLOGICAL ORIGIN

Following gastrulation in the embryo, the previously simple hollow ball of cells, or blastula, becomes multilayered, and these layers eventually form the outer germ layer of the embryo, the ectoderm, the inner germ layer, the endoderm, and the cells lying in between the two layers, the mesoderm. Whereas the mesoderm generates the connective, skeletal, and hemopoietic tissues, it is the ectoderm and endoderm that generate the epithelial layers. Two exceptions, which are mesodermally derived, are the collecting duct-lining cells of the kidney and the mesothelial cells, which line body cavities like the peritoneum and pleura. Although mesodermally derived, both cell types express characteristic cytokeratin intermediate filaments; mesothelium lacks desmosomes, however.

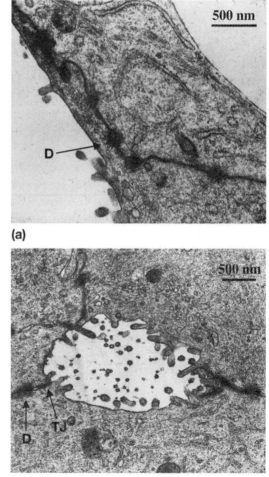

Fig 1.1. Junctions between epithelial cells. Transmission EM of sections through CA-KD cells grown on gas-permeable membrane Petri dish (Heraeus). (a) Desmosomes [D] show as dark blobs on the dark-staining opposed membranes of adjacent cells. (b) Canaliculus that formed in the same culture at an area of high cell density, showing junctional complexes (desmosomes and tight junctions [TJ]). Culture and photographs courtesy of C.M. MacDonald. Reproduced from Freshney [2000].

4. STEM CELLS AND MATURATION

In common with the hemopoietic system, and distinct from the supporting tissues, epithelial cells are constantly regenerated. This process may be quite rapid, as in the intestine and epidermis, or quite slow, as in liver and pancreas. Although as yet unidentified, stem cells exist in the basal layer of the epidermis (possibly localized in the outer root sheath of the hair follicles), in the crypts of the intestine, and possibly in the junction of the bile duct epithelium and bile canaliculi, constantly regenerating the functional epithelium as the terminally differentiated cells senesce, die, and are shed. These cells, plus the proliferating precursor cell compartment, make up the bulk of the cells in a proliferating culture. The distribution of the population among the stem cell, precursor cell, and differentiated cell compartments will influence the functional capacity and reproductive potential of the culture and create a degree of heterogeneity that is difficult to avoid in this type of regenerative tissue. Greater homogeneity can be achieved by isolating different stages in the lineage by physical techniques (see below), or by inducing proliferation and inhibiting differentiation (see Section 8, Differentiation), thereby increasing the proportion of stem and precursor cells. The longevity of the stem cell compartment is what will ultimately determine the lifespan of the culture.

Heterogeneity is not only derived from the disposition of cells within one differentiating pathway or lineage but may also be generated by differentiation down more than one pathway. Usually the environmental conditions will favor one particular lineage, but in some cases, particularly with cell lines derived from tumors, multiple phenotypes may be present within the culture, or even within one cell.

5. ISOLATION AND CULTURE

5.1. Disaggregation

As epithelial layers are closely associated in vivo and are strongly self-adherent, it is not surprising to find that they tend to survive better in vitro as clusters or sheets of cells. Dissociation techniques that have been found to be most successful tend to exploit this observation and do not try to reduce the population to a single cell suspension. For this reason, cultures have been derived either by gentle mechanical disaggregation or collagenase digestion in preference to trypsinization. Collagenase, in particular, appears to give good survival as it does not completely dissociate the epithelium but frees it from the surrounding stroma. The clusters of epithelium formed by this technique can often be collected preferentially by allowing them to sediment through the more finely dispersed fibroblastic stromal cells or by filtration through nylon gauze (see Chapter 4).

However, it is very difficult to eliminate all the fibroblasts by physical methods and, because of their more rapid growth rate, they will tend to overgrow the culture. This is caused by the stimulation of the fibroblasts by platelet-derived growth factor (PDGF) and by the cytostatic effect on the epithelium of transforming growth factor type α (TGF-α), released from platelets during the preparation of serum. It is also due partly to the design of the media, many of which were developed for fibroblastic cells (e.g., the NCTC Strain L).

5.2. Selective Attachment

Several methods have been developed, with varying degrees of sophistication and success, in the attempt to repress fibroblastic overgrowth. One simple method that is sometimes effective, at least for short periods of culture, is to seed the cell mixture into a flask for a short time (e.g., 30 min or 1 h) and then transfer the unattached cells into a fresh flask. This is repeated at intervals of 1–3 h up to 24 h or 48 h, and it is often found that the fibroblasts tend to stick down first, whereas the epithelial cells remain in suspension and attach in the later-seeded flasks. This is probably due to a combination of circumstances, some mechanical (the size of the epithelial aggregates) and some physiologic (the greater need for extracellular matrix regeneration for epithelial attachment). In general, selective adhesion methods such as these have limited success but may be of value in combination with other techniques or for short periods of culture.

5.3. Selective Detachment

Selective detachment has also been employed, and enzymes such as dispase can release epithelial sheets before the fibroblasts [Bevan et al., 1997]. Again, like selective attachment, it is effective in certain conditions, for example, releasing epithelial patches of colonic epithelial cells, but it is not universally successful and may select or alter the epithelium released [Poumay et al., 1993; Tomson et al., 1995; Schaefer et al., 1996]. EDTA can also be used to remove fibroblasts selectively from mixed cultures of keratinocytes (see Protocol 3.4).

5.4. Substrate Modification

To exploit the principle of selective attachment, some groups have attempted to modify the substrate to favor epithelial attachment. Collagen coating, particularly native or undenatured collagen, has been used to select epidermal cells [Freeman et al., 1976] and breast epithelium [Yang et al., 1980]. Collagen and laminin separately or combined, particularly in Matrigel, have also been found to encourage the expression of the differentiated phenotype in many epithelial cells [Seely and Aggeler, 1991; Kibbey et al., 1992; Darcy et al., 1995] (see also Chapters 2, 4, and 6), although this may limit their proliferative capacity. Becton Dickinson produces a modified plastic, Primaria, that has a net positive charge claimed to favor epithelial growth in preference to fibroblasts (see Chapter 13).

5.5. Feeder Layers

The most popular substrate modification is to preplate with a monolayer of fibroblasts, or other cells, that can be irradiated to prevent their further growth. A preformed layer of irradiated [Rheinwald, 1980] or mitomycin C-treated [Macpherson and Bryden, 1971] 3T3 cells enhances the survival of many epithelial cells, including keratinocytes (see Chapter 3), cervical epithelium (see Chapter 5), and breast epithelium (see Chapter 4) and appears to repress the further growth of fibroblasts. This may be caused, partly, by the ability of epithelium to attach to the fibroblasts, whereas normal fibroblasts are unable to do so, but is also probably caused by release by the feeder cells of paracrine factors that enhance epithelial survival and may block the action of TGF-β. It is probably the most generally successful method of enhancing epithelial growth and inhibiting fibroblastic overgrowth.

5.6. Cell Separation

It is possible to separate many cell types by physical methods, such as density gradient centrifugation, centrifugal elutriation, and flow cytometry [Freshney, 2000a]. Of these, flow cytometry has the greatest resolution, but it has a relatively low yield; centrifugal elutriation gives the highest yield but is only effective when there are clear distinctions in cell size. Both of these methods are technically complex to use and involve expensive equipment, but they have been used very successfully with many different cell systems [Lutz, 1992; Lag et al., 1996; Aitken et al., 1991; Boxberger et al., 1997; Swope et al., 1997].

Density gradient centrifugation is a cheaper system that has been very popular for many years and is moderately effective [Pretlow and Pretlow, 1989]. The purification achieved is seldom complete but may suffice for the generation of a purified population for immediate use; it seldom has a lasting effect, as the contaminating stromal cells usually proliferate more rapidly in standard media with serum supplementation.

Magnetic separation has become increasingly effective. Specific antibodies conjugated to iron-containing coated beads (see Appendix: Sources of Materials) have been used to isolate different cell types magnetically, either by a positive sort for epithelium [Formanek et al., 1998; Carr et al., 1999] or a negative sort for contaminating fibroblasts [Saalbach et al., 1997]. A cell suspension, previously incubated with antibody-conjugated beads, is passed down a glass cylinder, and the cells bound to the beads are trapped at the side of the tube by placing an electromagnet outside the cylinder. Turning off the current allows the beads to be eluted with the attached cells, which can be separated from the beads by trypsinization. Some systems (e.g., Miltenyi) used magnetizable microbeads that permit subsequent culture without requiring removal of the beads and have antibody conjugations suitable for both positively sorting epithelial cells and negatively sorting fibroblasts.

5.7. Selective Culture

The ideal method of purifying a population of cells is by cloning. Used in conjunction with a feeder layer, this method permits many epithelial cells to be cloned quite successfully, but unfortunately the culture may senesce before sufficient cells are generated. However, if relatively few cells are required, if the clones can be pooled, or if the line has been immortalized, cloning may prove to be the ideal method (see Chapter 10).

Selective media have become one of the principal methods for growing epithelial cells preferentially. Several media have been developed (see Chapters 3–8) capable of supporting different types of epithelial cells. They are serum-free, eliminating TGF-β and PDGF, which favor fibroblastic growth, and they often incorporate hormones and growth factors, such as hydrocortisone, isoproterenol (isoprenaline), and epidermal growth factor (EGF), which stimulate epithelial proliferation. They have the advantage that they do not depend on one selective event but continue to exert a selective pressure in a nutritionally optimized environment. Many of these media are available commercially (see Appendix: Sources of Materials) but do not always support the same plating efficiency, cell proliferation and longevity as achieved by media prepared in the laboratory or with the feeder layer system (see relevant chapters for further discussion).

6. CHARACTERIZATION

Validating selected epithelial cell lines requires the adoption of specific criteria for identifying the cells as epithelial. The time-honored method is by morphology, as most epithelial cultures have a characteristic tight pavementlike appearance with cells growing in well-circumscribed patches. However, not all epithelia grow in this manner; some show greater plasticity in shape, particularly when derived from tumors, and some mesenchyme-derived cells such as endothelium and mouse embryo fibroblasts like 3T3 cells (which are probably primitive mesenchyme rather than committed fibroblasts) can look quite epithelial at confluence. For these reasons, reliable epithelial identification has come to depend on the recognition of certain specific markers. The intermediate filament proteins have long been recognized for their tissue specificity [Lane, 1982; Moll et al., 1982; Taylor-Papadimitriou and Lane, 1987], and among these the cytokeratin group are found predominately in epithelia. Vimentin, the intermediate filament protein of fibroblasts and other mesenchymal cells, can also be expressed in epithelial cells in culture, particularly when the epithelium is derived from a tumor [Hunt and Davis, 1990], but cytokeratins are rarely seen in other cells.

Unlike the other intermediate filament proteins, the cytokeratins are a large group with considerable diversity. This means that different anti-cytokeratin antibodies may have differing specificities, enabling distinctions to be made among different types of epithelia or between different stages of differentiation. This is discussed in more detail in individual chapters but a summary is provided in Table 1.1.

When the culture reaches confluence, desmosome junctions, which are also specific to epithelia, can be detected by electron microscopy and desmosomal proteins, like desmoplakin [Moll et al., 1986], can be demonstrated by immunostaining. Where cultures of ductal cells are able to differentiate, it may also be possible to see junctional complexes with desmosomes and tight junctions in a characteristic association. Because of this ability to form tight junctions, and their ability to transport water and ions, epithelial monolayers sometime generate so-called domes, formed when the cell layer blisters off the substrate because of fluid and ion transport from the medium to the subcellular space (Fig. 1.2). This activity is characteristic of ductal and secretory epithelia.

A number of cell surface antigens have been shown to be specific to epithelium. These are often from one group of transmembrane mucinlike glycoproteins and include epithelial membrane antigen (EMA) [Heyderman et al., 1985], human milk fat globule (HMFG)-1 and HMFG-2 [Burchell et al., 1983], and Spl [Burchell et al., 1987]. These antigens are most strongly expressed in differentiated ductal epithelium, where they may become polarized to the apical surface, but present to varying degrees in many different epithelia. There are also a number of more specific markers such as involucrin in keratinocytes (see Chapters 2 and 3), which are dealt with in more detail in the appropriate chapters.

7. CROSS-CONTAMINATION

Apart from the need to determine the tissue of origin of a culture, it is also important to be able to guard against cross-

TABLE 1.1. Cytokeratins in Epithelial Cell Characterization

Cell type		Cytokeratin Expressed		Ref.
		In vivo	In vitro	
Epidermal keratinocytes	All	K5, K14	K5, K14	(See Chapter 2)
	All suprabasal	K1, K10	K1, K10	(See Chapter 2)
	Stratum granulosum	K2e	K2e	(See Chapter 2)
Cervical kertinocytes	Ectocervix	K5, K19	K5, K19	(See Chapter 5)
	Endocervix	K18	K18	(See Chapter 5)
Mammary	TDLU*	K19	K19	(See Chapter 4)
	Basal		K5, K7, K14 K18 (postelection)	(See Chapter 4)
Prostate	Basal	K5, K14	K5, K14	(See Chapter 6)
	Luminal	K8, K18	K8, K18	(See Chapter 6)
Intestine		K8, K18	K8, K18	(See Chapter 10)
Urothelium	General	K7, K8, K18, K19	K7, K8, K17, K18 and	(See Chapter 12)
	Basal	K5, K17	K19 (all cells)	(See Chapter 12)
	All but superficial	K13		(See Chapter 12)
	Superficial	K20		(See Chapter 12)

*TDLU = terminal ductal lobular units

contamination from other cell lines. This is particularly true where a continuous cell line is formed, as many continuous epithelial cell lines are morphologically similar. If any other continuous epithelial cell line is being maintained in your laboratory, or in the laboratory where the cell line originated, particularly if it prolif-

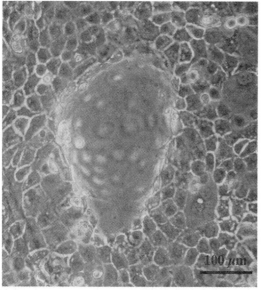

(a)

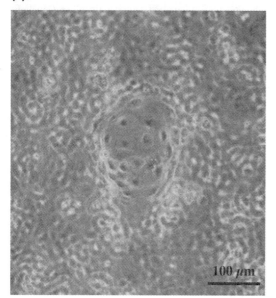

(b)

Fig 1.2. Domes forming in a monolayer of epithelial cells. Cell line CA-KD, derived from a secondary adenocarcinoma in the brain, from an unknown primary, forming domes when kept at confluence. (a) Focused on monolayer, (b) focused on top of dome. Culture and photographs courtesy of C.M. MacDonald. Reproduced from Freshney [2000].

erates rapidly, there is always the risk that is has contaminated your stock. In the late 1960s and the 1970s, Gartler [1967], Nelson Rees and Flandermeyer [1977], and others [e.g., Lavappa, 1978] proved that the majority of cultured lines in current use were HeLa-derived. Unfortunately, despite the publicity that this received at the time, cross-contamination remains a severe problem, and many cell lines submitted to cell banks have been shown to be cross-contaminated [Kneuchel and Masters, 1999; Stacey et al., 1999; MacLeod et al., 1999]. Periodically, the American Type Culture Collection (ATCC) issue bulletins on their web page (*www.ATCC.org*) highlighting where cross-contaminations have been detected.

The best method of guarding against cross-contamination is by DNA fingerprinting [Thacker et al., 1988] or DNA profiling [MacLeod et al., 1999; Thomson et al., 1999]. A DNA fingerprint may be stored as a photograph, and DNA profiling gives a digital output that can be stored in a database along with cell line records. Where new cell lines are being created, it is essential to store a sample of DNA, blood, or solid tissue from the donor at $-70°C$ or in liquid nitrogen at the time of isolation. When a successful line is generated, the DNA fingerprint or profile from the cell line can be compared with that of the donor and identity confirmed. If the technology for DNA fingerprinting or profiling is not available in your laboratory, it is possible to have it done commercially (see Appendix: Sources of Materials). Historically, several other tests have been used to validate cell lines. Of these, karyotype analysis and isoenzyme electrophoresis are probably the most effective [Freshney, 2000b]. If the contaminant is HeLa, the glucose-6-phosphate dehydrogenase isoenzyme pattern and the presence of certain marker chromosomes are diagnostic [Hay, 1986].

8. DIFFERENTIATION

The traditional problem of the early attempts to grow epithelium was the loss of the specialized properties of the tissue from which they were derived. In a significant proportion of these, the overgrowth was by stromal fibroblasts, as discussed above, but in some cases (e.g., in liver) the overgrowth was by epithelial cells that were not differentiated hepatocytes. The problem was described as *dedifferentiation* and has two likely causes, not necessarily mutually exclusive: (1) selection of the wrong lineage (e.g., stromal fibroblasts or endothelium instead of epithelium) and (2) propagation of cells from the early, proliferative, undifferentiated stage of the correct lineage. Elimination of the first of these has been dealt with above and depends on the development of selective media and culture conditions; correcting the second depends on the induction of differentiation. This is not reinduction, as it is presumed that most terminally differentiated cells do not dedifferentiate but become overgrown by precursor cells (not unduly surprising, as it is widely accepted that differentiation and proliferation are mutually exclusive in epithelial cells).

There are two main conclusions from this: (1) If specialized functions are required, they will require the correct inductive environment, and (2) propagation is likely to be carried out under a different set of conditions from the expression of differentiation. This may mean two distinct modes of culture depending on the required endpoint, but it can also mean that the culture may be heterogeneous, with cells at different phases of differentiation, much as would be found in vivo. It is often assumed that the population is homogeneous in either its differentiated or proliferative phase. In practice it is difficult to achieve complete homogeneity, and even under conditions of maximum stimulation of differentiation there is likely to be an equilibrium between the stem cells, the precursor cell compartment, and terminally differentiated cells. If a homogeneous population of cells is essential, it may be necessary to resort to a cell separation technique (see Section 5.6).

8.1. Induction of Differentiation

The induction of differentiation can be regarded as being under the control of four main parameters whose effects are interactive. These are (1) soluble inducers, (2) cell-cell interaction, (3) cell-matrix interaction, and (4) polarity and cell shape. Some of these, particularly in category (4), are probably permissive rather than directly inductive, but a distinction is not made in the present discussion, on the assumption that this is an attempt to define elements of the microenvironment that will favor differentiation rather than to analyze the regulatory processes per se.

8.1.1. Soluble Inducers

The substances that have been found to have differentiation-inducing activity are listed in Table 1.2. They include classical hormones such as hydrocortisone, vitamins such as retinoic acid, vitamin D_3, E, and K, and paracrine factors, mostly cytokines and growth factors (see Section 8.1.2). The prostaglandins have also been found to be active, for example, prostaglandin (PGE_2) in breast [Rudland et al., 1982]. With the exception of the sex steroids, these agents do not have a great deal of target specificity.

There is also a group of compounds the physiologic action of which is still far from clear. These are the planar-polar com-

TABLE 1.2. Examples of Factors Controlling Differentiation

Agent	Cells	Reference
Diffusible, physiologic:		
Ca^{2+}	Keratinocytes	Boyce and Ham, 1983
KGF	Keratinocytes	Marchese et al., 1990
KGF	Prostatic epithelium	Thomson et al., 1997
HGF	MDCK cells	Montesano et al., 1997
TGF-β	Bronchial epithelium	Masui et al. [1986]
		(See also Chapter 8)
Hydrocortisone, OSM, IL-6, lung fibroblast-conditioned medium	A549 cells	Speirs et al., 1991; McCormick et al., 1995; McCormick and Freshney, 2000
Retinoic acid	Tracheo-bronchial epithelium	Kaartinen, 1993
Vitamin D_3	IEC-6 cells	Jeng et al., 1994
Vitamin K	Kidney epithelium	Cancela et al., 1997
Insulin, prolactin, and hydrocortisone	Mammary epithelium	Marte et al., 1994
Epimorphin	Kidney epithelium	Hirai et al., 1992
Diffusible, nonphysiologic:		
Sodium butyrate	HT29 cells	Velcich et al., 1995
PMA (TPA)	Bronchial epithelium	Willey et al., 1984
PMA	HT29, CaCo-2 cells	Pignata et al., 1994; Velcich et al., 1995
DMSO	Mammary epithelium	Rudland et al., 1992
	Hepatocytes	Hino et al., 1999
		(See also Chapter 11)
Matrix:		
Collagen	Keratinocytes	(See Chapters 2, 5)
Collagen	Hepatocytes	Sattler et al., 1978
		(See also Chapter 11)
Collagen	Mammary epithelium	Berdichevsky et al., 1992
Laminin	Mammary epithelium	Blum and Wicha, 1988
Matrigel	Mammary epithelium	(See Chapter 4)
Heparan SO_4	Enterocytes	Simon-Assmanne at al., 1986
Heparan SO_4	A549 cells	Yevdokimova and Freshney, 1997
Indirect hormone action via stromal fibroblasts:		
Hydrocortisone	Intestine	Simon-Assmann et al., 1986
Hydrocortisone	Lung	Post et al., 1984
Androgen	Prostate	Cuhna, 1984; Thomson et al., 1997
Estrogen	Breast	Coletta et al., 1990
Estrogen	Uterus	Taguchi et al., 1983

pounds, or polar solvents, like dimethyl sulfoxide (DMSO), hexa-methylene bisacetamide (HMBA), sodium butyrate (NaBt), and N-methyl- and dimethylformamide (NMF, DMF), the former being the main metabolite of the latter. Their activities have been demonstrated chiefly in tumor cells [Schroy et al., 1988], for example, induction of alkaline phosphatase, a marker for differentiation, in A549 cells, derived from a putative alveolar type II adenocarcinoma of lung (Fig. 1.3), but they have also been shown to be active in some normal cells [Rudland et al., 1992; Hino et al., 1999; see also Chapter 11].

Ca^{2+} concentration influences differentiation in some epithelia [Boyce and Ham, 1983], with concentrations above 3 mM favoring differentiation and low concentrations favoring cell proliferation. This was demonstrated first for mouse skin (see Chapters 2 and 3), and it may also apply to other epithelia (see Chapter 13).

8.1.2. Cell-Cell Interaction

There is evidence of homotypic interaction in developing epithelial monolayers, and a high-density monolayer of secretory cells is more likely to become differentiated than a low-density culture. This may be due partly to the establishment of gap junc-

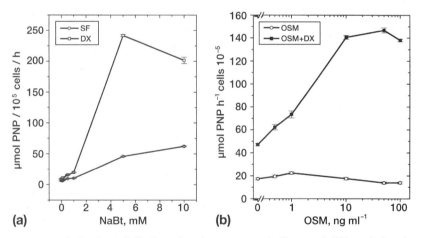

Fig 1.3. Induction of alkaline phosphatase, as an indicator of differentiation, in A549 cells. Cells were grown to confluence in Ham's F10:DMEM, 50:50, with 10% FBS, and then grown on for 3 days in serum-free F10:DMEM. Inducer was added for a further 3 days, and the alkaline phosphatase was assayed colorimetrically by release of p-nitrophenol from p-nitrophenol phosphate. (a) Inducer, sodium butyrate. Reprinted from Methods of Tissue Engineering, Ed. Atala and Lanza: Maintenance of primary and early passage cultures, R.I. Freshney, pp 37–53, 2002, Figure 3.5, by permission of the publisher Academic Press. (b) oncostatin M [Evans, McCormick, and Freshney, unpublished data].

tions between adjacent cells allowing the transfer of signal transducers such as cyclic AMP, partly to the decrease in cell proliferation at high cell density, and partly to the shape change achieved as a result of crowding at high cell densities, as discussed below (see Section 8.1.4).

Organogenesis in the embryo occurs by the interaction of developing epithelium from the endoderm or ectoderm with adjacent mesenchymal cells [Spooner and Wessells, 1970; Thesleff et al., 1977; Rutter et al., 1978]. This interaction is highly specific, and the source of the mesenchyme determines the fate of the epithelium. The maintenance of this heterotypic interaction in the adult is harder to demonstrate, but there is now good evidence for dermal interaction in epidermal differentiation (discussed in Chapter 2). It is also likely that at least part of the failure of differentiation in tumor cells is due to the breakdown in interaction with the appropriate stromal cells. Similarly, the failure to differentiate in culture is often due to elimination of stromal interaction. This presents a particular problem, because, as we have seen above, the production of cell lines from epithelial tissues requires selective conditions that suppress the stromal fibroblasts, whereas induction of differentiation may depend on them. As suggested above, this is a situation that may require proliferative conditions to be distinct from those conditions that favor differentiation.

One of the more interesting aspects of heterologous cell interaction is the participation of the stroma in the induction of differentiation by steroids. Prostatic differentiation is under the control of androgens, but their action is independent of epithelial receptors. Cunha [1984] and others showed that it is the presence of receptors in the stromal fibroblasts that is critical. Similarly, estrogen binds to stromal receptors in the uterus to induce maturation of the uterine epithelium [Taguchi et al., 1983]. In the lung just before birth a factor released by lung fibroblasts induces pulmonary surfactant production in the type II pneumocyte of the alveolus. The synthesis of this factor, fibrocyte-pneumonocyte factor (FPF), was shown to be positively regulated by cortisol [Post et al., 1984] and negatively regulated by TGF-β [Torday and Kourembanas, 1990]. Dexamethasone increases the inductive effect of lung fibroblasts on the A549 type II pneumocyte tumor cell line, cocultured in a filter well system [Speirs et al., 1991], although, at least part of this response is caused by a direct effect on the epithelial component (see below) [Yevdokimova and Freshney, 1997].

Many of the factors released by fibroblasts, and active in paracrine control of differentiation and morphogenesis, are cytokines and growth factors such as keratinocyte growth factor (KGF) in prostate [Yan et al., 1992; Thomson et al., 1997; Planz et al., 1998] and hepatocyte growth factor (HGF) in kidney [Montesano et al., 1997], salivary gland [Furue and Saito, 1997], and mammary gland [Soriano et al., 1995]. Both of these factors are classically paracrine in action as they are only produced by fibroblasts and their receptors are only found on epithelial cells. Screening of candidate growth factors for the response seen in A549 cocultured with fibroblasts (see above) showed that cytokines of the interleukin-6 (IL-6) family were most active, with oncostatin M having the greatest potency [McCormick et al., 1995; McCormick and Freshney, 2000] (Fig. 1.3b). However, disabling antibodies to OSM and IL-6 did not inhibit the activity found in medium conditioned by lung fibroblasts [McCormick and Freshney, 2000]. KGF was found to be inactive in this system, although others (see Chapter 9) have found that KGF mimics the effect of fibroblasts with freshly isolated type II pneumocytes.

Hence, complete differentiation of many types of epithelium is under the control of the fibroblasts (or, more correctly, fibrocytes) normally associated with the epithelium in vivo, and the activity of the fibrocytes may in turn be regulated by proximity to the epithelium as well as by systemic hormones. This requirement for heterologous cell interaction adds a degree of complexity to differentiated epithelial culture, as yet essential for full functional expression of some cell types. It is to be hoped that this interaction may be shown to depend on soluble paracrine factors like those described for lung and prostate [Post et al., 1984; Thomson, et al., 1997], as this would allow substitution of a defined factor for the more complex combined culture.

8.1.3. Cell-Matrix Interaction

Many, if not all, soluble paracrine factors may require binding to specific elements of the extracellular matrix (ECM) to become active. ECM is made up of the products of the cells associated with it; hence the matrix generated between a monolayer of fibroblasts and tissue culture plastic will be different from the matrix generated by endothelial or epithelial cells, and the matrix generated between two fibroblasts, two epithelial cells, or heterologous combinations of epithelium and fibroblasts, epithelium and endothelium, and so on, will in turn all be different. Hence, although it is treated here as a separate parameter, cell-matrix interaction is really another dimension of cell-cell interaction, where the stimulus is contact-mediated or made via soluble paracrine factors bound to the matrix

[Neufeld and Gospodarowicz, 1987], as demonstrated in bone marrow for GM-CSF [Cross and Dexter, 1991]. The activity of OSM and IL-6 on inducing differentiation in A549 cells was dependent on dexamethasone (DX), which was shown to induce the synthesis of a relatively low-charge-density heparan sulfate, designated HS1, by the A549 cells (Fig. 1.4a). A semipurified preparation of HS1 had a dose-dependent effect on induction of alkaline phosphatase in A549 cells by lung fibroblast-conditioned medium (Fig. 1.4b) and was able to replace DX in the activation of OSM and IL-6 (Fig. 1.4c) [Yevdokimova and Freshney, 1997].

There are several ways that matrix can vary. The common constituents are collagen, fibronectin, laminin, and proteoglycans. Not only can the proportions of each vary, but the type may also vary. Collagen is present in matrix in 4 common forms, and up to 12 in total [Vuorio and Crombrugghe, 1990]. Basement membrane, underlying the epithelium and separating it from the mesodermally derived compartment, contains predominately type IV. Fibronectin and laminin are fairly constant, but the proteoglycans are very heterogeneous. They are made up of proteins conjugated to four main types of GAGs: heparan sulfate, chondroitin sulfate, dermatan sulfate, and nonsulfated hyaluronan. Within each group, particularly heparan sulfate, there is heterogeneity in molecular size, charge, degree of branching, number and position of sugar residues, position and type of GAGs, and so on [Jalkamen, 1987].

Many matrix molecules contain the so-called RGD sequence of amino acids (arginine, glycine, aspartic acid), which is responsible for binding to the integrin class of receptors. RGD-containing peptides alone antagonize the biological effects of matrix, and it appears that receptor activation is dependent on RGD anchorage to, or spatial organization within, the matrix macromolecules.

The extracellular matrix is therefore a very complex and variable biosystem and, if one is attempting to control the microenvironment of the cells, something best to avoid. Nevertheless, many cells require being grown on matrix to express differentiated properties (see Chapters 2, 5, 8, 9). It is therefore an indispensable element of the microenvironment for some epithelial differentiation and may be the basis for the contact-mediated effect of some cell-cell interactions [Simon-Assmann et al., 1986].

8.1.4. Cell Shape and Polarity

The typical histologic appearance of secretory cells shows the nucleus located in the lower third of the cytoplasm, a basal lamina on the basal surface, microvilli on the apical surface, and junc-

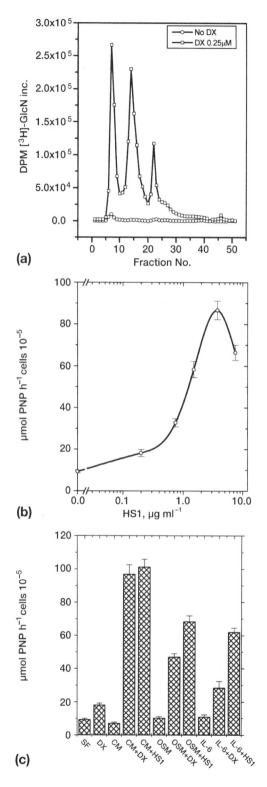

Fig 1.4. Effect of semi-purified heparan sulfate from A549 cells on induction of alkaline phosphatase. (a) Purification of [³H]glucosamine-labeled glycosaminoglycans from A549 cells on DEAE cellulose. The third peak is heparan sulfate and was isolated and termed HS1. (b) Dose-response curve of the effect of HS1 on the induction of alkaline phosphatase by lung fibroblast conditioned medium, which normally requires dexamethasone for activity. (c) Effect of HS1, 5 µg/ml, or dexamethasone, 0.25 µM, on induction of alkaline phosphatase by lung fibroblast conditioned medium, oncostatin M, or interleukin-6. SF, serum-free control; DX, 0.25 µM dexamethasone, CM, lung fibroblast conditioned medium; OSM, oncostatin M; IL-6, interleukin-6; PNP, *p*-nitrophenol. Reprinted from British Journal of Cancer 76(3), Yevdokimova and Freshney: Activation of paracrine growth factors by heparan sulphate induced by glucocorticoid in A549 lung carcinoma cells, pp 281–289, 1977, Figures 1B, 5, 7, by permission of the publisher Churchill Livingstone.

tional complexes on the apicolateral surfaces. Cell surface antigens like HMFG and P-glycoprotein become polarized to the apical surface and peptide hormone receptors to the basal surface. These are examples of the differentiated properties of epithelium, and it is a little teleological to say that they cause differentiation. However, unless the cell is cultured in such a way as to allow this polarity to develop, complete differentiation is not expressed.

One of the best examples is thyroid epithelium, where cells grown on plastic become only partially polarized. Grown on collagen in a filter well, the filter surface, in contact with the medium, develops thyroid-stimulating hormone (TSH) receptors, transports iodine into the cell, and secretes triiodothyronine (T_3) into the medium. The apicolateral surfaces, in contact with adjacent cells, develop complexes of tight junctions and desmosomes, and the apical surface develops microvilli, secretes thyroglobulin and iodine, and takes up newly synthesized T_3 to be transported to the basal surface [Chambard et al., 1987].

Many other epithelia, grown in filter wells, also acquire polarity. Colonic cells will transport amino acids from the apical to the basal surface [Hidalgo and Borchardt, 1990], that is, from the filter well to the underlying medium, and transport toxins from the basal to the apical surface by virtue of the concentration of the efflux protein P-glycoprotein on the apical surface [Meyers et al., 1991].

It is therefore important for many epithelial cells, to achieve maximum expression of differentiation, to be grown on a floating raft of collagen (see Chapter 5) or in a filter well (see Chapter 2). Filter wells have the additional advantage that a high cell density can be generated locally, which is necessary for the cell to change in shape from a flattened proliferative cell to a cuboid or columnar nonproliferative cell but maintains a nonlimiting amount of medium. Furthermore, vectorial transport can be modeled effectively and the significance of cell interactions can be studied by direct contact, by transfilter combination, or by separated coculture with cells in the bottom of the dish interacting with those in the filter well by diffusion of signaling molecules. By the last of these methods, it has been possible to show that lung fibroblasts will induce surfactant synthesis in type II pneumocytes (see Chapter 9) and in A549 alveolar carcinoma cells, particularly when treated with glucocorticoid [Speirs and Freshney, 1991].

9. TRANSFORMATION

Typically, a cell line isolated from a normal tissue will complete a set number of generations in vitro, stop growing, and eventually die out. Cell lines from tumors, however, often undergo a crisis in which most of the cells are overgrown by a minority population of smaller, faster-growing cells that are no longer anchorage-dependent for growth. These cells give rise to a continuous cell line that may be already, or may become, tumorigenic.

There are also a number of otherwise normal epithelial cell lines that have become immortal, like the MDCK dog kidney epithelium, various monkey kidney cell lines, and the mink lung epithelial cell line MvlLu (Table 1.3). There are also reports of immortalized human cell lines, like HB 100 from breast [Gaffney et al., 1976], and HaCaT epidermal keratinocytes [Boukamp et al., 1988, 1990]. However, spontaneous immortalization is still a rare event, and still disputed, so many laboratories have now developed techniques for inducing immortalization by transfection with oncogenic or viral DNA such as the large T-antigen gene from SV40 [Linder and Marshall, 1990] or human papillomavirus (see Chapters 3, 4, and 5). A number of cell lines have been produced that retain some specific functionality, survive indefinitely, and are free of transmissible viruses. This offers considerable potential to the biotechnology industry for the production of biopharmaceuticals and is a rapidly expanding area of interest.

The events involved in transformation are, of course, of major interest to cancer biologists, and it is from their efforts that much of the information regarding the mechanisms involved in transformation are emerging. Like carcinogenesis, transformation is a multistage process, and it undoubtedly shares some of the steps involved in carcinogenesis. Probably the first event to be observed in vitro is immortalization, and this is the feature that most people would associate with the term in vitro transformation. Secondly, and not necessarily simultaneously, there is an alteration in growth

TABLE 1.3. Examples of "Spontaneously" Immortalized Epithelial Cell Lines From Normal Tissue

Cell line	Source	Tumorigenicity	Reference
HaCaT	Human epidermia	No	Boukamp et al., 1988, 1990
MvlLu	Mink lung	Low	ATCC CCL64
MDCK	Dog kidney	No	Rindler et al., 1979
HB100	Human breast	No	Gaffney et al., 1976
LLC-PK$_1$	Pig kidney	No	Hull et al., 1976
BS-C-1	Monkey kidney	No	ATCC CCL26
COMMA-D	Mouse mammary gland	No	Danielson et al., 1984
Various	Rat liver	Yes	Yeoh et al., 1990
Various	Mouse liver	No	Paul et al., 1988

control, which produces a more rapidly growing cell that is no longer anchorage-dependent. The mink lung epithelial cell line Mv1Lu became immortalized during the early stages of its evolution, but, like the 3T3 cell, it can become more rapidly growing, anchorage-independent, and tumorigenic by transfection with the *Ha-ras* or other oncogenes [Khan et al., 1991].

Hence, the term *transformation* should be used with caution and preferably as a binomial, for example, *malignant transformation* to imply a change from a nontumorigenic line to one that forms invasive tumors; *morphologic transformation* where only morphologic change has been observed; and *in vitro transformation* to imply immortalization combined with an alteration in growth control (e.g., anchorage-independent growth, loss of contact inhibition of cell migration, and loss of density limitation of cell proliferation or *topoinhibition*). Where no alteration in growth control is implied (e.g., in contact-inhibited 3T3 cell lines), it is better to use the term *immortalization* and reserve *in vitro transformation* for cells that show altered growth control. Usually, but not always, the development of autonomous growth control (lower serum growth factor dependence), loss of contact inhibition and topoinhibition, and anchorage independence correlate with malignancy and they may be the same as, or at least a major component of, malignant transformation.

From a practical standpoint, it is likely that the higher cloning efficiencies of transformed cells and continuous cell lines derive from their acquisition of autonomous growth control. Although cell proliferation in a tissue may usually be under paracrine control, which is unavailable to cloning cells, growth of transformed cells is more likely to be under autocrine control, and hence independent of cell density and cell-cell interaction. Transformed cells will therefore tend to show higher plating efficiencies and reduced serum dependence.

Because of the frequent correlation of in vitro transformation (loss of growth control) with malignancy, the characteristics used to recognize transformed cells are often used to identify tumor cells in vitro. It should be realized, however, that tumor cells freshly explanted from a tumor and grown in early-passage culture need not necessarily express all the characteristics of a cell line that has transformed, or has been transformed, in vitro. However, it is useful to summarize these for the benefit of those who wish to culture tumor cells. Few are diagnostic alone, and simultaneous expression of several properties may be required to be at all certain:

1. *Aneuploidy.* The chromosomal constitution of continuous cell lines is usually abnormal and unstable. It may be by virtue of this instability that the cell line has become immortal. Evidence of aneuploidy may be seen in chromosome changes such as deletions, polysomy, and translocations revealed by conventional karyotyping or by the use of specific molecular probes or chromosome paints [Croce, 1991].

2. *Heteroploidy.* This is also the result of genetic instability, and it implies that the population contains a range of cells with differing chromosome numbers.

3. *Contact inhibition.* This is the inhibition of cell movement at confluence brought about by cell contact, and it produces a regular monolayer [Abercrombie et al., 1967]. Some cells may become multilayered in an ordered manner without losing contact inhibition (e.g., keratinocytes before desquamation), but this should be distinguished from a disorderly array of cells with a high rate of motility and proliferation in the upper layers.

4. *Density limitation of cell proliferation (topoinhibition).* As cells become crowded in a confluent monolayer, they change shape and occupy less of the substrate. Normal cells will cease to divide at this stage, known as saturation density, but transformed cells will continue to divide [Stoker and Rubin, 1967], generating a higher saturation density and exhibiting a higher labeling index with [^{3}H]TdR or cycle-specific probes such as proliferating cell nuclear antigen (PCNA) or Ki67.

5. *Anchorage independence.* Transformed cells will generally form colonies in suspension in agar with a higher efficiency than untransformed cells.

6. *Proteases.* Transformed cells often exhibit higher proteolytic activity than untransformed cells [Mahdavi and Hynes, 1979], owing frequently to elevated plasminogen activator activity, usually of the urokinase type [Markus et al., 1980].

7. *Angiogenesis.* Tumors grow beyond about 1 mm in diameter only by inducing their own vascularization. They do so by secreting angiogenesis factors, and these may be assayed by absorbing a cell extract on filter paper and placing it on the chorioallantoic membrane of the hen's egg [Ausprunk et al., 1975].

8. *Invasiveness.* It is possible to assay invasiveness by coculturing aggregates of cells with precultured 10-day chick embryo heart fragments [Mareel et al., 1979]. Invasive cells penetrate the chick heart tissue, cause degeneration, and ultimately re-

place it. It is also possible to place the cells in a chemotaxis chamber on Matrigel with a chemoattractant in the lower chamber [Hendrix et al., 1987] or to seed tumor cells on the lower side of a filter well and monitor invasion into Matrigel in the upper compartment by confocal microscopy [Brunton et al., 1997].

9. *Tumorigenesis.* Transformed cells will produce tumors in an isologous host or, as xenografts, in immuno-incompetent mice, such as the nude mouse [Giovanella et al., 1974; Pretlow et al., 1991]. Technically, these tumors should be invasive to be malignant, but often cells isolated from a patently malignant human tumor form tumors in nude mice but do not invade or metastasize.

The following chapters deal with some of the more commonly used epithelia and present specific protocols for their cultivation and characterization.

REFERENCES

Abercrombie M, Heaysman JEM (1954): Observations on the social behaviour of cells in tissue culture. II. "Monolayering" of fibroblasts. Exp Cell Res 6: 293–306.

Aitken ML, Villalon M, Verdugo P, Nameroff M (1991): Enrichment of sub-populations of respiratory epithelial cells using flow cytometry. Am J Respir Cell Mol Biol 4: 174–178.

Ausprunk DH, Knighton DR, Folkman J (1975): Vascularization of normal and neoplastic tissues grafted to the chick chorioallantois: Role of host and pre-existing graft blood vessels. Am J Pathol 79: 597–628.

Berdichevsky F, Gilbert C, Shearer M, Taylor-Papadimitriou J (1992): Collagen-induced rapid morphogenesis of human mammary epithelial cells: The role of the alpha 2 beta 1 integrin. J Cell Sci 102: 437–446.

Bevan S, Woodward B, Ng RL, Green C, Martin R (1997): Retroviral gene transfer into porcine keratinocytes following improved methods of cultivation. Burns 23: 525–532.

Blum JL, Wicha MS (1988): Role of the cytoskeleton in laminin induced mammary expression. J Cell Physiol 135: 13–22.

Boukamp P, Petrusevska RI, Breitkreutz D, Hornung J, Markham A, Fusenig NE (1988): Normal keratinization in a spontaneously immortalized aneuploid human keratinocyte cell line. J Cell Biol 106: 761–771.

Boukamp P, Stanbridge EJ, Foo DY, Cerutti PA, Fusenig NE (1990): *c-Ha-ras* oncogene expression in immortalized human keratinocytes (HaCaT) alters growth potential in vivo but lacks correlation with malignancy. Cancer Res 50: 2840–2847.

Boxberger HJ, Meyer TF, Grausam MC, Reich K, Becker HD, Sessler MJ. (1997): Isolating and maintaining highly polarized primary epithelial cells from normal human duodenum for growth as spheroid-like vesicles. In Vitro Cell Dev Biol Anim 33: 536–545.

Boyce ST, Ham RG (1983): Calcium-regulated differentiation of normal human epidermal keratinocytes in chemically defined clonal culture and serum-free serial culture. J Invest Dermatol 81(Suppl): 33s–40s.

Brunton V, Ozanne B, Paraskeva C, Frame M (1997): A role for epidermal growth factor receptor, c-Src and focal adhesion kinase in an in vitro model for the progression of colon cancer. Oncogene. 14: 283–293.

Burchell J, Durbin H, Taylor-Papadimitriou J (1983): Complexity of expression of antigenic determinants, recognized by monoclonal antibodies HMFG-1 and HMFG-2 in normal and malignant human mammary epithelial cells. J Immunol 131: 508–513.

Burchell J, Gendler S, Taylor-Papadimitriou J, Girling A, Lewis A, Millis R, Lamport D (1987): Development and characterization of breast cancer reactive monoclonal antibodies directed to the core protein of the human milk mucin. Cancer Res 47: 5476–5482.

Cancela ML, Hu B, Price PA (1997): Effect of cell density and growth factors on matrix GLA protein expression by normal rat kidney cells. J Cell Physiol 171: 125–134.

Carr T, Evans P, Campbell S, Bass P, Albano J (1999): Culture of human renal tubular cells: positive selection of kallikrein-containing cells. Immunopharmacology 44: 161–167.

Chambard M, Mauchamp J, Chaband O (1987): Synthesis and apical and basolateral secretion of thyroglobulin by thyroid cell monolayers on permeable substrate: Modulation by thyrotropin. J Cell Physiol 133: 37–45.

Colletta AA, Wakefield LM, Howell FV, van Roozendaal KEP, Danielpour D, Ebbs SR, Sporn MB, Baum M (1990): Anti-oestrogens induce the secretion of active transforming growth factor beta from human fetal fibroblasts. Br J Cancer 62: 405–409.

Croce CM (1991): Genetic approaches to the study of the molecular basis of human cancer. Cancer Res (Suppl) 51: 5015s–5018s.

Cross M, Dexter TM (1991): Growth factors in development, transformation and tumorigenesis. Cell 64: 271–280.

Cunha GR (1984): Androgenic effects upon prostatic epithelium are mediated via tropic influences from stroma. In Kimball FA, Buhl AE, Carter DB (eds): "New Approaches to Benign Prostatic Hyperplasia." New York, Alan R. Liss, pp 81–102.

Danielson KG, Oborn CJ, Durban EM, Buetel IS, Medina D (1984): Epithelial mouse mammary cell line exhibiting normal morphogenesis in vivo and functional differentiation in vitro. Proc Natl Acad Sci USA 81: 3756–3760.

Darcy KM, Shoemaker SF, Lee P-PH, Vaughan MM, Black JD, Ip MM (1995): Prolactin and epidermal growth factor regulation of the proliferation, morphogenesis, and functional differentiation of normal rat mammary epithelial cells in three dimensional primary culture. J Cell Physiol 163: 346–364.

Formanek M, Temmel A, Knerer B, Willheim M, Millesi W, Kornfehl J (1998): Magnetic cell separation for purification of human oral keratinocytes: An effective method for functional studies without prior cell subcultivation. Eur Arch Oto-Rhino-Laryngol 255: 211–215.

Freeman AE, Igel HG, Herrman BJ, Kleinfeld KL (1976): Growth and characterization of human skin epithelial cells. In Vitro 12: 352–362.

Freshney RI (2000a): "Culture of Animal Cells, a Manual of Basic Technique." 4th ed. New York: Wiley, pp 215–217.

Freshney RI (2000b): "Culture of Animal Cells, a Manual of Basic Technique." 4th ed. New York: Wiley, pp. 241–254.

Furue M, Saito S (1997): Synergistic effect of hepatocyte growth factor and fibroblast growth factor-1 on the branching morphogenesis of rat submandibular gland epithelial cells. Tissue Cult Res Commun 16: 189–194.

Gaffney EV, Polanowski FP, Blackburn SE, et al. (1976): Origin concentration and structural features of human mammary cells cultured from breast secretions. Cell Tissue Res 172: 269–279.

Gartler SM (1967): Genetic markers as tracers in cell culture. In: "Second Biennial Review Conference on Cell Tissue and Organ Culture." NCI Monographs, pp 167–195.

Giovanella BC, Stehlin IS, Williams LI (1974): Heterotransplantation of human malignant tumors in "nude" mice. II. Malignant tumors induced by injection of cell cultures derived from human solid tumors. J Natl Cancer Inst 52: 921–930.

Hay RJ (1986): Cell preservation and authentication. In Masters JRW (ed): "Animal Cell Culture, a Practical Approach." Oxford: Oxford University Press, pp 69–103.

Hendrix MI, Seftor EA, Seftor RE, Fidler II (1987): A simple quantitative assay for studying the invasive potential of high and low human metastatic variants. Cancer Lett 38: 137–147.

Heyderman E, Strudley I, Powell G, Richardson TC, Cordell IL, Mason DY (1985): A new monoclonal antibody to epithelial membrane antigen (EMA)E29. A comparison of its immunocytochemical reactivity with polyclonal anti-EMA antibodies and with another monoclonal antibody, HMFG-2. Br J Cancer 52: 355–361.

Hidalgo IJ, Borchardt RT (1990): Transport of a large neutral amino acid (phenylalanine) in a human intestinal epithelial cell line: Caco-2. Biochim Biophys Acta 1028: 25–30.

Hino H, Tateno C, Sato H, Yamasaki C, Katayama S, Kohashi T, Aratani A, Asahara T, Dohi K, Yoshizato K (1999):. A long-term culture of human hepatocytes which show a high growth potential and express their differentiated phenotypes. Biochem Biophys Res Commun 256: 184–191.

Hirai Y, Takebe K, Takashina M, Kobayashi S, Takeichi M (1992): Epimorphin: A mesenchymal protein essential for epithelial morphogenesis. Cell 69: 471–481.

Hull RN, Cherry WR, Weaver GW (1976): The origin and characteristics of a pig kidney cell strain, LLC-PK1. In Vitro 12: 670–677.

Hunt RC, Davis AA (1990): Altered expression of keratin and vimentin in human retinal pigment epithelial cells in vivo and in vitro. Cell Physiol 145: 187–199.

Jalkamen M (1987): Biology of cell surface heparan sulfate proteoglycans. Med Biol 65: 41–47.

Jeng Y-J, Watson CS, Thomas ML.(1994): Identification of vitamin D-stimulated phosphatase in IEC-6 cells, a rat small intestine crypt cell line. Exp Cell Res 212: 338–343.

Kaartinen L, Nettesheim P, Adler KB, Randell SH (1993): Rat tracheal epithelial cell differentiation in vitro. In Vitro Cell Dev Biol 29A: 481–492.

Khan MZ, Spandidos DA, McNicol AM, Lang IC, Kerr DI, DeRidder I, Freshney RI (1991): Oncogene transfection of mink lung cells: Effect on growth characteristics in vitro and in vivo. Anticancer Research 11: 1343–1348.

Kibbey MC, Royce LS, Dym M, Baum BJ, Kleinman HK (1992) Glandular-like morphogenesis of the human submandibular tumour cell line A253 on basement membrane components. Exp Cell Res 198: 343–351.

Kneuchel R, Masters JRW (1999): Bladder cancer. In Masters JRW, Palsson B (eds): "Human Cell Culture." Vol. I. Dordrecht: Kluwer, pp 213–230.

Lag M, Becher R, Samuelsen JT, Wiger R, Refsnes M, Huitfeldt HS, Schwarze PE (1996): Expression of CYP2B1 in freshly isolated and proliferating cultures of epithelial rat lung cells. Exp Lung Res 22: 627–649.

Lane EB (1982): Monoclonal antibodies provide specific intramolecular markers for the study of epithelial tonofilament organization. J Cell Biol 92: 665–673.

Lavappa KS (1978) Survey of ATCC stocks of human cell lines for HeLa contamination. In Vitro 14(5): 469–475.

Linder S Marshal H (1990): Immortalization of primary cells by DNA tumor viruses. Exp Cell Res 191: 1–7.

Lutz MP, Gaedicke G, Hartmann W (1992): Large-scale cell separation by centrifugal elutriation. Anal Biochem 200: 376–380.

MacLeod RA, Dirks WG, Matsuo Y, Kaufmann M, Milch H, Drexler HG (1999): Widespread intraspecies cross-contamination of human tumor cell lines arising at source. Int J Cancer 83: 555–563.

Macpherson I, Bryden A (1971): Mitomycin C treated cells as feeders. Exp Cell Res 69: 240–241.

Mahdavi V, Hynes RO (1979): Proteolytic enzymes in normal and transformed cells. Biochim Biophys Acta 583: 167–178.

Marchese C, Rubin I, Ron D, Faggioni A, Torrisi MR, Messina A, Frati M, Aaronson SA (1990); Human keratinocyte growth factor activity on proliferation and differentiation of human keratinocytes: Differentiation response distinguishes KGF from EGF family. J Cell Physiol 144: 326–332.

Mareel M, Kint I, Meyvisch C (1979): Methods of study of the invasion of malignant C3H mouse fibroblasts into embryonic chick heart in vitro. Virchows Arch B Cell Pathol 30: 95–111.

Markus G, Takita H, Camiolo SM, Corsant, J, Evers JL, Hobika JH (1980): Content and characterization of plasminogen activators in human lung tumours and normal lung tissue. Cancer Res 40: 841–848.

Marte BM, Meyer T, Stabel S, Standke GJR, Jaken S, Fabbro D, Hynes NE (1994): Protein kinase C and mammary cell differentiation: involvement of protein kinase C alpha in the induction of beta-casein expression. Cell Growth Differ 5: 239–247.

Masui T, Wakefield LM, Lechner JF, LaVeck MA, Sporn MB, Harris CC (1986): Type beta transforming growth factor is the primary differentiation-inducing serum factor for normal human bronchial epithelial cells. Proc Natl Acad Sci USA 83: 2438–2442.

McCormick C, Freshney RI (2000): Activity of growth factors in the IL-6 group in the differentiation of human lung adenocarcinoma. Br J Cancer 82: 881–890.

McCormick C, Freshney RI, Speirs V (1995): Activity of interferon alpha, interleukin 6 and insulin in the regulation of differentiation in A549 alveolar carcinoma cells. Br J Cancer 71: 232–239.

Meyers BM, Scotto KW, Sirotnak FM (1991): P-glycoprotein content and mediation of vincristine efflux: Correlation with the level of differentiation in luminal epithelium of mouse small intestine. Cancer Commun 3: 159–165.

Moll R, Cowin P. Kapprell H-P, Franke WW (1986): Desmosomal proteins: New markers for identification and classification of tumors. Lab Invest 54: 4–25.

Moll R, Franke WW, Schiller DL (1982): The catalog of human cytokeratins: Patterns of expression in normal epithelia, tumors, and cultured cells. Cell 31: 11–24.

Montesano R, Soriano JV, Pepper MS, Orci L (1997): Induction of epithelial branching tubulogenesis in vitro. J Cell Physiol 173: 152–161.

Nelson-Rees W, Flandermeyer RR (1977): Inter- and intraspecies contamination of human breast tumor cell lines HBC and BrCaS and other cell cultures. Science 195: 1343–1344.

Neufeld G, Gospodarowicz D (1987): Protamine sulfate inhibits mitogenic activities of the extracellular matrix and fibroblast growth factor, but potentiates that of epidermal growth factor. J Cell Physiol 132: 287–294.

Paul D, Hohne M, Pinkert C, Piasecki A, Ummelmann E, Brinster RL (1988): Immortalized differentiated hepatocyte cell lines derived from transgenic mice harboring SV-40 T-antigen genes. Exp Cell Res 175: 354–362.

Pignata S, Maggini L, Zarrilli R, Rea A, Acquaviva AM(1994): The enterocyte-like differentiation of the Caco-2 tumour cell line strongly correlates with responsiveness to cAMP and activation of kinase A pathway. Cell Growth Differ 5: 967–973.

Planz B, Wang Q, Kirley SD, Lin CW, McDougal WS (1998): Androgen responsiveness of stromal cells of the human prostate: regulation of cell proliferation and keratinocyte growth factor by androgen. J Urol 160: 1850–1855.

Post M, Floros I, Smith BT (1984): Inhibition of lung maturation by monoclonal antibodies against fibroblast-pneumonocyte factor. Nature 308: 284–285.

Poumay Y, Boucher F, Leclercq-Smekens M, Degen A, Leloup R (1993): Basal cell adhesion to a culture substratum controls the polarized spatial organization of human epidermal keratinocytes into proliferating basal and terminally differentiating suprabasal populations. Epithelial Cell Biol 2: 7–16.

Pretlow TG, Pretlow TP (1989): Cell separation by gradient centrifugation methods. Methods Enzymol 171: 462–482.

Pretlow TG, Delmoro CM, Dilley GG, Spadafora CG, Pretlow TP (1991): Transplantation of human prostatic carcinoma into nude mice in Matrigel. Cancer Res 51: 3814–3817.

Rheinwald IG (1980): Serial cultivation of normal human epidermal keratinocytes. Methods Cell Biol 12A: 229–254.

Rindler MI, Chuman LM, Shaffer L, Saier MH Jr (1979): Retention of differentiated properties in an established dog kidney epithelial cell line (MDCK). J Cell Biol 81: 635–648.

Rudland PS, Davies AT, Warburton MI (1982): Prostaglandin induced differentiation: Reduction of the neoplastic potential of a rat mammary tumor stem cell line. J Natl Cancer Inst 69: 1083–1093.

Rudland PS (1992): Use of peanut lectin and rat mammary stem cell lines to identify a cellular differentiation pathway for the alveolar cell in the rat mammary gland. J Cell Physiol 153:157–168.

Rutter WI, Pictet RL, Harding ID, Chirgwin IM, MacDonald RI, Przybyla AE (1978): An analysis of pancreatic development: Role of mesenchymal factor and other extracellular factors. In Papaconstantinou I, Rutter WI (eds): "Molecular Control of Proliferation and Differentiation." New York: Academic Press, p 205.

Saalbach A, Aust G, Haustein UF, Herrmann K, Anderegg U (1997): The fibroblast-specific MAb AS02: A novel tool for detection and elimination of human fibroblasts. Cell Tissue Res 290: 593–599.

Sattler CA, Michalopoulos G, Sattler GL, Pitot HC (1978): Ultrastructure of adult rat hepatocytes cultured on floating collagen membranes. Cancer Res 38: 1539–1549.

Schaefer BM, Reinartz J, Bechtel MJ, Inndorf S, Lang E, Kramer MD (1996): Dispase-mediated basal detachment of cultured keratinocytes induces urokinase-type plasminogen activator (uPA) and its receptor (uPA-R, CD87). Exp Cell Res 228: 246–253.

Schroy PC, Carnright K, Winawer SI, Friedman EA (1988): Heterogeneous responses of human colon carcinomas to hexamethylene bisacetimide. Cancer Res 48: 5487–5494.

Seely KA, Aggeler J (1991): Modulation of milk protein synthesis through alteration of the cytoskeleton in mouse mammary epithelial cells cultured on a reconstituted basement membrane. J Cell Physiol 146: 117–130.

Simon-Assmann P, Kedinger, M, Haffen, K (1986): Immunocytochemical localization of extracellular matrix proteins in relation to rat intestinal morphogenesis. Differentiation 32: 59–66.

Soriano V, Pepper MS, Nakamura T, Orci L, Montesano R (1995): Hepatocyte growth factor stimulates extensive development of branching duct-like structures by cloned mammary gland epithelial cells. J Cell Sci 108: 413–430.

Speirs V, Ray KP, Freshney RI (1991): Paracrine control of differentiation in the alveolar carcinoma, A549, by human foetal lung fibroblasts. Br J Cancer 64: 693–699.

Spooner BS, Wessells NK (1970): Mammalian lung development: interactions in primordium formation and bronchial morphogenesis. J Exp Zool 175: 445–454.

Stacey GN, Masters JRM, Hay RJ, Drexler HG, MacLeod RAF, Freshney RI (2000): Cell contamination leads to inaccurate data: We must take action now. Nature 403: 456.

Stoker MGP, Rubin H (1967): Density dependent inhibition of cell growth in culture. Nature 215: 171–172.

Swope VB, Supp AP, Cornelius JR, Babcock GF, Boyce ST (1997): Regulation of pigmentation in cultured skin substitutes by cytometric sorting of melanocytes and keratinocytes. J Invest Dermatol 109: 289–295.

Taguchi O, Cunha GR, Robboy SJ (1983): Experimental study of the effect of diethylstilbestrol on the development of the human female reproductive tract. Biol Res Pregnancy 4: 56–70.

Taylor-Papadimitriou J, Lane EB (1987): Keratin expression in the mammary gland. In Neville MC, Daniel CW (eds): "The Mammary Gland." New York, Plenum, pp 181–215.

Thacker I, Webb MBT, Debenham PG (1988): Fingerprinting cell lines: Use of human hypervariable DNA probes to characterize mammalian cell cultures Somatic Cell Mol Genet 14: 519–525.

Thesleff I, Lehtonen E, Wartiovaara I, Saxen L (1977): Effect of interposed 0.1 μm, 0.2 μm and 0.6 μm Nuclepore filters on epithelio-mesenchymal interaction in embryonic mouse tooth. Dev Biol 58: 197–203.

Thomson AA, Foster BA, Cunha GR (1997): Analysis of growth factor and receptor mRNA levels during development of the rat seminal vesicle and prostate. Development 124: 2431–2439.

Thomson JA, Pilotti V, Stevens P, Ayres KL, Debenham PG (1999): Validation of short tandem repeat analysis for the investigation of cases of disputed paternity. Forensic Sci Int 100: 1–16.

Tomson AM, Scholma J, Blaauw EH (1995): The effect of detachment of cultured epithelial sheets on cellular ultrastructure and organization. Epithelial Cell Biol 4: 43–51.

Torday JS, Kourembanas S (1990): Fetal rat lung fibroblasts produce a TGF-β homolog that blocks alveolar type II cell maturation. Dev Biol 13: 35–41.

Velcich A, Palumbo L, Jarry A, Laboisse C, Racevskis J, Augenlicht L (1995): Patterns of expression of lineage-specific markers during the in vitro induced differentiation of HT29 colon carcinoma cells. Cell Growth Differ 6: 749–757.

Vuorio E, Crombrugghe B (1990): The family of collagen genes. Ann Rev Biochem 59: 837–872.

Willey JC, Saladino Al, Ozanne C, Lechner IF, Harris CC (1984): Acute effects of 1 2-O-tetradecanoylphorbol-13-acetate, teleocidin B, or 2,3,7,8-tetrachlorodibenzo-*p*-dioxin on cultured normal human bronchial cells. Carcinogenesis 5: 209–215.

Yan G, Fukabori Y, Nikolaropoulost S, Wang F, McKeehan WL (1992): Heparin binding keratinocyte growth factor is a candidate stromal to epithelial cell andromedin. Mol Endocrinol 6, 2123–2128.

Yang I, Richards I, Guzman R, Imgawa W, Nandi S (1980): Sustained growth in primary cultures of normal mammary epithelium embedded in collagen gels. Proc Natl Acad Sci USA 77: 2088–2092.

Yeoh GCT, Hilliard C, Fletcher S, Douglas A (1990): Gene expression in clonally derived cell lines produced by in vitro transformation of rat fetal hepatocytes: Isolation of cell lines which retain liver-specific markers. Cancer Res 50: 7593–7602.

Yevdokimova N, Freshney RI (1997): Activation of paracrine growth factors by heparan sulphate induced by glucocorticoid in A549 lung carcinoma cells. Br J Cancer 76: 261–289.

APPENDIX: SOURCES OF MATERIALS

Materials	Supplier
Collagenase	GIBCO/BRL; Sigma
Dispase	Roche (Boehringer); GIBCO/BRL
DNA fingerprinting or profiling	ATCC; ECCAC; LGC
Immunomagnetic sorting beads	Dynal; Miltenyi Biotech
Selective serum-free media	Biofluids; BioWhittaker; GIBCO/BRL; Sigma

2

Cell Interaction and Epithelial Differentiation

Nicole Maas-Szabowski, Hans-Jürgen Stark, and
Norbert E. Fusenig*

*Division of Carcinogenesis and Differentiation, German Cancer Research
Center (Deutsches Krebsforschungszentrum), Im Neuenheimer Feld 280,
D-69120 Heidelberg, Germany*

To whom correspondence should be addressed: n.fusenig@dkfz-heidelberg.de

Culture of Epithelial Cells, pages 31–63

I. INTRODUCTION

Epithelial cells of most organs can be grown and studied in tissue culture because of the progress made in basic cell culture technology and the improvement in our understanding of the distinct culture requirements of the various epithelia (see other chapters in this volume). Among these cells, the stratified squamous epithelia covering external or internal surfaces have received particular attention (see Chapters 3 and 5) because of their frequent involvement in disease.

The development of an orderly, structured, and well-organized epithelium during embryogenesis as well as the maintenance of the homeostasis of epithelia in vivo strictly depends on epithelial interactions with appropriate connective tissue. Accordingly, in skin the formation and maintenance of the mature epidermis, consisting of basal, spinous, granular, and cornified strata, a continuous process involving keratinocyte proliferation and terminal differentiation, is regulated by mesenchymal influences (Fig. 2.1)

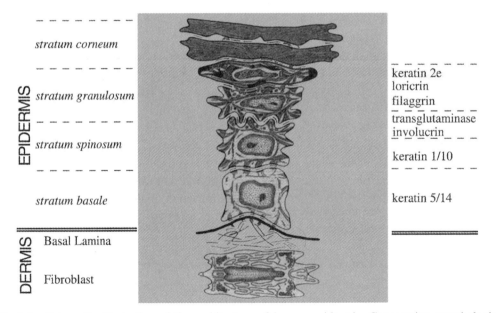

Fig 2.1. Schematic illustration of the architecture of human epidermis. Consecutive morphologic changes during tissue differentiation are paralleled by the spatial expression and modification of differentiation products [for details see Fusenig, 1986 and Bowden et al., 1987; modified from Fusenig, 1986].

[for review, see Fusenig, 1994]. Transplantation studies have revealed that the underlying mesenchyme profoundly influences morphogenesis and differentiation of adult epithelia. Normalization of epithelial development, including formation of a structured basement membrane, is independent of direct contact between epithelial and mesenchymal cells, as shown by a 1- to 2-mm-thick diffusible collagen gel lattice that served as matrix for keratinocytes and separated the epithelial cells from the mesenchyme [Fusenig et al., 1982; Bohnert et al., 1986; Boukamp et al., 1990]. This indicated that the epidermal homeostasis and the differentiation program are regulated by diffusible factors provided by the mesenchyme.

In vitro, the deficiency of keratinocyte growth and epithelialization is due to the absence of mesenchymal influences [Breitkreutz et al., 1984; Fusenig, 1992; Smola et al., 1993]. However, in coculture with mesenchymal cells, isolated and cultured epithelial cells realize their intrinsic potential for tissue-specific differentiation and still respond to appropriate extracellular regulatory stimuli [Maas-Szabowski et al., 2000]. On the basis of these observations, culture models have been developed in vitro to study epithelial-mesenchymal interactions and to identify the regulating diffusible factors. Organ culture preparations, on the other hand, are of limited use because of their relatively short culture life and their heterogeneous cellular composition.

An early attempt at establishing in vitro models to study the influence of mesenchymal cells on proliferation and differentiation of epithelial cells was the feeder-layer coculture method developed by Rheinwald and Green [1975] to expand primary keratinocytes. With this method keratinocytes grow in coculture with postmitotic fibroblasts (feeder cells) submerged in culture medium (see Chapters 3 and 5); the growth arrest of fibroblasts is indispensable to prevent the mesenchymal cells from overgrowing the epithelial cells. In these cocultures it was demonstrated that keratinocyte growth strongly depends on the presence of the mesenchymal cells. Because direct cell-cell contact of both cell types is not required, growth stimulation of epithelial cells is provided by soluble factors produced by the fibroblasts [Waelti et al., 1992]. Feeder cells, rendered postmitotic by irradiation with γ-rays or mitomycin C treatment, are still functionally competent and able to react to external stimuli and to upregulate growth factor production necessary for keratinocyte proliferation [Maas-Szabowski and Fusenig, 1996]. Thus the often-used term "lethally irradiated cells" is misleading and should be replaced by "permanently postmitotic cells."

However, in these two-dimensional feeder-layer cocultures, keratinocyte differentiation is still compromised and thus incomplete, in that properly stratified and keratinizing epithelia are not formed. Only in three-dimensional in vitro culture systems or transplantation assays in vivo will keratinocytes develop well-ordered epithelia allowing analysis of the differentiation process and its regulation. To examine this process, organotypic cocultures were established and further refined consisting of normal epithelial and mesenchymal cells, neoplastically transformed epithelial cells, immortalized cell lines, combinations of both, or even combinations of cells from different species (e.g., human/mouse). The use of heterologous models facilitates the identification of the source of diffusible factors involved in epithelial-mesenchymal interactions. In general, organotypic cocultures offer the following opportunities:

(i)   To study the influence of known local and systemically acting growth factors, hormones, and vitamins
(ii)   To characterize the altered growth and differentiation features of transformed cells
(iii) To understand the characteristic behavior of malignant cells such as loss of histotypic architecture, tumor formation, and invasion.

Although epithelial-mesenchymal interactions are operative in in vitro culture model systems, the biological significance and in vivo relevance of the effects observed in vitro should always be confirmed under more physiologic, i.e., in vivo conditions. Along with the examination of altered gene function in knock-out mice or transgenic mice [see Bajou et al., 1998], the surface transplantation assay is considered the most reliable test to identify normal epithelial physiology [Fusenig, 1983; Breitkreutz et al., 1998] as well as alterations in growth and differentiation associated with malignant transformation [Skobe et al., 1997; Bajou et al., 1998]. Both the transplantation assay and in vitro culture models used to study epithelial-mesenchymal interaction are outlined below.

2. TRANSPLANTATION MODELS FOR SURFACE EPITHELIA

Whether cultivated epithelial cells have preserved their capability to differentiate and to reorganize into structured epithelia should be tested under physiologic, i.e., in vivo, conditions. For human keratinocytes the method of choice is orthotopic transplantation onto the back muscle fascia of nude mice [Fusenig et al., 1983, 1994]. This surface transplantation assay is also useful to monitor the tumorigenic potential of transformed keratinocytes to develop a malignant phenotype and to grow invasively [Skobe et al., 1997; Fusenig et al., 2000].

The particular technique presented here exploits hat-shaped silicone transplantation chambers (see Appendix: Sources of Materials) that protect the graft from desiccation and isolate it from contiguous host epidermis. In general, there are two alternatives for inserting keratinocytes into the transplantation chamber: (1) as a single cell suspension directly onto the host dorsal muscle fascia (Fig. 2.2, left) and (2) as a preformed monolayer or even organotypic culture on an intermediate matrix separating epithelium and mesenchyme (Fig. 2.2, right). The latter version is preferred because it provides more controlled conditions of cell take and thus reproducibility of the graft take. To produce these grafts, normal

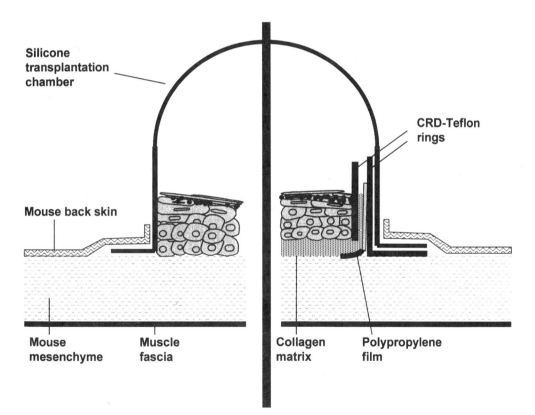

Fig 2.2. Schematic cross sections through a transplantation system of keratinocytes either directly inoculated as single cells onto the host mesenchyme (left) or implanted as intact organotypic culture on a collagen gel (mounted in CRD) that separates epithelium and mesenchyme (right).

or transformed keratinocytes (typically 2×10^5/graft) are precultivated in vitro on a collagen type I gel layer (1–2 mm thick) prepared as described in Protocol 2.3(A), either with or without incorporated fibroblasts. To achieve higher stability and better handling, the collagen gels are mounted into two concentric Teflon rings of the Combi-Ring-Dish-system (CRD) described by Noser and Limat [1987]. which exactly fit into the silicone transplantation chambers. Keratinocytes are seeded onto the collagen surface and incubated submerged for 24–48 h. These organotypic CRD-cultures are then covered with the silicone chamber and subsequently implanted onto the dorsal muscle fascia of nude mice (for details see Protocol 2.2).

The advantages of this grafting assay for cultured cells are:

(i) A low cell number is required (1–2 $\times 10^5$ per graft) for a high take rate (95–100%).

(ii) Because the cells are transplanted as preformed cultures attached to the matrix, no cell loss caused by lack of attachment in vivo (as encountered after injection of cell suspensions) occurs.

(iii) Transplants across histocompatibility barriers remain vital for at least 4 weeks. This lack of early rejection is most probably caused by the low number of allogenic cells and the virtual absence of a larger number of dead cells that might act as immunogens [Fusenig et al., 1983, 2000].

(iv) The graft is protected from overgrowth by host keratinocytes and can be easily recognized and dissected en bloc.

(v) Because of the interposed collagen gel, early mesenchymal reactions (e.g., granulation tissue formation, angiogenesis) can be studied in detail.

(vi) Finally, these surface transplants maintain a stable geometry typical for a surface epithelium and allow the analysis of epithelial-mesenchymal interactions in the same configuration as established in organotypic cocultures in vitro.

Protocol 2.1. Transplantation of Keratinocyte Suspensions

Reagents and Materials

Sterile or Aseptically Prepared

❑ Ketanest
❑ Rompun
❑ Medium: DMEM with 10% fetal bovine serum (FBS)
❑ Keratinocyte suspension, 1×10^6–2×10^7 cells/ml

❑ Silicone transplantation chamber (without CRD)
❑ Scalpels, #11
❑ Scissors, fine
❑ Syringe, 1 ml, with a needle (2 gauge)
❑ Cannula (size 0.40 × 21 mm)

Nonsterile

❑ Mice for implantation

Protocol

(a) Implant the silicone transplantation chamber onto the mouse back muscle fascia as follows:
   i) Anesthetize the mice by i.p. injection of 0.1 mg per g body weight Ketanest and 0.015 mg per g body weight Rompun.
   ii) Make a sagittal incision in the back of an anesthetized nude mouse. Transfer the transplantation chamber unit onto the muscle fascia.
   iii) Keep in place by closing the skin above the ring of the silicone chamber.
   iv) Fix the wound margins tightly with wound clips.
(b) Inoculate the cells directly into the chamber. Usually 1 × 10^5–2 × 10^6 cells in 100 μl of medium are applied by syringe with a needle pricked through the roof of the silicon chamber, while a second needle (0.40 × 21 mm) is inserted to avoid overpressure (Fig. 2.2, left).
(c) Take care to keep the mice anesthetized and immobilized for about half an hour, so that the chambers can remain horizontal for cell attachment to the muscle fascia and to prevent cell outflow from the chamber thus leading to irregular cell distribution or failure of take.

Protocol 2.2. Transplantation of Keratinocytes on a Collagen Matrix

Reagents and Materials

Sterile

❑ Culture medium: DMEM with 10% FBS
❑ CRD assembly, 8-mm internal diameter (see Fig. 2.2, right)
❑ Collagen gel solution prepared according to Protocol 2.3(A) (see below)

- ❏ Multiwell plates, 24 wells
- ❏ Polypropylene film, 20-m thickness (available from Renner, Germany), 3 × 3-cm pieces with a central circular perforation corresponding to the inner diameter of the inner Teflon ring of the CRD assembly. Sterilized in 70% ethanol.
- ❏ Stanzen Petri dishes
- ❏ Forceps, fine

Protocol

(a) Pour collagen gel solution into 24-well plates, 500 μl per well (16-mm diameter), to fabricate gels of appropriate size to fit into the CRD assembly.

(b) Allow 1 h at 37°C in a humidified incubator for gelation to take place.

(c) Cover the gels with 1 ml of culture medium.

(d) Detach gels from wells and place on a piece of polypropylene film. This is an important auxiliary tool for mounting that prevents the gel from being ruptured while being mounted between the concentric Teflon rings of the CRD.

(e) Center the gel and polypropylene film carefully above the outer ring of the CRD.

(f) Place the inner ring centrally on top of the collagen gel and push the gel on the film gently into the outer ring so that the gel now stretches over the lower open end of the CRD assembly (see Fig. 2.2, right).

(g) Equilibrate assembled CRDs with culture medium in Stanzen Petri dishes providing free medium access from below.

(h) Incubate at 37°C.

(i) Plate 2 × 10^5 epithelial cells, in 100 μl of medium, onto the collagen gel in the inner ring of the CRD.

(j) Allow to attach for 12–24 h.

(k) Rinse the cells with medium.

(l) Aspirate the medium covering the cells from the CRD.

(m) Cover the CRD with the silicone transplantation chamber, fitting the outer Teflon ring tightly.

(n) Insert a cannula (size 0.4 × 21 mm) into the dome-shaped roof of the transplantation chamber to release the pressure, to prevent the risk of damaging the collagen matrix by mechanical distortion or by creating overpressure inside the chamber.

(o) Lift the chamber with this cannula onto the CRD and push gently down with forceps.

Maas-Szabowski, Stark, and Fusenig

(p) For transplantation,
  i) Anesthetize mice by i.p. injection of 0.1 mg per g body weight Ketanest and 0.015 mg per g body weight Rompun.
  ii) Make a sagittal incision in the back of the anesthetized nude mice.
  iii) Transfer the complete CRD-transplantation chamber unit onto the muscle fascia.
  iv) Keep in place by closing the skin above the ring of the silicone chamber and tightly fix the wound margins with wound clips.
(q) Transplants are excised en bloc at desired time points and further processed for histology and cryotome sectioning (see Protocol 2.3, Analysis (ii), below).

Both methods are suited for reconstitution of epithelial tissue with characteristic differentiation features by grafted cells within 1 week [Breitkreutz et al., 1984, 1997]. In addition, this transplantation assay represents a reliable method to discriminate benign (noninvasive) and malignant phenotypes of epithelial cells. Although various degrees of epidermal dysplasia are common to transplants of transformed keratinocytes in different stages of neoplastic conversion, the malignant cells exclusively display invasive growth in such transplants, whereas premalignant cells form stratified epithelia on top of a newly formed granulation tissue. Primarily in cancer research, this transplantation assay is an indispensable tool to evaluate altered cell regulation in the context of a physiologic environment that, so far, cannot be provided by in vitro models [for review see Fusenig et al., 2000].

3. ORGANOTYPIC COCULTURES OF EPITHELIAL AND MESENCHYMAL CELLS

The molecular mechanisms of epithelial-mesenchymal interactions are difficult to study under in vivo conditions because of the many variables involved and the lack of properly controlled experimental conditions. Consequently, suitable in vitro models for studying epithelial-mesenchymal interaction have been developed.

3.1. Organotypic Epithelial Cultures

All surface epithelia, including the epidermis, are exposed with their upper cell sheets to the outer or inner environment while being nourished from the basal side attached to the stroma. This in vivo situation is completely altered in conventional culture systems: the epithelial cell population grows submerged in medium, devoid of specific extracellular matrix and mesenchymal influence, making it difficult to achieve the correct cellular polarity. To render the culture more like in vivo conditions, organotypic culture models have been developed [Bell et al., 1981; Prunieras et al., 1983].

The simplest way to study the effect of mesenchymal cells on epithelial cell growth and differentiation is to add a piece of structured mesenchyme (e.g., dermis) to such cultures by placing it beneath the collagen gel matrix [Fusenig et al., 1983; Fusenig, 1992]. The piece of mesenchyme can either be vital or devitalized by repeated freezing and thawing (at least $3\times$ freezing in liquid nitrogen and thawing at 37°C). However, the use of living dermis under a gel matrix, as well as epithelia cultured directly on dermis, could create the following problems, (1) Because of the thickness of the mesenchyme, cells in the center will soon degenerate when incubated in medium under regular culture conditions. (2) Remnants of epithelial cells from skin appendages (hair follicles, sweat glands) will rapidly repopulate the surface of the mesenchyme and influence the mesenchymal-epithelial interaction [Fusenig et al., 1991].

Recombinant organotypic cultures of isolated epidermal cells grown directly on devitalized dermis result in the formation of well-structured epithelia within 8–10 days. The multilayered epithelia express characteristic differentiation products such as keratins, involucrin, and lipids [Prunieras et al., 1983; Grinnell, 1987; Fartasch and Ponec, 1994; Hertle et al., 1995; see also Section 5.2]. The complex tissue of an intact dermis, even if devitalized by freezing and thawing or by irradiation, still contains large amounts of active soluble factors, possibly immobilized in the matrix, able to exert short-term regulatory effects on the epithelial cells growing on the upper surface [Regnier and Darmon, 1989].

Moreover, organotypic culture systems with devitalized dermis are difficult to standardize, because pieces of dermis with reproducible quality (in structure, age, or body site) are difficult to produce and even more difficult to analyze for causal factors and their mechanisms of action. Therefore, simplified organotypic recombinant culture models with isolated mesenchymal cells represent a preferable way to analyze the function of connective tissue elements.

In such organotypic cultures, human epidermal keratinocytes grow exposed to air in special filter inserts (see Appendix: Sources of Materials) on a matrix of collagen type I, which is isolated from rat tail tendon or calf skin (Fig. 2.3). To become functional dermal equivalents, the collagen gels contain dermal fibroblasts that may proliferate in the collagen gel and eventually reorganize this matrix by producing extracellular matrix components comparable to the wound situation [Coulomb et al., 1984; Smola et al., 1993]. While contracting the gels to a densely structured lattice with oriented collagen fibrils, the fibroblasts reduce their proliferative activity, alter their protein synthesis, and acquire a resting state comparable to that of dermis [Coulomb et al., 1984]. Furthermore, in this model, the contact of the cultures with medium is restricted to the base of the gel so that fibroblasts and keratinocytes are nourished by diffusion from below. Optionally, cultures can be grown in serum-containing medium or under more defined conditions in defined medium (Stark et al., 1999; see Section 4.2).

When plated on the upper surface of collagen gels containing embedded fibroblasts, epithelial cells rapidly attach and form confluent layers within 1–2 days. Subsequently, keratinocytes reconstitute an epithelial tissue architecture resembling the epidermis (Figs. 2.4, 2.5a–f) and expressing characteristic epidermal differentiation markers [Parenteau et al., 1991; Contard et al., 1993; Fusenig, 1994; Stark et al., 1999]. In the absence of fibroblasts only thin epithelia arise with rapid loss of proliferation and incomplete differentiation (Fig. 2.4a) [Smola et al., 1993; Fusenig, 1994; Maas-Szabowski et al., 2000].

In cocultures of mesenchymal and epithelial cells, the function of diffusible factors mediating epithelial-mesenchymal interactions and the dynamics of basement membrane formation (Fig. 2.6) has been demonstrated [Smola et al., 1998; Maas-Szabowski et al., 2000]. Furthermore, many aspects of epidermal biology depending on regular keratinocyte differentiation became acces-

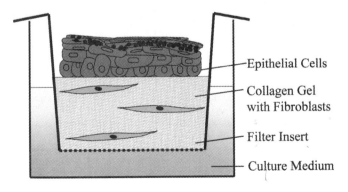

Epithelial Cells

Collagen Gel
with Fibroblasts

Filter Insert

Culture Medium

Fig 2.3. Schematic illustration of the organotypic culture system. Keratinocytes growing air-exposed on a fibroblast-containing collagen gel nourished by medium from underneath.

sible, e.g., the reepithelialization in wound closure, the relation of proliferation and integrin pattern, the expression of human papillomavirus promoters, and the development of the stratum corneum barrier [Garlick and Taichman, 1994; Nuss Parker et al., 1997; Ponec et al., 1997; Rikimaru et al., 1997]. These aspects can be analyzed in organotypic cocultures for up to 3 weeks. with maximum effects usually discernible by 1–2 weeks and a decline thereafter. Morphologic criteria can be visualized by histologic (Figs. 2.4, 2.5a–f) and electron microscopic techniques (Fig. 2.6) as well as the spatial expression of differentiation products by immunohistochemistry. The expression patterns of interacting molecules can be analyzed by RNA and protein levels according

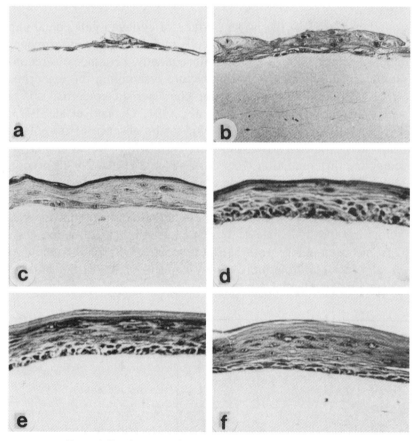

Fig 2.4. Effect of fibroblast numbers on epidermal tissue regeneration in organotypic cocultures. Histologic sections of 7-day-old organotypic cultures with no (A), 1×10^4 (B), 2×10^5 (C), 5×10^4 (D), 1×10^5 (E), and 2×10^5 (F) postmitotic fibroblasts per ml in the collagen matrix. (H and E staining) [see also Maas-Szabowski et al., 2000].

Maas-Szabowski, Stark, and Fusenig

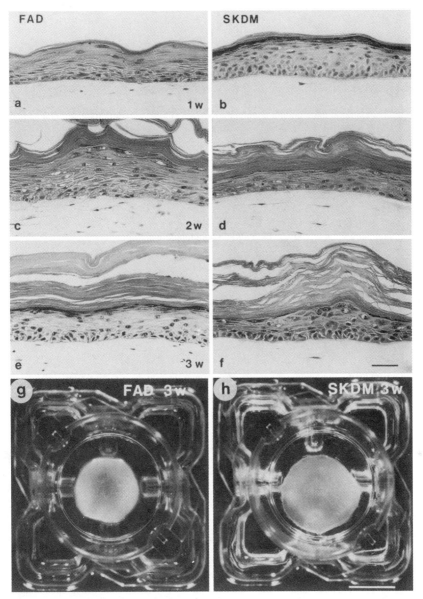

Fig 2.5. Epithelial morphogenesis in organotypic cocultures of keratinocytes and mitotic fibroblasts. Keratinocytes are cultured air-exposed on fibroblast-containing collagen lattices in serum-containing medium (FAD; a, c, e) and defined medium (SKDM; b, d, f) and processed for histology at 1 wk (a, b), 2 wk (c, d), and 3 wk (e, f). There is a large increase in stratifying cell layers during the first week (a, b), whereas later viable layers approach an equilibrium with the thickening stratum corneum (H and E staining; scale bar: 50 μm). (g, h) Macroscopic views of 3-wk-old organotypic cocultures in serum-containing FAD medium (g) and defined SKDM medium (h) illustrate the different degrees of retraction performed by the fibroblasts. (Scale bar: 1cm) [taken from Stark et al., 1999].

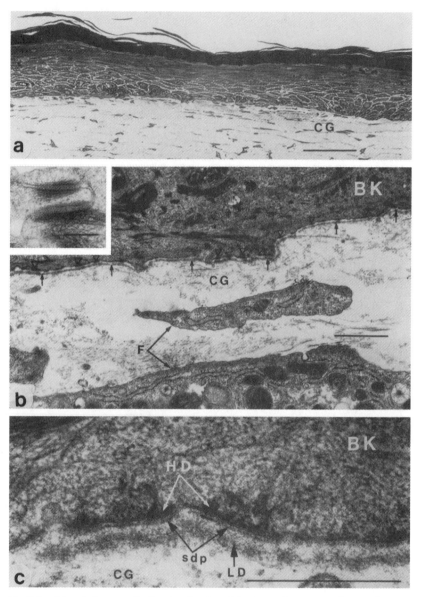

Fig 2.6. Morphology and ultrastructural architecture of organotypic cocultures at 3 wk. (a) Semi-thin section showing the overall morphology of the developing epidermis, (b, c) different magnifications of the basal aspects of basal keratinocytes (BK) on top of fibroblast (F)-containing collagen gels (CG). Straight arrows depict the lamina lucida (LD) of the newly formed basement membrane, which also contains mature hemidesmosomes (HD) and subbasal dense plates (sdp). Inset in (b), desmosomal junctions between adjacent keratinocytes reinforced by attached tonofilament bundles. [Bars 100 μm in (a), 200 nm in (b) and (c), 40 nm in inset in (b)] [for details see Smola et al., 1998].

to appropriate molecular methods [Smola et al., 1993, 1998; Maas-Szabowski et al., 2000].

3.2. Dermal Equivalents

Besides collagen type I, other extracellular matrices have been utilized in organotypic cultures such as mixtures of collagen type I and III [Lillie et al., 1988] or basal lamina constituents (e.g., laminin, collagen type IV, fibronectin) [Tinois et al., 1991]. A widely used material is Matrigel, a mixture of ECM components extracted from tumor stroma [Kleinman et al., 1986] (see also Appendix: Sources of Materials).

In the organotypic culture system with mesenchymal cells dispersed in the gel, direct cell-cell contact between the surface epithelium and the matrix-embedded fibroblasts cannot be strictly excluded because of the tendency of mesenchymal cells to migrate and accumulate beneath the epithelium. To generate a more defined localization of both cell types, epithelial and mesenchymal cells can be separated by addition of a cell-free matrix on top of the fibroblast-containing collagen gel consisting of collagen type I, other specific matrix components, or a mixture of ECM components (Matrigel). With a similar sandwich technique it is even possible to introduce a third cell type, e.g., endothelial cells, in a gel below the fibroblast matrix. To prevent early mesenchymal-epithelial cell contact, fibroblasts are plated on the surface of a filter insert and, after attachment, a cell-free gel is poured above. Alternatively, fibroblasts are plated on the lower membrane surface of a filter insert containing a cell-free collagen gel and, after attachment, keratinocytes are plated on top of the cell-free matrix. Within 1–3 weeks of culture, mesenchymal cells continue to multiply and progressively repopulate the collagen lattice, usually maintaining horizontal orientation but remaining separated from the epithelium for 2–3 weeks.

In addition to the problem of direct cell-cell contact, the fluctuating number and different proliferative state of fibroblasts cause further variations influencing the dynamics of the epidermal-dermal cell interplay because of the variable increase in cell number depending on seeding density [Coulomb et al., 1989; Stark et al., 1999]. To standardize the fibroblast compartment, the organotypic culture system was further improved by using fibroblasts rendered permanently postmitotic by high-dose X irradiation. As demonstrated in two-dimensional cultures, in which feeder layer cocultures are used to promote expansion of the keratinocytes, the irradiated fibroblasts are still functionally active, as far as cellular integrity, expression and secretion of growth factors and cytokines, and the response to specific inducers are concerned [Limat et al., 1989; Waelti et al., 1992; Smola et al., 1993, 1994; Bumann et al., 1995; Maas-Szabowski and Fusenig, 1996].

For organotypic cocultures, the use of postmitotic cells offers several advantages. (1) The fibroblast number is kept constant throughout extended culture periods, at least for to 3 weeks. In contrast, proliferating fibroblasts, depending on the culture system and collagen concentration, multiply at different rates in the matrix, eventually populating the filter surface as well and thus causing considerable variation in cell numbers. (2) Based on a stably maintained fibroblast population, it is possible to determine reliable cell numbers required for sustaining minimal or promoting optimal epidermal growth and differentiation (Fig. 2.4). This allowed establishment of organotypic cultures with subthreshold cell numbers to study the effect of added specific growth factors at given time points [Maas-Szabowski et al., 1999]. (3) Importantly, the irradiated postmitotic fibroblasts more closely resemble the resting stage exhibited by the majority of fibroblasts in normal dermis. (4) Finally, the resting fibroblasts also reduced the collagen gel contraction (see Fig. 2.5g, h), a problem usually encountered with proliferating fibroblasts in collagen gels [Stark et al., 1999].

Protocol 2.3. Preparation of Organotypic Skin Cocultures

Reagents and Materials

Sterile or aseptically prepared

- ❑ Epithelial cells, e.g., human skin keratinocytes
- ❑ Dermal fibroblasts
- ❑ FBS
- ❑ Culture media: DMEM with 10% FBS or, particularly for normal human keratinocytes, FAD (Ham's F12 and DMEM, 1 +3) with 10% FBS; alternatively serum-free, defined formulations such as SKDM [see Stark et al., 1999]; all media supplemented with 50 μg L-ascorbic acid per ml)
- ❑ Type I collagen
- ❑ Hanks' balanced salt solution, 10×
- ❑ NaOH, I N
- ❑ Acetic acid, 0.1% (0.17 M)

❑ Filter well inserts, 2.5 cm (see Appendix: Sources of Materials; see also Fig. 2.3)

❑ Multiwell plate, 6-well, deep wells

Nonsterile

❑ Ice

Protocol

(A) Dermal equivalents

(a) Resolubilize the collagen at the desired concentration (2–4 mg/ml; dry weight) in 0.1% acetic acid and keep at 4°C. (Collagen solutions above 6 mg/ml are very viscous and difficult to handle.)

(b) Mix ice-cold collagen solution (80% of total volume, 4 mg/ml) with 10× Hanks' salt solution (10% of total volume) and adjust it to pH 7.4 by adding 20–60 μl of 1 N NaOH while stirring on ice.

(c) The number of fibroblasts necessary for the desired concentration in the gel (1×10^5–1×10^6 per ml) is resuspended in FBS (10% of total volume), or, in the case of cell-free gels, FBS alone (10% of total volume) is mixed with the gel solution on ice with gentle stirring.

(d) Starting with 4 mg/ml collagen solution in acetic acid the final concentration of the collagen solution is then ~3.2 mg/ml.

(e) Using cooled pipettes, dispense 2.5-ml aliquots of the complete collagen solution into each 2.5-cm filter insert.

(f) Place the filter inserts into a deep six-well plate and incubate for 1 h at 37°C in a humidified incubator for gelation.

(g) Place glass rings corresponding to the diameter of the filter inserts (internal diameter 18 mm, wall thickness 2 mm, height 8 mm) on the gel and gently push down by mild pressure with forceps to compress the gel and to delineate the area for seeding the keratinocytes.

(h) Place gels with the glass rings for 1 h at 37°C in a humidified incubator.

(i) Gently aspirate the excess liquid pressed out without touching the glass ring.

(j) Equilibrate the gels by complete immersion in culture medium for 24 h.

(B) Epithelial cells

(k) Plate epithelial cells, e.g., human skin keratinocytes, (1×10^6 cells in 1 ml of medium for 2.5-cm inserts) inside the inner ring. They attach within 12–24 h and form a nearly confluent layer on top of the collagen gel.

(l) Rinse the keratinocyte cell layer with 1 ml of medium 24–30 h after seeding.

(m) Remove the glass rings, avoiding any mechanical distortion of the epithelial cell sheet. Occasionally, the margin of the cell layer must be detached from the glass rings with a scalpel before the ring is removed.

(n) Change the culture medium, and, by lowering the medium level to the lower parts of the gels, raise the cultures to the air-liquid interphase, restricting nourishment to diffusion from below.

Analysis

The regulation of directional processes such as secretory functions or apical differentiation mechanisms can be studied in such polarized cultures. Furthermore, it is possible to investigate the effects of agents applied either "topically" (to the upper surface of the epithelial cultures) or "systemically" (added to the culture medium and, after diffusion through the collagen lattice, coming into contact first with the basal-layer epithelial cells).

(i) Specific effectors can be added to the medium and replaced by medium changes every 2–3 days to act as "local" or "systemic" factors after diffusion through the dermal compartment.

(ii) For histologic analysis (see Figs. 2.4, 2.5a–f) or immunohistochemistry, embed the organotypic cocultures in agar (2%) to prevent dislodgment of the epidermal and dermal compartment during further preparation, fix in formaldehyde (3.7%), and then process en bloc in paraffin or prepare as specimens for cryosectioning by embedding in Tissue Tek-OTC compound and subsequent snap freezing in liquid nitrogen.

(iii) For expression studies RNA or proteins can be extracted from the epithelial and mesenchymal compartments separately, after simple mechanical separation, without incurring cross contamination. Possible contamination of the epidermal compartment by fibroblasts is excluded by RT-PCR analysis of KGF mRNA (produced exclusively by stromal cells) and, vice versa, by checking the fibroblast compartment for expression of keratins (epithelial exclusive).

(iv) Cell numbers in the dermal equivalent can be quantitated by counting cells after their release from the collagen lattice by dissolving the gels in PBSA for 2–4 min at 60°C and collecting cells by centrifugation. Alternatively, gels can be digested by incubation in collagenase, 2 μg/ml, at 30°C for 35 min, although this is a more cumbersome and less accurate procedure, usually restricted to the recovery of living cells.

(v) Analysis of cell numbers in the reconstituted epithelium is more difficult because dissociation of the epithelial layers into single cells is problematic. Assessment of epithelial cell numbers may be achieved by determining total DNA content and calculating the number of nucleated cells based on standard curves established with monolayer cultures (see Section 5.1).

(vi) At different time points the culture medium is collected and stored at −80°C for determination of secreted proteins (ECM components, growth factors, proteases, etc.) by ELISA and Western blot analysis [see Maas-Szabowski et al., 1999, 2000; Szabowski et al., 2000].

4. MODIFICATIONS OF ORGANOTYPIC COCULTURES

Various modifications of the recombinant culture model described above have been designed to study different aspects of skin biology such as the effects of specific cell types and matrix compositions.

4.1. Variations of Epithelial and Mesenchymal Cells

Both isologous and heterologous combinations of epithelial and mesenchymal cells from different species have been used. Examples for epithelia-derived cells and cell lines used in cocultures and/or transplantation assays can only be listed here without further details, e.g., mouse skin keratinocytes [Breitkreutz et al., 1984; Mackenzie and Fusenig, 1993; Mackenzie et al., 1983], human epidermal keratinocytes [Fusenig et al., 1983; Fusenig, 1992], outer root sheet cells of hair follicles [Noser and Limat, 1987], squamous cell carcinoma line SCC-13 [Kopan and Fuchs, 1989], normal foreskin keratinocytes and virus transformed keratinocytes [Kaur and Carter, 1992], hair matrix and follicular keratinocytes [Detmar et al., 1993], the spontaneously immortalized keratinocyte cell line HaCaT [Breitkreutz et al., 1998; Schoop et al., 1999], H-ras transformed HaCaT cells [Vaccariello et al., 1999]; conjunctival epithelial cells [Chen et al., 1994], human ovarian epithelial cells [Gregoire et al., 1998], and mucosa epithelial cells [Tomakidi et al., 1998]. Nonkeratinocyte cell types of the epidermis such as melanocytes and Langerhans cells have also been incorporated into the epithelial compartment of organotypic cocultures [Regnier et al., 1997; Laning et al., 1999]. The insertion of melanocytes makes it possible to investigate the regulation of skin pigmentation as well as its modulation by cosmetic or medical treatment. On the other hand, an in vitro skin model including mature and functional Langerhans cells could become a valuable device for testing of skin sensitization by contact allergens, provided a meaningful end point marker can be established.

Dermal cell type mouse 3T3 fibroblasts [Kopan et al., 1987; Kaur and Carter, 1992; Chen et al., 1995], human dermal fibroblasts [Fusenig et al., 1983; Asselineau and Pruniéras, 1984; Noser and Limat, 1987; Breitkreutz et al., 1998; Stark et al., 1999; Maas-Szabowski et al., 2000], scleroderma fibroblasts [Mauch et al., 1992], or even SCC tumor-derived fibroblasts [Atula et al., 1997] have been incorporated into the matrix depending on the experimental purpose. Different approaches have also exploited devitalized dermis to establish recombinant cultures [Ponec et al., 1997; Eming et al., 1998]. With endothelial cells included in cultured skin equivalents, an in vitro reconstruction of capillary-like structures could be achieved [Black et al., 1998, 1999]. This might have important implications for angiogenesis studies as well as graft acceptance supported by improved vascularization. Most recently, by including mouse fibroblasts from knock-out mice, even if the genetic modifications are lethal at the embryonic stage, novel aspects of epithelial-mesenchymal interactions with these genetically modified fibroblasts and normal keratinocytes have become accessible for molecular functional studies [Szabowski et al., 2000].

4.2. Variations of Extracellular Matrix and Culture Media

The most common matrices for organotypic cocultures are collagen type I gels used at different collagen concentrations (1–4 mg/ml) and obtained from different species and organs (e.g., rat, bovine, tendons, skin, placenta). Alternatively, dermal equivalents were reconstituted from collagen type IV, Matrigel, soft agar, or mixtures of collagen and glycosaminoglycans [Dawson et al., 1996; Supp et al., 2000; Takahashi and Nogawa, 1991; Zheng and

Vaheri, 1995]. It is even possible to examine mesenchymal-epithelial interaction without direct cell-cell contact of both cell populations in two-chamber transfilter systems without any exogenous extracellular matrix component [Axel et al., 1997; Gharary et al., 1998, 1999].

The majority of cell culture experiments are performed in conventional culture media (e.g., DMEM or other formulations) containing serum and additional supplements (such as insulin, EGF, cholera toxin either alone or in combination; see also Chapters 3 and 5). More defined culture conditions have become available by the development of serum-free culture media (Fig. 2.5) [see also Stark et al., 1999]. Under those defined conditions it is possible to examine the intrinsic mesenchymal-epithelial interaction free of ill-defined serum constituents and to evaluate more precisely the responses of cells to addition or depletion of growth factors, hormones, vitamins, and other compounds in the culture medium.

5. CRITERIA FOR EVALUATION OF GROWTH AND DIFFERENTIATION

The criteria for the analysis of the performance of epithelial cells in mesenchymal cocultures are applicable to most cell types but are particularly focused on skin epithelial cells (keratinocytes), which have been studied most extensively in these in vitro model systems.

5.1. Proliferation Parameters

Cell proliferation can be analyzed in tissue sections by established methods such as mitotic index or immunolabeling. Some of the conventional methods for studying cell proliferation in normal cell culture systems, such as cell counting and cloning efficiency, cannot be applied to these complex model systems, in which keratinocytes form keratinizing epithelia so that a complete dissociation into single cells is no longer feasible.

Biochemically, proliferation can be assessed by measuring changes in total DNA content, which usually parallel the number of nucleated cells. However, this technique is not reliable for determining the total cell number of the epidermis, because the DNA is degraded during the differentiation process in the stratum corneum. Measurement of protein content as a criterion of cell proliferation is also not reliable because of changing cellular protein levels during keratinocyte maturation. Determination of proliferating cells has been done conventionally by incorporation of radioactive thymidine and analysis by autoradiography. The most frequently used method today is labeling with the thymidine analog BrdU (bromodeoxyuridine) and subsequent detection of the proliferating cells on paraffin or frozen sections by specific anti-BrdU antibodies. Positive nuclear reaction in cells that were in S phase during the BrdU pulse can be recorded relative to the total number of nuclei counterstained by a DNA dye. Alternatively, immunohistochemical monitoring of proliferation in tissue or cell culture sections, without any prelabeling, is possible with anti-Ki-67 or anti-Mib1 antibodies specific for nuclear antigens in cycling cells [Gerdes et al., 1984; Cattoretti et al., 1992].

5.2. Differentiation Markers

Characterization of epithelial differentiation in vitro by identifying expression and localization of specific differentiation products of the relevant tissue can be performed by conventional biochemical, histochemical, and molecular biological methods. The data obtained must be compared with established standards such as the profile of differentiation markers in epidermis in vivo. However, under experimental in vitro conditions, differentiation parameters that are usually coexpressed in vivo can become uncoupled, indicating inappropriate or altered differentiation processes [Stark et al., 1999].

Morphology, as the most important qualitative parameter of epidermal tissue reconstitution, is evaluated by light and electron microscopy. The formation of a regular tissue architecture usually is paralleled by normal expression patterns of differentiation products. On tissue sections RNA expression can be visualized and localized by in situ hybridization. In addition, histochemical analysis of frozen or fixed tissue sections will demonstrate specific differentiation products and their distribution in the tissue. Antibodies to tissue-specific differentiation proteins, to cell surface structures, to desmosomal or junctional proteins, or to basement membrane components and various others are available for most tissue types [see, e.g., Smola et al., 1998; Stark et al., 1999].

For evaluation of the differentiation process in epidermis-like organotypic cultures, the following marker proteins are suggested as useful hallmarks:

(i) Keratins as the predominant differentiation products of keratinocytes and constituents of tonofilaments. Although keratins 5 and 14 are present in all keratinocytes, keratins 1 and 10 predominate in all suprabasal layers and keratin 2e predominates in the stratum granulosum.

(ii)   Cornified envelope proteins such as involucrin and loricrin are also located in the stratum granulosum.

(iii) Filaggrin, the major constituent of the keratohyalin granules, and transglutaminase are localized in the stratum granulosum as well.

6. FACTORS CONTROLLING TISSUE REGENERATION

Important questions in the study of epithelial-mesenchymal interactions are directed toward the molecular mechanisms and factors involved in the permissive and/or inductive effects of the tissue compartments involved. Cell-cell interactions via diffusible factors and cell-matrix interactions via integrins have been shown to modulate epithelial morphogenesis [Werner et al., 1992; Smola et al., 1993; Breitkreutz et al., 1997]. Maintenance of tissue homeostasis requires the proper functioning of these epithelial-mesenchymal control mechanisms, which are predominantly mediated by diffusible factors [Fusenig, 1994; Maas-Szabowski et al., 2000]. Although not all of these factors are defined yet, the following principles must be considered as essential:

(i)   Tissue homeostasis is controlled by the concerted action of multiple factors regulating proliferation and differentiation.

(ii)   Different factors originating from the mesenchymal and epithelial compartment and acting in paracrine and/or autocrine loops may interact with and influence each other.

(iii) Superimposed on these local factors are the systemic effects of hormones, vitamins, and other mediators delivered by the circulation and acting synergistically or antagonistically on epithelial and mesenchymal tissue elements.

(iv)   The relative concentrations of interacting factors are important for a balanced development and maintenance of tissue architecture.

In this multifactorial interaction, polypeptide growth factors are important mediators of intercellular communication and play an important role in maintaining tissue homeostasis, outlined here for the skin. Several growth factors and interleukins have been detected in skin as well as in keratinocyte and fibroblast cultures, such as IL-1, IL-6, IL-8, GM-CSF, TGF-α and -β, NGF, and PDGF as well as several members of the FGF family [Luger and Schwarz, 1995; Kupper and Groves, 1995; Schröder, 1995]. They are primarily understood as potent mediators of immune reactions and inflammatory processes [Luger and Schwarz, 1990, 1995] but are also actively involved in skin repair after wounding [Werner, 1998]. As yet the control mechanisms of expression and the interplay of these factors still remain largely unknown.

In the simplest coculture system, originally developed just to expand keratinocytes and composed of growth arrested fibroblasts and proliferating keratinocytes [Rheinwald and Green, 1975], the functional role of several cytokines has been studied [Waelti et al., 1992; Smola et al., 1993]. It has been determined that cocultured fibroblasts produce and secrete KGF after stimulation by IL-1 released by keratinocytes, representing a novel type of keratinocyte-fibroblast interplay via a double paracrine pathway [Maas-Szabowski et al., 1996, 1999]. Subsequently, under the more physiologic conditions of organotypic cocultures using postmitotic fibroblasts and a defined culture medium, we have demonstrated that this novel growth control mechanism functions as well in the more in vivo-like skin equivalent [Fig. 2.7; see also Maas-Szabowski et al., 2000]. It might thus be of central importance in vivo in skin regeneration and homeostasis.

The induction of KGF expression in fibroblasts by keratinocytes via release of IL-1 was confirmed and its functional significance documented by application of IL-1-neutralizing antibodies and an IL-1 receptor antagonist, respectively (Fig. 2.7). Blocking of IL-1 signaling inhibited KGF release, keratinocyte prolifera-

Fig 2.7. Schematic illustration of the double paracrine pathways of keratinocyte growth regulation in organotypic cocultures with fibroblasts involving IL-1, KGF, and GM-CSF as well as their receptors [see also Maas-Szabowski et al., 2000; Szabowski et al. 2000].

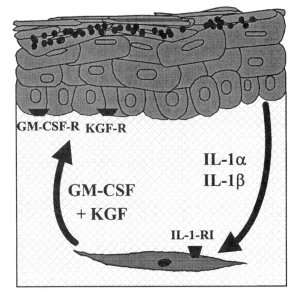

tion, and tissue formation, an effect comparable to that produced by KGF-blocking antibodies. On the other hand, IL-1 itself had no effect on keratinocyte proliferation in monocultures. Moreover, addition of KGF to cocultures with inactivated IL-1 pathway completely reversed growth inhibition. Furthermore, in organotypic cocultures with subthreshold fibroblast numbers, addition of either IL-1 or KGF restored the impaired epidermal morphogenesis. Thus the results demonstrate the functional significance of this novel growth regulatory pathway as a major control mechanism for keratinocyte proliferation and epidermal tissue formation [Maas-Szabowski et al., 2000].

However, the characterization of paracrine-acting factors between fibroblasts and keratinocytes is sometimes difficult in a homologous skin model system containing human cells in both compartments. A heterologous skin equivalent harboring cell types of different species of origin would have the advantage that the source of the respective gene products can be more easily and unequivocally distinguished. Heterologous three-dimensional coculture systems containing human keratinocytes and nonhuman fibroblasts have already been used [Kaur and Carter, 1992; Turksen et al., 1991; Choi and Fuchs, 1994]. In those studies, however, the fibroblasts were supposed to act merely as producers of matrix components. Recently, an advanced heterologous coculture system was established exploiting various mouse fibroblast lines derived from *c-jun*$^{-/-}$ or *junB*$^{-/-}$ mouse embryos [Szabowski et al., 2000]. This paved the way to address in more detail the role of fibroblasts in skin tissue homeostasis and to study in particular the role of c-Jun- and JunB-regulated genes in fibroblasts acting in *trans* on proliferation and differentiation of keratinocytes. The *c-jun* and *junB* gene products are members of the immediate-early transcription factor family AP-1 and are expressed in many organs during development and in the adult. Functional proof for this assumption was provided by loss of function in *c-jun* and *junB* knock-out mice, resulting in embryonic lethality [Hilberg et al., 1993; Schorpp-Kistner et al., 1999]. However, embryonic fibroblast cell lines have been established and successfully cocultured with human keratinocytes in organotypic cultures. Whereas wild-type (normal) mouse fibroblasts as well as human fibroblasts support proliferation and differentiation of keratinocytes, *c-jun*$^{-/-}$ fibroblasts have lost this competence. On the contrary, keratinocyte growth and differentiation were enhanced by *junB*$^{-/-}$ fibroblasts. Responsible target genes of AP-1 in fibroblasts were identified as GM-CSF and KGF, the latter already known as a paracrine-acting mediator in this system.

The active regulation of KGF and GM-CSF in fibroblasts via AP-1 is triggered by IL-1 released by keratinocytes (Fig. 2.7).

KGF has been identified as a typical paracrine-acting growth factor, produced by mesenchymal cells such as fibroblasts, stimulating epithelial cell proliferation via KGF receptors only expressed in these target cells [for review see Marchese, 1995; Werner, 1998]. An IL-1/KGF loop has already been identified in homologous skin equivalents [Maas-Szabowski et al., 2000] and discussed in the context of the early wound healing process [Werner, 1998]. The other factor, GM-CSF, has been associated primarily with the hematopoietic cell system, where it promotes the proliferation of progenitors in the erythroid, eosinophil, and megakaryocyte lineage on one hand and the differentiation of hematopoietic progenitor cells toward mature granulocytes and macrophages on the other [Metcalf, 1998]. In skin, GM-CSF has been shown to stimulate keratinocyte proliferation after in vivo application, however, without any mechanistic interpretation [Braunstein et al., 1994]. We now have strong evidence from studies in organotypic cocultures that GM-CSF is involved as a positive stimulus in the regulation of epidermal proliferation and differentiation.

Moreover, AP-1 seems to be an essential switch in the mechanisms regulating the cross talk between keratinocytes and fibroblasts in organotypic cocultures and is critically involved in the double paracrine loop controlling epidermal growth and differentiation. KGF and GM-CSF are the first known AP-1-dependent genes that are antagonistically regulated by c-Jun and JunB. Obviously, a fine-tuned balance between KGF and GM-CSF is necessary for epithelial regeneration and homeostasis in skin. Interestingly, KGF and GM-CSF alone are not sufficient to support keratinocyte growth in the absence of fibroblasts, indicating that further mediators, or at least one more c-jun-independent survival factor, are involved in these tissue interactions.

These studies clearly indicate that the appropriate in vitro models reflecting the major cell types and structural characteristics of the tissue in the organism not only allow reconstitution of the tissue specific structures but provide useful and biologically relevant model systems to study the molecular mechanisms regulating cell proliferation and differentiation in a tissue-type context.

REFERENCES

Asselineau D, Prunieras M (1984): Reconstruction of simplified skin: Control of fabrication. Br J Dermatol 111(27): 219–222.

Atula S, Grenman R, Syrjänen S (1997): Fibroblasts can modulate the phenotype of malignant epithelial cells in vitro. Exp Cell Res 235: 180–187.

Axel DI, Riessen R, Athanasiadis A, Runge H, Koveker G, Karsch KR (1997): Growth factor expression of human arterial smooth muscle cells and endothelial cells in a transfilter coculture system. J Mol Cell Cardiol 29(11): 2967–2978.

Bajou K, Noel A, Gerard RD, Masson V, Brunner N, Holst-Hansen C, Skobe M, Fusenig NE, Carmeliet P, Collen D, Foidart JM (1998): Absence of host plasminogen activator inhibitor 1 prevents cancer invasion and vascularization. Nat Med 4(8): 923–928.

Bell E, Ehrlich HP, Buttle DJ, Nakatsuji T (1981): Living tissue formed in vivo and accepted as skin-equivalent tissue of full thickness. Science 211: 1052–1054.

Black AF, Berthold F, L'Heureux N, Germain L, Auger FA (1998): In vitro reconstruction of a capillary-like network in a tissue-engineered skin equivalent. FASEB J 12: 1311–1340.

Black AF, Hudon V, Damour O, Germain L, Auger FA (1999): A novel approach for studying angiogenesis: A human skin equivalent with a capillary-like network. Cell Biol Toxicol 15(2): 81–90.

Bohnert A, Hornung J, Mackenzie IC, Fusenig NE (1986): Epithelial-mesenchymal interactions control basement membrane production and differentiation in cultured and transplanted mouse keratinocytes. Cell Tissue Res 244: 413–429.

Boukamp P, Breitkreutz D, Stark HJ, Fusenig NE (1990): Mesenchyme-mediated and endogenous regulation of growth and differentiation of human skin keratinocytes derived from different body sites. Differentiation 44: 150–161.

Bowden PE, Stark HJ, Breitkreutz D, Fusenig NE (1987): Expression and modification of keratins during terminal differentiation of mammalian epidermis. Curr Top Dev Biol 22: 35–68.

Braunstein S, Kaplan G, Gottlieb AB, Schwarz M, Walsh G, Abalos RM, Fajardo TT, Guido LS, Krueger JG (1994): GM-CSF activates regenerative epidermal growth and stimulates keratinocyte proliferation in human skin in vivo. J Invest Dermatol 103: 601–604.

Breitkreutz D, Bohnert A, Herzmann E, Bowden PE, Boukamp P, Fusenig NE (1984): Differentiation specific functions in cultured and transplanted mouse keratinocytes: Environmental influences on ultrastructure and keratin expression. Differentiation 26: 154–169.

Breitkreutz D, Stark HJ, Mirancea N, Tomakidi P, Steinbauer H, Fusenig NE (1997): Integrin and basement membrane normalization in mouse grafts of human keratinocytes—implications for epithelial homeostasis. Differentiation 61: 195–209.

Breitkreutz D, Schoop VM, Mirancea N, Baur M, Stark HJ, Fusenig NE (1998): Epidermal differentiation and basement membrane formation by HaCaT cells in surface transplants. Eur J Cell Biol 75: 273–286.

Bumann J, Santo-Holtje L, Loffler H, Bamberg M, Rodemann HP (1995): Radiation-induced alterations of the proliferation dynamics of human skin fibroblasts after repeated irradiation in the sub-therapeutic dose range. Strahlenther Oncol 171(1): 35–41.

Cattoretti G, Becker MHG, Key G, Duchrow M, Schlüter C, Galle J, Gerdes J (1992): Monoclonal antibodies against recombinant parts of the Ki-67 antigen (Mib1 and Mib3) detect proliferating cells in microwave-processed formalin-fixed paraffin sections. J Pathol 168: 357–363.

Chen CSJ, Lavker RM, Rodeck U, Risse B, Jensen P (1995): Use of a serum-free epidermal culture model to show deleterious effects of epidermal growth factor on morphogenesis and differentiation. J Invest Dermatol 104: 107–112.

Chen YQ, Mauviel A, Ryynanen J, Sollberg S, Uitto J (1994): Type VII collagen gene expression by human skin fibroblasts and keratinocytes in culture: Influence of donor age and cytokine responses. J Invest Dermatol 102(2): 205–209.

Choi Y, Fuchs E (1994): TGF-ß and retinoic acid: Regulators of growth and modifiers of differentiation in human epidermal cells. Cell Regul 1: 791–809.

Contard P, Bartel RL, Jacobs L 2d, Perlish JS, MacDonald ED 2d, Handler L, Cone D, Fleischmajer R: (1993) Culturing keratinocytes and fibroblasts in a three-dimensional mesh results in epidermal differentiation and formation of a basal lamina-anchoring zone. J Invest Dermatol 100: 35–39.

Coulomb B, Dubertret L, Merrill C, Touraine R, Bell E (1984): The collagen lattice: A model for studying epidermalization in vitro. Br J Dermatol 114: 91–101.

Coulomb B, Lebreton C, Dubertret L (1989): Influence of human dermal fibroblasts on epidermalization. J Invest Dermatol 92: 122–125.

Dawson RA, Goberdhan NJ, Freedlander E, MacNeil S (1996): Influence of extracellular matrix proteins on human keratinocyte attachment, proliferation and transfer to a dermal wound model. Burns 22(2): 93–100.

Detmar M, Schaart FM, Blume U, Orfanos CE (1993): Culture of hair matrix and follicular keratinocytes. J Invest Dermatol 101: 130–134.

Dinarello CA (1996): Biologic basis for interleukin-1 in disease. Blood 87: 2095–2107.

Eming SA, Medalie DA, Tompkins RG, Yarmush ML, Morgan JR (1998): Genetically modified human keratinocytes overexpressing PDGF-A enhance the performance of a composite skin graft. Hum Gene Ther 9(4): 529–539.

Fartasch M, Ponec M (1994): Improved barrier structure formation in air-exposed human keratinocyte culture systems. J Invest Dermatol 102: 366–374.

Fusenig NE, Breitkreutz D, Dzarlieva RT, Boukamp P, Herzmann E, Bohnert A, Pöhlmann J, Rausch C, Schutz S, Hornung J (1982): Epidermal cell differentiation and malignant transformation in culture. Cancer Forum 6: 209–240.

Fusenig NE, Breitkreutz D, Dzarlieva RI, Boukamp P, Bohnert A, Tilgen W (1983): Growth and differentiation of transformed keratinocytes from mouse and human skin in vitro and in vivo. J Invest Dermatol 81: 168–175.

Fusenig NE (1986): Mammalian epidermal cells in culture. In Breiter-Hahn J, Matoltsy AG, Richards KS (eds): "Biology of the Integument." Berlin: Springer Verlag, pp 409–442.

Fusenig NE, Breitkreutz D, Boukamp P, Bohnert A, Mackenzie IC (1991): Epithelial mesenchymal interaction in tissue homeostasis and malignant transformation. In Johnson NW (ed.):"Oral Cancer: Detection of Patients and Lesions at Risk." Cambridge: Cambridge University Press, pp 218–256.

Fusenig NE (1992): Cell interaction and epithelial differentiation. In RI Freshney (ed.). "Culture of Epithelial Cells." New York: Wiley-Liss Inc, pp 25–57.

Fusenig NE (1994): Epithelial-mesenchymal interactions regulate keratinocyte growth and differentiation in vitro. In Leigh IM, Lane EB WattFM, (eds.) "The Keratinocyte Handbook." Cambridge: Cambridge University Press, pp 71–94.

Fusenig NE, Skobe M, Vosseler S., Hansen M, Lederle W, Airola K, Tomakidi P, Stark HJ, Boukamp P, Breitkreutz D: Tissue models to study tumor-stroma interactions. In Muschel RJ, Foidard JM (eds.). "Proteases and Their Inhibitors in Cancer Metastasis." Kluwer Academic Press, in press.

Garlick JA, Taichman LB (1994): Fate of human keratinocytes during reepithelialization in an organotypic culture model. Lab Invest 70(6): 916–924.

Gerdes J, Lemke H, Balsch H, Wacker HH, Schwab U, Stein H (1984): Cell cycle analysis of cell proliferation-associated human nuclear antigen defined by the monoclonal antibody Ki-67. J Immunol 133: 1710–1715.

Ghahary A, Tredget EE, Chang IJ, Scott PG, Shen Q (1998): Genetically modified dermal keratinocytes express high levels of transforming growth factor-beta 1. J Invest Dermatol 110(5): 800–805.

Ghahary A, Tredget EE, Shen Q (1999): Insulin-like growth factor-II/mannose 6 phosphate receptors facilitate the matrix effects of latent transforming growth factor-beta 1 released from genetically modified keratinocytes in a fibroblast/keratinocyte co-culture system. J Cell Physiol 180(1): 61–70.

Gregoire L, Munkareh A, Rabah R, Morris RT, Lancaster WD (1998): Organotypic culture of human ovarian surface epithelial cells: A potential model for ovarian carcinogenesis. In Vitro Cell Dev Biol Anim 34(8): 636–639.

Grinnell F, Toda KI, Lamke-Seymour C (1987): Reconstitution of human epidermis in vitro is accompanied by transient activation of basal keratinocyte spreading. Exp Cell Res 172: 439–449.

Hertle MD, Jones PH, Groves RW, Hudson DL, Watt FM (1995): Integrin expression by human epidermal keratinocytes can be modulated by interferon-gamma, transforming growth factor-beta, tumor necrosis factor-alpha and culture on a dermal equivalent. J Invest Dermatol 104: 260–265.

Herzhoff K, Sollberg S, Huerkamp C, Krieg T, Eckes B (1999): Fibroblast expression of collagen integrin receptors alpha1beta1 and alpha2beta1 is not changed in systemic scleroderma. Br J Dermatol 141(2): 218–223.

Hilberg F, Aguzzi A, Howells N, Wagner EF (1993): c-jun is essential for normal mouse development and hepatogenesis. Nature 365: 179–181.

Kaur P, Carter WG (1992): Integrin expression and differentiation in transformed human epidermal cells is regulated by fibroblasts. J Cell Sci 103: 755–763.

Kleinman HK, McGarvey ML, Hassell JR, Star VL, Cannon FB, Laurie GW, Martin GR (1986): Basement membrane complexes with biological activity. Biochemistry 25: 312–318.

Kopan R, Traska G, Fuchs E (1987): Retinoids as important regulators of terminal differentiation: Examining keratin expression in individual epidermal cells at various stages of keratinization. J Cell Biol 105(1): 427–440.

Kopan R, Fuchs E (1989): The use of retinoic acid to probe the relation between hyperproliferation-associated keratins and cell proliferation in normal and malignant epidermal cells. J Cell Biol 109(1): 295–307.

Kupper TS, Groves RW (1995): The interleukin-1 axis in cutaneous inflammation. J Invest Dermatol 105: 62–66.

Laning JC, DeLuca JE, Hardin-Young J (1999): Effects of immunoregulatory cytokines on the immunogenic potential of the cellular components of a bilayered living skin equivalent. Tissue Eng 5(2): 171–181.

Lillie JH, MacCullum DK, Jepsen A (1988): Growth of stratified squamous epithelium on reconstituted extracellular matrices: Longterm culture. J Invest Dermatol 90(2): 100–109.

Limat A, Hunziker T, Boillat C, Bayreuther K, Noser F (1989): Post-mitotic human dermal fibroblasts efficiently support the growth of human follicular keratinocytes. J Invest Dermatol 92: 758–762.

Luger TA, Schwarz T (1990): Evidence for an epidermal cytokine network. J Invest Dermatol 95: 100–104.

Luger TA, Schwarz T (1995): The role of cytokines and neuroendocrine hormones in cutaneous immunity and inflammation. Allergy 50: 292–302.

Maas-Szabowski N, Fusenig NE (1996): Interleukin 1 induced growth factor expression in postmitotic and resting fibroblasts. J Invest Dermatol 107: 849–855.

Maas-Szabowski N, Shimotoyodome A, Fusenig NE (1999): Keratinocyte growth regulation in fibroblast cocultures via a double paracrine mechanism. J Cell Sci 112: 1843–1853.

Maas-Szabowski N, Stark HJ, Fusenig NE (2000): Keratinocyte growth regulation in defined organotypic cultures through IL-1-induced KGF expression in resting fibroblasts. J Invest Dermatol 114: 1075–1084.

Mackenzie IC, Fusenig NE (1983): Regeneration of organized epithelial structure. J Invest Dermatol 81(1): 189–194.

Mackenzie I, Rittman G, Bohnert A, Breitkreutz D, Fusenig NE (1993): Influence of connective tissues on the in vitro growth and differentiation of murine epidermis. Epithelial Cell Biol: 2: 107–119.

Madison KC, Swartzendruber DC, Wertz PW, Downing DT (1998): Lamellar granule extrusion and stratum corneum intercellular lamellae in murine keratinocyte cultures. J Invest Dermatol 90: 110–116.

Marchese C, Chedid M, Dirsch OR, Csaky KG, Santanelli F, Latini C, La-Rochelle WJ, Torrisi MR, Aaronson SA (1995): Modulation of keratinocyte growth factor and its receptor in reepithelializing human skin. J Exp Med 182: 1369–1376.

Mauch C, Kozlowska E, Eckes B, Krieg T (1992): Altered regulation of collagen metabolism in scleroderma fibroblasts growth within three-dimensional collagen gels. Exp Dermatol 1(4): 185–190.

Metcalf D, Mifsud S, Di Rago L, Robb L, Nicola NA, Alexander W (1998): The biological consequences of excess GM-CSF levels in transgenic mice also lacking high-affinity receptors for GM-CSF. Leukemia 12(3): 353–362.

Noser FK, Limat A (1987): Organotypic culture of outer root sheath cells from human hair follicles using a new culture device. In Vitro Cell Dev Biol 23(8): 541–545.

Nuss Parker J, Zhao W, Askins KJ, Broker TR, Chow LT (1997): Mutational analyses of differentiation-dependent human papillomavirus type 18 enhance elements in epithelial raft cultures of neonatal foreskin keratinocytes. Cell Growth Differ 8: 751–762.

Parenteau NL, Nolte CM, Bilbo P, Rosenberg M, Wilkins LM, Johnson EW, Watson S, Mason VS, Bell E (1991): Epidermis generated in vitro: Practical considerations and applications. J Cell Biochem 45: 245–251.

Ponec M., Gibbs S, Weerheim A, Kempenaar J, Mulder A, Mommaas AM (1997): Epithelial growth factor and temperature regulate keratinocyte differentiation. Arch Dermatol Res 289: 317–326.

Pruniéras M, Régnier M, Fougère S, Woodley D (1983): Keratinocytes synthesize basal-lamina proteins in culture. J Invest Dermatol 81(1): 74–81.

Regnier M, Darmon D (1989): Human epidermis reconstructed in vitro: a model to study keratinocyte differentiation and its modulation by retinoic acid. In Vitro Cell Dev Biology 25(11): 1000–1008.

Regnier M, Staquet MJ, Schmitt D, Schmidt R (1997): Integration of Langerhans cells into a pigmented reconstructed human epidermis. J Invest Dermatol 109(4): 510–512.

Rheinwald JG, Green H (1975): Serial cultivation of strains of human epidermal keratinocytes: the formation of keratinizing colonies from single cells. Cell 6: 331–344.

Rikimaru K, Moles JP, Watt FM (1997): Correlation between hyperproliferation and suprabasal integrin expression in human epidermis reconstituted in culture. Exp Dermatol 6: 214–221.

Schoop VM, Mirancea N, Fusenig NE (1999): Epidermal organization and differentiation of HaCaT keratinocytes in organotypic cocultures with human dermal fibroblasts. J Invest Dermatol 112: 343–353.

Schorpp-Kistner M, Wang ZQ, Angel P, Wagner EF (1999): JunB is essential for mammalian placentation. EMBO J 18: 934–948.

Schröder JM (1995): Cytokine networks in the skin. J Invest Dermatol 105: 20–24.

Schürer NY, Monger DJ, Hincenbergs M, Williams ML (1989): Fatty acid metabolism in human keratinocytes cultivated at an air-medium interface. J Invest Dermatol. 92(2): 196–202.

Skobe M, Rockwell P, Goldstein N, Vosseler S, Fusenig (1997): Halting angiogenesis suppresses carcinoma cell invasion. Nat Med 3(11): 1222–1227.

Smola H, Thiekötter G, Fusenig NE (1993): Mutual induction of growth factor gene expression by epidermal-dermal cell interaction. J Cell Biol 122(2): 417–429.

Smola H, Thiekötter G, Baur M, Stark H-J, Breitkreutz D, Fusenig NE (1994): Organotypic and epidermal-dermal co-cultures of normal human keratinocytes and dermal cells: Regulations of transforming growth factor α, $\beta1$ and $\beta2$ mRNA levels. Toxicol Vitr 8(4): 641–650.

Smola H, Stark HJ, Thiekötter G, Mirancea N, Krieg T, Fusenig NE (1998): Dynamics of basement membrane formation by keratinocyte-fibroblast interactions in organotypic skin culture. Exp Cell Res 239: 399–410.

Stark HJ, Baur M, Breitkreutz D, Fusenig NE (1999): Organotypic keratinocyte cocultures in defined medium with regular epidermal morphogenesis and differentiation. J Invest Dermatol 112: 681–691.

Supp DM, Supp AP, Bell SM, Boyce ST (2000): Enhanced vascularization of cultured skin substitutes genetically modified to overexpress vascular endothelial growth factor 1. J Invest Dermatol 114(1): 5–13.

Szabowski A, Maas-Szabowski N, Andrecht S, Kolbus A, Schorpp-Kistner M, Fusenig NE, Angel P (2000): c-Jun and JunB antagonistically control cytokine-regulated mesenchymal-epidermal interaction in skin. Cell 103: 745–755.

Takahashi Y, Nogawa H (1991): Branching morphogenesis of mouse salivary epithelium in basement membrane-like substratum separated from mesenchyme by the membrane filter. Development 111(2): 327–335.

Takei T, Kito H, Du W, Mills I, Sumpio BE (1998): Induction of Interleukin-1α and -β gene expression in human keratinocytes exposed to repetitive strain: Their role in strain-induced keratinocyte proliferation and morphological change. J Cell Biochem 69: 95–103.

Tinois E, Tiollier J, Gaucherande M, Dumas H, Tardy M, Thivolet J (1991): In vitro and post-transplantation differentiation of human keratinocytes grown on the human type IV collagen film of a bilayered dermal substitute. Exp Cell Res 193: 310–319.

Tomakidi P, Breitkreutz D, Fusenig NE, Zoller J, Kohl A, Komposch G (1998): Establishment of oral mucosa phenotype in vitro in correlation to epithelial anchorage. Cell Tissue Res 298: 355–366.

Turksen K, Choi Y, Fuchs E (1991): Transforming growth factor alpha induces collagen degradation and cell migration in differentiating human epidermal raft cultures. Cell Regul 2(8): 613–625.

Vaccariello M, Javaherian A, Wang Y, Fusenig NE, Garlick JA (1999): Cell interactions control the fate of malignant keratinocytes in an organotypic model of early neoplasia. J Invest Dermatol 113: 384–391.

Waelti ER, Inaebnit SP, Rast HP, Hunziker T, Limat A, Braathen L, Wiesmann U (1992): Co-culture of human keratinocytes on post-mitotic human dermal fibroblast feeder cells: production of large amounts of interleukin 6. J Invest Dermatol 98: 805–808.

Werner S, Peters KG, Longaker MT, Fuller-Pace F, Banda MJ, Williams LT (1992): Large induction of keratinocyte growth factor expression in the dermis during wound healing. Proc Natl Acad Sci USA 89: 6896–6900.

Werner S (1998): Keratinocyte growth factor: a unique player in epithelial repair processes. Cytokine Growth Factor Rev 9: 153–165.

Zheng, J, Vaheri A (1995): Human skin fibroblasts induce anchorage-independent growth of HPV-16-DNA-immortalized cervical epithelial cells. Int J Cancer 61(5): 658–665.

APPENDIX: SOURCES OF MATERIALS

Item	Varieties	Catalog #	Supplier
Collagen: commercially available preparations used for gel formation as extracellular matrix substitutes	a) Vitrogen-100 bovine dermal collagen (type I), e.g., see Madison et al. [1988]; Grinnell et al. [1987]	—	Collagen Corp.
	b) Type I collagen, calf skin, e.g., see Asselineau and Pruniéras [1984] Herzhoff et al. [1999]	C-9791	Sigma, IBFB
	c) Type I collagen, rat tail tendons	C-7661	Sigma
	d) Type I collagen, e.g., Kopan et al. [1987]	—	Seikagaku America Inc
	e) Type I collagen, bovine cornea	—	Funakoshi Pharmaceutial Company
	f) Matrigel EHS solution, basal membrane extract from transplantable mouse tumor EHS	—	Serva
Collagenase		C-9891	Sigma-Aldrich
Rompun		—	Bayer Vital
DMEM	With stabilized L-glutamine	FG 0435	GIBCO-BRL, Biochrom
DMEM/Ham's F12 (to prepare FAD)	With stabilized L-glutamine	FG 4815	Biochrom
Supplemented keratinocyte defined medium (SKDM), modified on the base of keratinocyte basal medium	see Stark et al. [1999]	CC-3101	Clonetics/Bio Whittaker

Appendix continues

Item	Varieties	Catalog #	Supplier
Membrane filter holders for support of organotypic cultures (filter well inserts)	a) Millicell-HA filter holder inserts with Millipore membranes (pore size: 0.456 μm) to be placed in 6-well tissue cultures plates	—	Millipore
	b) Transwell, cell culture chamber insert, with Nucleopore membranes (pore size: 0.4 μm) designed for use in 6-well- and 24-well cluster dishes	—	Corning
	c) Nunc 25-mm tissue culture inserts	137435	Nalge Nunc
	d) Nyaflo membranes	—	Gelman Sciences
	e) Falcon cell culture inserts 1.0-μm pores 3.0-μm pores	#3102 #3091	Becton Dickinson Labware
Biocoat 6-well, deep well plate (which allows a sufficient medium volume of 10 ml in air-exposed configuration), see also Stark et al. [1999]		#5467	Beckton Dickinson Labware
Combi Ring dish (CRD): culture chamber consisting of pairs of concentric Teflon rings of different diameters for mounting extracellular matrices between the tightly fitting Teflon rings	Teflon ring type b Teflon ring type c′	#30907 (inner) #30910 (outer)	Renner; Germany
Stanzen Petri dishes: 35-mm tissue culture Petri dishes with 4 (8-mm-diameter) rings with a height of 1 mm on the culture surface of the dish		—	Fa. Greiner and Söhne (also supplied by Renner KG)
Transplantation chamber: made of silicone with a dome-shaped central part and a broad, thin rim, available in different sizes	Type F2U	#30268	Renner; Germany (exclusive supplier)
Tissue Tek-O.T.C™-compound		4583	Sakura Finetek Europe, Zoeterwoude, The Netherlands

3

The Epidermis

E. Kenneth Parkinson and W. Andrew Yeudall

*The Beatson Institute for Cancer Research, Garscube Estate,
Switchback Road, Bearsden, Glasgow G61 1BD, United Kingdom.
K.Parkinson@beatson.gla.ac.uk*

Culture of Epithelial Cells, pages 65–94

I. INTRODUCTION

Most early attempts at keratinocyte culture involved explant or organ culture in which the keratinocytes were contaminated by fibroblast growth as well as other nonkeratinocyte epidermal cells [Fell, 1964; Prose et al., 1967; Flaxman et al., 1967]; later on there were several attempts to culture disaggregated epidermal keratinocytes as monolayers [Cruickshank et al., 1960; Briggaman et al., 1967; Yuspa et al., 1970; Karasek and Charlton, 1971; Fusenig, 1971; Fusenig and Worst, 1974]. These studies showed that the cultures grew only to a limited extent and could not be satisfactorily subcultured. Plating similar suspensions on collagen-coated Petri dishes [Liu and Karasek, 1978] or reducing the pH of the growth medium [Eisinger et al., 1979] enabled limited subculturing, but it was the discovery by Rheinwald and Green [1975] that led to successful in vitro studies on keratinocytes. They demonstrated that a feeder layer of irradiated mouse 3T3 mesenchymal cells permitted the clonal growth of keratinocytes but not other cell types. This subsequently led to the development of serum-free culture media in which the keratinocytes could grow without feeders [Macaig et al., 1981; Boyce and Ham, 1983; Wille et al., 1984] and permitted the partial purification of one keratinocyte growth factor from the hypothalamus [Gilchrest et al., 1984] and the purification [Rubin et al., 1989] and cloning [Finch et al., 1989] of another from a human fibroblast cell line.

The 3T3 feeder technique has been widely used to study keratinocyte biology, and it is this technique that is described in detail in this chapter. The historical development of the technique and the characterization of human epidermal cultures were reviewed by Rheinwald [1980]; that article is strongly recommended as complementary reading material to this chapter. Other widely used keratinocyte culture methods are also mentioned here and the relative merits of the different techniques are discussed (see also Chapter 2).

2. PREPARATION OF REAGENTS AND MEDIA

2.1. Media

2.1.1. Growth Medium

DMEM	3 parts
Ham's F12	1 part
HEPES	20 mM
Fetal bovine serum (selected batch)	10% v/v
Penicillin (if required)	100 U/ml
Streptomycin (if required)	100 μg/ml

Add $NaHCO_3$, 26 mM, to give pH 7.4 at 37°C under 5% CO_2. If used under 10% CO_2, 44 mM $NaHCO_3$ will be required and the HEPES is omitted.

2.1.2. Complete Growth Medium

Add the following supplements to growth medium from Section 2.1.1 to make complete growth medium:

Transferrin	5 μg/ml	6.4×10^{-8} M
Insulin	5 μg/ml	8.7×10^{-7} M
Triiodothyronine	1.4 ng/ml	2×10^{-9} M
[Allen-Hoffman and Rheinwald, 1984]		
Cholera toxin	8.4 ng/ml	1×10^{-10} M
[Green, 1978]		
Adenine hydrochloride	31 mg/ml	1.8×10^{-4}
Hydrocortisone, hemisuccinate	0.4 μg/ml	8.3×10^{-7} M
[Rheinwald and Green, 1975]		

Add to complete growth medium, 3–4 days after seeding:

Epidermal growth factor	10 ng/ml	$\sim 2 \times 10^{-9}$ M

2.2. Preparation of Medium Supplements

2.2.1. Cholera toxin (CT)

(i) To make a master stock add 1.18 ml of sterile UPW to 1 mg of powder to give $\sim 1 \times 10^{-5}$ M solution (mol wt 84,000).

(ii) Store at 4°C.

(iii) To prepare a 1×10^{-7} M (1,000×) working stock add 100 μl of 1×10^{-5} M CT to 10 ml of growth medium.

(iv) Filter sterilize and store at -20°C.

(v) Dilute 0.5 ml working stock to 500 ml in complete growth medium for use at a final concentration of 1×10^{-10} M.

(vi) Use immediately or store at -20°C.

2.2.2. Hydrocortisone hemisuccinate (sodium salt)

(i) Dissolve at 4 mg/ml in 95% ethanol.

(ii) Dilute 1:10 (v/v) in growth medium to make 8.3×10^{-4} M, a 1,000× stock.

(iii) Store at -20°C.

(iv) Dilute stock 1:1000 (v/v) in complete growth medium to make 8.3×10^{-7} M.

(v) Use immediately or store at -20°C.

2.2.3. Epidermal growth factor

(i) Dissolve in UPW at 100 μg/ml to make 1,000× stock.

(ii) Store at -20°C.

(iii) Dilute stock 1:1000 to give 10 ng/ml, 2×10^{-9} M, in complete growth medium.

(iv) Use immediately or store at -20°C.

2.2.4. Transferrin (Bovine) and Triiodothyronine, Sodium Salt

(i) Dissolve transferrin 5 mg/ml (6.4×10^{-5} M) in PBSA.

(ii) Dissolve triiodothyronine 1.3 mg/ml (2×10^{-3} M) in PBSA and dilute 1:1000 into transferrin solution to give 2×10^{-6} M.

This makes a 1000× combined stock.

(iii) Sterilize by filtration at 0.22 μm.

(iv) Store at -20°C.

(v) Dilute 1:1000 (v/v) for use in complete growth medium.

2.2.6. Insulin

(i)   Dissolve at 5 mg/ml in 0.05 M HCl in UPW.
(ii)   Dilute 1:10 in PBSA to make stock.
(iii)   Filter sterilize, 0.22-μm, low-protein-binding filter.
(iv)   Store at $-20°C$.
(v)   Dilute stock 1:100 in complete growth medium for use at 5 μg/ml, 8.7×10^{-7} M.

2.3. Trypsin/EDTA

(i)   Trypsin, 0.5%, in UPW.
(ii)   Sterilize by filtration, 0.22-μm filter
(iii)   Store at $-20°C$.
(iv)   For use, mix 1:1 with 2× PBSA and then 1:1 with EDTA, 0.7 mM (0.02%), in PBSA to give 0.125% trypsin in 0.35 mM (0.01%) EDTA.
(v)   Store at 4°C.

3. CULTIVATION OF NORMAL HUMAN EPIDERMAL KERATINOCYTES

3.1. Sample Collection and Storage

To collect samples of human skin we normally contact plastic surgeons, who perform "bat ear" correction operations that result in two thin strips of flat skin from behind the ear. Alternatively, we contact surgeons who perform circumcisions. Material from both these sources is sterile and disease-free, and the donors are usually in the range of 0–10 years of age. Plastic universals each containing 10–15 ml of Dulbecco's modification of Eagle's medium (DMEM) supplemented with 10% v/v bovine serum, 100 U/ml penicillin, and 100 μg/ml streptomycin are regularly supplied to the operating theater senior nurse or assistant surgeon, who telephone when the tissue is ready. The tissue is very robust and can be mailed from the theater to the laboratory if no suitable operating list can be found locally. Reasonable cultures have been obtained from samples that have been stored in serum-containing medium for up to 1 wk at 4°C.

Δ*Safety note.* Human samples should be regarded as potentially infected with human pathogens. They should be handled in the laboratory in a Class II microbiological safety cabinet, and all materials used with them should be discarded into disinfectant and/or autoclaved or incinerated.

3.2. Cell Dispersal Techniques

After dissection, samples of skin can be disaggregated by short incubation in warm trypsin or by prolonged incubation in cold trypsin.

Protocol 3.1. Disaggregation of Skin by Warm Trypsin

Reagents and Materials

Sterile

- ❏ PBSA: Ca^{2+}- and Mg^{2+}-free phosphate-buffered saline
- ❏ Trypsin, 0.25%, in PBSA
- ❏ Growth medium: DMEM with 10% FBS, 100 U/ml penicillin, and 100 μg/ml streptomycin
- ❏ Trypsinization flask
- ❏ Stirring bar (magnetic follower)
- ❏ Scalpels, #11
- ❏ Scissors, fine, curved
- ❏ Culture flasks, 25 cm^2 or 75 cm^2

Nonsterile

- ❏ Magnetic stirrer

Protocol

- (a) Rinse the sample several times with PBSA to remove any blood and serum.
- (b) Place the tissue in a 9-cm dish and remove most of the subcutaneous fat and membranous material with either a scalpel blade or a sharp pair of curved scissors. The skin from behind the ear normally needs very little trimming.
- (c) Wash the skin once more with PBSA.
- (d) Chop the sample into fine pieces approximately 1–2 mm^3.
- (e) Add to a flask containing a sterile stirring bar and 0.25% trypsin in PBSA, approximately 1 ml of trypsin per mg tissue.
- (f) Stir the tissue at 100 rpm at 37°C for 30–45 min.
- (g) Collect the trypsinate and centrifuge to obtain the released cells.
- (h) Resuspend the cells in growth medium and store at 4°C.
- (i) Add fresh trypsin solution to the flask and repeat (f)–(h).
- (j) Repeat this cycle several times for 4–5 h or until the tissue is completely digested [Rheinwald, 1980].

(k) Pool the cell fractions, and count the cells.

(l) Seed into flasks at 2×10^4 cells/cm^2, 1×10^5/ml in growth medium.

(m) Incubate at 37°C under 5% CO_2.

Minor variations on this technique include the addition of EDTA to the trypsin solution [Peehl and Ham, 1980a] at 0.3–1 mM. In our experience, the 37°C trypsinization procedure is very time consuming and does not give reproducibly high cloning efficiencies [Rheinwald and Green, 1975].

Protocol 3.2. Disaggregation of Skin by Cold Trypsin

Reagents and Materials

Sterile

❑ PBSA: Ca^{2+}- and Mg^{2+}-free phosphate-buffered saline

❑ Trypsin, 0.125%, in PBSA, freshly prepared and kept at 4°C [Parkinson et al., 1986]

❑ Growth medium: DMEM with 10% FBS, 100 U/ml penicillin, and 100 μg/ml streptomycin

❑ Scalpels, #11

❑ Scissors, fine, curved

❑ Culture flasks, 25 cm^2 or 75 cm^2

Nonsterile

❑ Ice bath

Protocol

(a) Rinse the sample several times with PBSA to remove any blood and serum.

(b) Place the tissue in a 9-cm dish and remove most of the subcutaneous fat and membranous material with either a scalpel blade or a sharp pair of curved scissors.

(c) Wash the skin once more with PBSA.

(d) Slice the skin into 0.5-cm-wide strips.

(e) Immerse each strip in a total of 50 ml of 0.125% trypsin at 4°C.

(f) Place at 4°C overnight ($\sim$16 h).

(g) Remove the trypsin and add 10 ml of growth medium at 37°C.

(h) Scrape the epidermis from the dermis with a scalpel.

(i) Gently triturate the skin with a wide-bore pipette to release the epidermal cells, allowing the undisaggregated dermis to settle to the bottom of the container.

(j) Pool the epidermal cells, and centrifuge at 80 g for 5 min.

(k) Resuspend in growth medium, and count the cells.

(l) Seed into flasks at 2×10^4 cells/cm^2, 1×10^5/ml in growth medium.

(m) Incubate at 37°C under 5% CO_2.

This technique is non-labor-intensive and results in keratinocyte suspensions consisting of at least 85% single cells without further processing. The cloning efficiency of around 4% is highly reproducible if donors of less than 10 years of age are used. Older donors may give lower cloning efficiencies than this [Rheinwald and Green, 1975].

3.3. Selective Growth Conditions and Preparation of 3T3 Feeder Layers

The cell suspensions generated by the cold trypsin method described above contain predominantly keratinocytes but also a few dermal fibroblasts as well as melanocytes, Langerhans cells, and Merkel cells. The fibroblasts represent the most serious source of contamination of the epidermal cultures, because Merkel cells and Langerhans cells do not survive in culture and melanocytes do not proliferate unless special culture conditions are used [Halaban et al., 1987, 1988; Naeyaert et al., 1991; Park et al., 2000].

Rheinwald and Green [1975] discovered that if epidermal suspensions are plated together with a fairly dense (one-third confluent) lethally irradiated feeder layer of mouse 3T3 mesenchymal cells, the keratinocytes form macroscopic colonies from single cells whereas the proliferation of any fibroblasts is suppressed. Swiss 3T3 (American Type Culture Collection No. CCL92) or Balb 3T3 A31 mouse mesenchyme cells have been shown to support the growth of human epidermal keratinocytes in our laboratory (see also Chapter 5, Protocol 5.4). The 3T3 cells are normally cultured in DMEM supplemented with 10% v/v bovine serum (a selected lot) in an atmosphere of 10% CO_2-90% air. If 5% CO_2-95% air is to be used, the sodium bicarbonate concentration of the medium should be reduced to 26 mM, about 60% of the recommended concentration for DMEM, to give optimum growth. When preparing for the first time, check an aliquot by incubating in an open dish for 2 h in the appropriate gas mixture.

The 3T3 cells are subcultured by exposing the cultures to a small amount ($\sim$20 μl/cm^2) of 0.1% trypsin for 3–4 min and dispersing the cells in growth medium ($\sim$200 μl/cm^2). The cells are centrifuged, resuspended, counted, and seeded at a density of 1×10^4 cells per 9-cm plate to give confluence after 2 wk. The medium is changed on Day 11, when the cells are becoming dense (for routine subculture, however, 3T3 should be subcultured when subconfluent to avoid spontaneous transformation). We set up two lots of cultures on alternate weeks to ensure a supply of feeder cells every week. Each week the confluent dishes are subcultured and the excess cells are irradiated in suspension with 60 Gy of γ-irradiation from either a ^{60}Co or a ^{37}Cs source (see Chapter 5, Protocol 5.4). The cells are then either used immediately or stored for up to 48 h at 4°C without any appreciable loss of feeding capacity. If desired, the feeder cells can be plated in advance of the keratinocytes, as they are at their optimum 48 h after seeding [Rheinwald, 1980], but normally for convenience we plate the lethally irradiated 3T3 feeder layer and the keratinocytes together.

Although 3T3 cells must not be allowed to reach confluence during serial propagation, it is important that they be allowed to reach confluence before being prepared for feeder layers and that they be routinely checked for mycoplasma contamination, because mycoplasma-contaminated feeders do not support the proliferation of keratinocytes. It is also important to freeze down stocks of 3T3 cells as soon as possible after receipt so that fresh cultures can be started every 10–12 wk, when the original 3T3 cells have increased their saturation density because of continuous selection for fast-growing variants. These variants do not survive as long after irradiation and they are inferior as feeders. The use of high-quality trypsin (see Appendix: Sources of Materials) and a selected batch of bovine serum (sometimes called donor calf serum) and application of the subcultivation protocol described above will minimize such problems. Do *not* use fetal bovine serum or newborn calf serum to grow the 3T3 cells.

Protocol 3.3. Culture of Keratinocytes on 3T3 Feeder Layers

Reagents and Materials

❑ Keratinocyte suspension from Protocol 3.2
❑ Preformed 3T3 feeder layer or growth-arrested feeder cells (see above and Protocol 5.4)

❏ Growth medium: supplemented DMEM:F12 (see Section 2.1.2)
❏ Epidermal growth factor, EGF, 1 μg/ml in DMEM with 10% bovine serum (see Section 2.2.3)

Protocol

(a) Seed the keratinocytes at 2×10^4 cells/cm², 1×10^5/ml in growth medium, minus EGF, onto a preformed feeder layer, or seed with the appropriate number of 3T3 cells to give 1×10^5 cells/cm².

(b) Change medium at 3–4 days after seeding.

(c) Add EGF to a final concentration of 10 ng/ml ($\sim 2 \times 10^{-9}$ M) at this first medium change, as addition at the time of seeding reduces plating efficiency [Rheinwald and Green, 1977].

In this growth medium the keratinocytes grow from single cells into macroscopic colonies containing several thousand cells that can be used for experiments or subcultured for at least 80 population doublings in the case of adults (unpublished data) and more than 140 population doublings in the case of newborn donors [Rheinwald and Green, 1977].

Hydrocortisone is essential to maintain growth rate, colony morphology, and differentiation when the keratinocytes are subcultured [Rheinwald and Green, 1975] and may also prevent deterioration of the 3T3 feeder layer [Pera and Gorman, 1984]. Cholera toxin, by raising cAMP levels, seems to oppose the tendency of keratinocytes to increase in cell size [Green, 1978] and may therefore oppose the onset of terminal differentiation [Sun and Green, 1976; Barrandon and Green, 1985]. EGF is much more potent in cultures derived from newborn donors [Rheinwald and Green, 1977; Sun and Green, 1977; Green, 1980] and appears to antagonize the effects of crowding in the centers of the keratinocyte colonies [Rheinwald and Green, 1977] by stimulating migration of the growing keratinocytes out of the center of the colonies [Barrandon and Green, 1987]. EGF appears to antagonize terminal differentiation and increase the size of the dividing and clonogenic populations by a mechanism that is distinct from that of cholera toxin [Rheinwald and Green, 1977; Green, 1978], and the effects of the two agents together exceed that of each alone [Green, 1978].

Together hydrocortisone, cholera toxin, and EGF combine to increase the clonogenic fraction, the population growth rate, and the culture lifespan [Rheinwald, 1980; Green, 1980], so that large numbers of cultured human keratinocytes can be obtained rapidly from even a small skin biopsy [Green et al., 1979; Allen-Hoffman and Rheinwald, 1984]. Insulin, transferrin, and triiodothyronine reduce the requirement for serum from 20% to 10% and, with poor or mediocre serum lots, also improve growth rate.

3.4. Subculture

The keratinocyte colonies can be subcultured by first removing the feeder layer and any contaminating cell types.

Protocol 3.4. Removing Fibroblasts from Primary Keratinocyte Cultures

Reagents and Materials

Sterile or Aseptically Prepared

❑ 3T3 cells, lethally irradiated, 1/30th of confluent density, i.e., ~3 × 10^3 cells/cm^2
❑ EDTA, 0.7 mM, (0.02%), in PBSA
❑ PBSA

Protocol

(a) Treat the culture with 0.02% (0.7 mM) EDTA for 15–30 s.
(b) Vigorously pipette streams of PBSA against the growth surface to detach the 3T3 cells and fibroblasts [Rheinwald and Green, 1975].
(c) Assess the contamination by dermal fibroblasts of the subcultured suspensions (if necessary) by replating a sample of the suspension onto a new, lethally irradiated, low-density 3T3 feeder layer.

Fibroblastic contamination was found to be less than 0.1% when the cold trypsin method was used (unpublished data) and less than 1% when the 37°C trypsin method was used [Parkinson and Newbold, 1980]. This level of contamination decreased with each passage of the keratinocytes. The contamination of the suspension by lethally irradiated mouse 3T3 cells can be assessed by the different fluorescent staining pattern of the nucleus after staining with Hoechst 33258 [Alitalo et al., 1982] or by reaction with the monoclonal antibody LP4N (see Fig. 3.2f), which reveals only human nuclei after indirect immunocytochemical staining [Boukamp et al., 1985]. The contamination is in the range 0.01–0.1% [Alitalo et al., 1982; E.K. Parkinson, unpublished data].

After removal of the 3T3 feeder layer, the keratinocyte colonies can be subcultured.

Protocol 3.5. Subculture of Keratinocytes on Feeder Layer

Reagents and Materials

- ❏ Complete growth medium minus EGF (see Section 2.1.2)
- ❏ Trypsin EDTA: trypsin, 0.1%, mixed 1:1 with EDTA, 0.02% (5.4 mM), to give 0.05% trypsin in 0.3 mM EDTA

Protocol

(a) Incubate with trypsin EDTA at 37°C.
(b) Disaggregate the colonies into single cells after about 40 min of incubation [Rheinwald and Green, 1975; Rheinwald, 1980]; the exact length of time will depend on the extent of confluence of the cultures.
(c) Count the cells in a hemocytometer.
(d) Dilute in any growth medium containing serum and replate in complete growth medium minus EGF at 2×10^4 cells/cm^2, 1×10^5/ml onto fresh lethally irradiated 3T3 feeder cells (see Protocol 3.3, above).
(e) Alternatively, cryopreserve in liquid nitrogen (see Protocol 3.6, below).

3.5. Cryopreservation

Keratinocyte suspensions can be frozen and stored in liquid nitrogen after subculture, using standard procedures.

Protocol 3.6. Cryopreservation of Keratinocytes

Reagents and Materials

Sterile

- ❏ Trypsin/EDTA: 0.05% trypsin in 0.3 mM EDTA
- ❏ Growth medium (see Section 2.1.1)
- ❏ Complete growth medium minus EGF (see Section 2.1.2)
- ❏ Freezing medium: complete growth medium containing 10% v/v glycerol [Rheinwald, 1980] or 10% v/v dimethyl sulfoxide as a cryopreservative

❑ Cryotubes, 1.2 ml, labeled and dated

Nonsterile

❑ Insulated storage box (sandwich box lined with cotton wool)

Protocol

Freezing

(a) Harvest keratinocyte monolayer by trypsin/EDTA (see Protocol 3.5).
(b) Centrifuge at 1000 rpm, (80–100 g).
(c) Resuspend in fresh growth medium, and centrifuge again.
(d) Resuspend in freezing medium at a concentration of 1×10^6 cells/ml [Rheinwald, 1980].
(e) Add 1 ml of the cell suspension to cryotubes.
(f) Keep the tubes on ice, then wrap in cotton wool, and place in the plastic sandwich box.
(g) Place the box in a $-20°C$ freezer for 30 min.
(h) Transfer to a $-70°C$ freezer overnight.
(i) Transfer the cryotubes to permanent storage in the liquid nitrogen storage facility.

△*Safety note.* Wear cryoprotective gloves, a face mask, and a closed lab coat when working with liquid nitrogen. Make sure the room is well ventilated to avoid asphyxiation from evaporated nitrogen.

Freezing rate. The cotton wool insulation ensures gradual cooling of the cryotubes and results in good viability of the cells on thawing. Alternatively, the cryotubes can be placed in an adjustable liquid nitrogen tank head. The tubes can then be gradually lowered toward the nitrogen surface at a suitable rate to achieve slow freezing, but we find the first method to be satisfactory.

Thawing

(a) Thaw the keratinocyte suspensions by placing the cryotubes in water at 37°C, preferably in a bucket with a lid to contain any potential explosion of the ampoule.

△*Safety note.* An ampoule that has been stored in liquid nitrogen can inspire liquid nitrogen if not properly sealed. The ampoule will then explode violently when warmed. To protect from potential explosion of ampoules, thaw in a covered container, such as a large plastic bucket with a lid, or store in the vapor phase. Wear gloves, a face mask, and a closed lab coat.

(b) Check the label on the cryovial to confirm identity, then flood the outside of the cryotube with 70% ethanol and blot dry with tissue.

(c) After the tubes are dry, withdraw the cells from the ampoule and dilute quickly in prewarmed (37°C) complete growth medium.

(d) Centrifuge for 2 min at 80–100 g.

(e) Resuspend in fresh growth medium minus EGF.

(f) Dilute the cell suspension, mix with irradiated 3T3 feeders, and seed at 2×10^4 keratinocytes and 2×10^4 3T3 cells/cm^2, 1×10^5 keratinocytes and 1×10^5 3T3 cells/ml.

(g) The recovery of the cells is in the range of 30–100% [Rheinwald, 1980]. If a high recovery is obtained routinely, the seeding concentration may be reduced.

(h) Add EGF, 1 μg/ml, at first feed.

3.6. Adaptation to Keratinocytes from Other Species and Sites

The methods described here have been used to grow epidermal keratinocytes from many species, including rabbits [Sun and Green, 1977], rats [Phillips and Rice, 1983], bovines [Kubilus et al., 1979], and Syrian hamsters [Newbold and Overell, personal communication]. The technique can readily be adapted to grow keratinocytes from various strains of mice, provided that the temperature of the incubator is reduced to 31°C and the concentration of hydrocortisone is increased to 1 μg/ml (2.8 μM) [Pera and Gorman, 1984; Parkinson et al., 1986, 1987; Appleby et al., 1989]. The in vitro lifespan of keratinocytes from other species, however, may be considerably shorter than that obtained with humans. Adult mouse epidermal keratinocytes can barely complete 15–20 population doublings in culture, whereas the cultures from adult humans last much longer [Green et al., 1979; unpublished data]. As with humans, newborn mouse keratinocytes have a longer in vitro lifespan (around 50 population doublings) than their adult counterparts [Pera and Gorman, 1984].

The 3T3 support system can also be used to culture epithelial cells from other sites, including oral cavity [Taichman et al., 1979], cervix [Stanley and Parkinson, 1979; see also Chapter 5], nasopharynx and trachea [Green, 1978], cornea and conjunctiva [Sun and Green, 1977], bladder (Wu et al., 1982], esophagus [Doran et al., 1980], colon [Paraskeva et al., 1984], and mammary gland [Taylor-Papadimitriou et al., 1977].

Many techniques have been described for keratinocyte culture, including explant culture [Fell, 1964; Prose et al., 1967; Flaxman et al., 1967] and high-density plating on collagen [Liu and Karasek, 1978], in low-pH medium [Eisinger et al., 1979], or in low-calcium (<0.1 mM) medium [Hennings et al., 1980]. Clonal growth has been described in medium 199 with 20% fetal bovine serum, 10 μg/ml hydrocortisone, and bovine pituitary extract [Peehl and Ham, 1980a] and also in medium 199 supplemented with 10 ng/ml EGF, 10 μg/ml transferrin, 1.4×10^{-6} M hydrocortisone, 2 mg/ml bovine serum albumin, and an extract from bovine hypothalamus, if the cells are plated onto dishes coated with fibronectin [Macaig et al., 1981; Gilchrest et al., 1984].

A complete chemical redefinition of the growth medium Ham's F12, including lowering the calcium concentrations [Peehl and Ham, 1980b; Tsau et al., 1982; Boyce and Ham, 1983], led to the development of the medium MCDB 153 [Wille et al., 1984], which, when supplemented with bovine pituitary extract, insulin, hydrocortisone, EGF, ethanolamine, and phosphoethanolamine, can give remarkably high cloning efficiencies of up to 56% [Wille et al., 1984]. This medium can now be obtained in a stabilized and easily usable form known as keratinocyte basal medium from Clonetics Corporation (BioWhittaker) and is supplied with supplements and full instructions for use (see also Chapter 7). In our hands, the Clonetics medium remains the most reliable source of MCDB 153 for the growth of mass cultures of keratinocytes. However, the commercial medium, although convenient to use, does not support proliferation at the very low densities supported by MCDB 153 [Wille et al., 1984] and is therefore unsuitable for isolating clones.

3.7. Relative Merits and Physiological Relevance of More Successful Techniques

The most widely used keratinocyte culture techniques are the low-calcium minimal essential medium technique supplemented with calcium-depleted fetal bovine serum for high-density mouse cultures [Hennings et al., 1980], the 3T3 feeder layer support system of Rheinwald and Green [Rheinwald and Green, 1975; Rheinwald, 1980; Green, 1980] for the clonal growth of keratinocytes from many species and sites, and low-calcium (0.15 mM) serum-free MCDB 153 medium [Boyce and Ham, 1983; Willie et al., 1984], which supports the clonal growth of human epidermal keratinocytes. The relative merits of these three systems are listed in Table 3.1.; the possible problems and solutions for them are listed in Table 3.2.

The 3T3 support system described in this chapter, while having the disadvantage of using undefined growth factors from serum and another cell type (the 3T3 cell), is the only clonal system in which proliferation is largely limited to the true basal cells [Rheinwald and Green, 1975; Barrandon and Green, 1985], and terminal differentiation proceeds to completion as the keratinocytes stratify. MCDB 153 can support the clonal proliferation of very mature suprabasal cells as efficiently as, if not more efficiently than, the true basal proliferating cells [Wilke et al., 1988], and also the culture lifespan in this medium is short, particularly in the case of adults (30 population doublings) [Wille et al., 1984]. MCDB 153 from commercial sources does not support proliferation at cell densities of <500 cells/cm^2.

3.8. Applications of Normal Keratinocyte Cultures

The most widespread early use for normal human keratinocyte cultures has been in the treatment of burns and skin ulcers with sheets of human epidermal cells cultured using 3T3 feeders [Clancy et al., 1988, Compton et al., 1989] and MCDB 153 [Pittelkow and Scott 1986]. The system has also been used to address dermatological questions such as contact dermatitis [Sainte-Marie et al., 1998] and inflammatory conditions [Cowan et al., 1998] including psoriasis. Keratinocyte culture has proved to be extremely valuable in the study of epithelial differentiation (see Section 6 and Chapter 2).

3.9. Generation of Immortal Human Keratinocyte Lines from Cultures of Normal Cells

Early attempts to generate cell lines from human keratinocyte cultures utilized DNA tumor viruses such as SV40 [Steinberg and Defendi 1979] or adenovirus 5 E1A [Barrandon et al., 1989], and cell lines were readily generated without any obvious sign of the crisis seen in fibroblast cultures. However, these cultures invariably have abnormal karyotypes and are therefore imperfect models of normal keratinocyte behavior, as is the established cell line HaCaT for the same reason [Boukamp et al., 1988] and keratinocyte lines immortalized by Id1 [Alani et al., 1999]. More recent attempts at immortalizing human keratinocytes have exploited the observation that the ectopic expression of telomerase, which maintains the telomeres at the ends of mammalian chromosomes,

TABLE 3.1. Comparison of Various Keratinocyte Culture Methods

Method	Advantages	Disadvantages
Explant culture	Relatively easy Maintains cell-cell interactions	Requires continuous supply of samples Culture life short Contamination with other cell types Rapid build-up of barriers to diffusible molecules Not clonal Subculture difficult
High-density culture	Relatively easy	As above
Low-Ca^{2-}, (<0.1 mM) medium	Cultures long-lived Cells have basal morphology Differentiation can be manipulated Cultures are homotypic Low contamination with other cell types Can be grafted onto syngeneic animals	Not clonal Subculture difficult
Low-Ca^{2-} (0.15 mM) serum-free medium	Cultures long-lived Subcultures possible Clonal Cells have basal morphology Differentiation can be manipulated Cultures are homotypic Low contamination with other cell types Serum-free Can be grafted onto humans or experimental animals	Designed for human keratinocytes; modifications required for other species Inappropriate proliferation of differentiating cells Expansion of numbers small
3T3 feeder layer	Cultures long-lived Subculture possible Clonal Large expansion of cell numbers possible Proliferating and differentiating cell types both present Proliferation largely confined to the basal layer Low contamination with other proliferating cell types Applicable to many species Applicable to many epithelia Applicable to tumors Can be grafted onto humans or experimental animals	Not homotypic Risk of contamination of human cells with mouse retroviruses or mouse genetic material

can extend the lifespan of a number of cell types and lead to immortalization [Bodnar et al., 1998]. When this idea is applied to human keratinocytes cultured either using 3T3 feeders [Dickson et al., 2000] or with MCDB153 [Kiyono et al., 1998] telomerase does block senescence, but the cells only become immortal following the epigenetic silencing of the p16^{INK4A} tumor suppressor gene. Nevertheless, these cells are often diploid and exhibit minimal alterations in their differentiation program [Farwell et al., 1999, Dickson et al., 2000], suggesting that these cultures will provide much better cell line models than previously produced. Similarly, the immortalization of human keratinocytes grown on 3T3 feeders has also been achieved by the retroviral delivery of 14-3-3σ antisense, and this too results in cell lines with a diploid karyotype [Dellambra et al., 2000]. In this study, however, the cells were blocked at an early stage of keratinocyte differentiation.

4. SELECTIVE CONDITIONS FOR PREFERENTIAL CULTIVATION OF KERATINOCYTE TUMOR CELLS

4.1. Reduced Dependence on Serum Growth Factors

The cells derived from human [Rheinwald and Beckett, 1981] and mouse [Pera and Gorman, 1984] squamous cell carcinomas all require far less fetal bovine serum (<5% v/v) for optimal growth than their normal counterparts. To select for the growth

TABLE 3.2. Troubleshooting Chart

Problem	Possible Cause	Remedy
No colonies	Mycoplasma	Check for mycoplasma. If positive discard and recover a new ampoule of 3T3
	Feeder layer too sparse	Recover a new ampoule of 3T3
	Feeder layer unhealthy	Recover a new ampoule of 3T3
	Batch of fetal bovine serum inappropriate	Rescreen fetal bovine serum
	pH too high	Check gassing and medium pH
Colonies not well spread and growing slowly	Feeder layer too dense	Plate fewer feeders
	Hydrocortisone ineffective	Prepare fresh hydrocortisone
	Mycoplasma	Check cells for mycoplasma
Poor cloning efficiency on transfer	Cultures too dense	Subculture before cells become confluent

of transformed keratinocytes on a 3T3 feeder layer we have used DMEM supplemented with 2% v/v fetal bovine serum and 0.4 μg/ml hydrocortisone. This medium prevents the growth of normal fibroblasts and of normal keratinocytes, both of which contaminate a tumor cell suspension. Epidermal growth factor [Rheinwald and Green, 1977] and cholera toxin [Green, 1978], which are potent mitogens for normal keratinocytes, can actually be inhibitory to squamous cell carcinoma cells [E.K. Parkinson, unpublished data; Gill and Lazar, 1981]. The morphologic appearance of a lingual tumor line developed by A. Yeudall in our laboratory (Fig. 3.1b) can be compared with that of normal human keratinocytes growing in fully supplemented growth medium (Fig. 3.1a). The tumor cells in this instance are flatter than normal and appear less stratified. However, morphologic criteria are not sufficient to determine whether keratinocytes are transformed, because a wide variety of squamous cell carcinoma morphologies have been noted [Rheinwald and Beckett, 1981].

4.2. Enhanced Resistance to Terminal Differentiation Stimuli and to Inhibitory Factors

When normal keratinocytes are placed in methocel-stabilized suspension cultures, they lose their capability to form colonies (their colony-forming half-life is 3 h) [Rheinwald and Green, 1977; Rheinwald, 1979], and most go on to terminally differentiate [Green, 1977]. Keratinocytes from tumors do not generally display anchorage-independent growth [Rheinwald and Beckett, 1981], but they do appear to terminally differentiate more slowly in this system than normal keratinocytes [Rheinwald and Beckett, 1980]. The tumor cells are also resistant to other terminal differentiation signals such as 1.2 mM calcium [Kulesz-Martin et al., 1980] under certain conditions and also to phorbol esters [Parkinson et al., 1983]. In addition, some keratinocyte cell lines derived from tumors are resistant to the effects of the growth inhibitors interferon α/β (Yaar et al., 1985] and transforming growth factor β [Shipley et al., 1986]. These properties might also be used to help the selection of squamous carcinoma cells in vitro.

4.3. Acquisition of Indefinite In Vitro Lifespan by Squamous Carcinoma Keratinocytes

A significant proportion of tumors from epidermis and tongue form established cell lines when placed in culture by the 3T3 feeder technique [Rheinwald and Beckett, 1981], and the acquisition of an indefinite in vitro lifespan is potentially a selectable as well as a diagnostic feature of transformed keratinocytes, particularly if the culture conditions are manipulated to give a short normal keratinocyte in vitro lifespan.

4.4. Tumor Formation in Nude Mice

In all cases, confirmation that the cultures are indeed epidermal tumor cells can be achieved by subcutaneous injection into nude mice [Rheinwald and Beckett, 1981] or by seeding the cells onto experimentally induced granulation tissue beds in nude mice [Boukamp et al., 1985]. Squamous cell carcinoma cells have been reported to form invading tumors in both cases. Basal cell carcinomas can also be cultured by methods very similar to those used for normal keratinocytes [Hernandez et al., 1985] and have also been reported to grow in nude mice when subcutaneously injected [Grimwood et al., 1985].

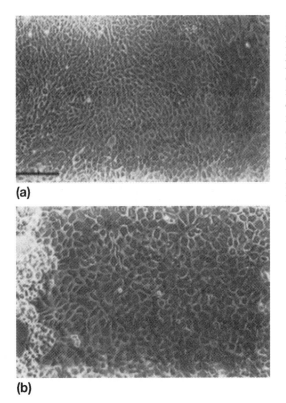

(a)

(b)

Fig 3.1. Phase-contrast micrographs of a formalin-fixed cells. **a.** Normal human keratinocyte colony after 10 days growth in complete growth medium (see text). **b.** Squamous cell carcinoma colony after 14 days growth in Dulbecco's medium containing 10% fetal bovine serum and 0.4 μg/ml hydrocortisone. Bar = 200 μm.

5. EPITHELIAL AND KERATINOCYTE MARKERS

Most epithelial cells have an intermediate filament cytoskeleton composed of keratin polypeptides [Sun et al., 1979; Franke et al., 1979] and/or possess desmosomal intercellular contacts [Cowin and Garrod, 1983]. Many monoclonal antibodies are now available, and some of them react specifically with stratified epithelial cells, that is, with true keratinocytes [Lane, 1982; Woodcock-Mitchell et al., 1982] (Fig. 3.2a,b). Polyclonal antisera raised against keratin extracts will react with all types of epithelial cells, as will polyclonal antisera raised against the desmoplakin (Fig. 3.2c) [Franke et al., 1981, 1982] and the desmocollin (Fig. 3.2d) [Cowin et al., 1984] proteins of the desmosome.

Polyclonal antisera against the envelope precursor protein involucrin [Rice and Green, 1979; Watt and Green, 1981] will react only with true keratinocytes in vivo, at least in primates and humans [Rice and Thacher, 1986], but in vitro (Fig. 3.2e) involucrin is eventually expressed in other epithelial cells, which undergo a process similar to metaplasia with longer-term in vitro cultivation [M. Stanley, personal communication].

6. INDUCTION OF COMPLETE DIFFERENTIATION

Like most cell types, in vitro keratinocytes proliferate very fast and are most likely to be in a state of regeneration rather than steady state. The cultured cells express many of the markers associated with the keratinocyte lineage such as keratin polypeptides [Sun and Green, 1978], desmosomal proteins [Franke et al., 1981, 1982; Cowin and Garrod, 1983; Cowin et al., 1984; Watt et al., 1984], and involucrin [Rice and Green, 1979; Watt and Green, 1981]. However, the spatial distribution of involucrin [Watt, 1983] and the expression of certain keratins [Kopan et al., 1987] is changed in vitro, and other markers such as keratohyaline granules, membrane-coated vesicles [Fuchs and Green, 1981], and certain keratins [Sun and Green, 1978] are not seen at all. Additionally, no proper stratum corneum is formed (Fig. 3.3a) and the cultures shed nucleated squames [Green, 1977], which is a phenomenon normally restricted to wet-surfaced squamous epithelia [Frost, 1979] and to certain pathological epidermal conditions such as psoriasis [Mescon and Grots, 1974]. A proper stratum corneum that is similar to the in vivo epithelium (Fig. 3.3b) and stratum granulosum, with the associated keratins, keratohyaline granules, and membrane-coated vesicles, can be restored in hu-

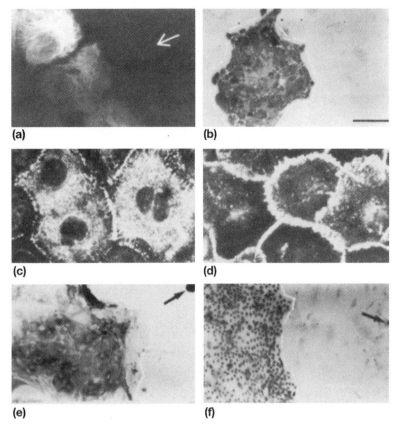

Fig 3.2. Immunostaining of cultured keratinocytes. **a.** A 10-day old normal human epidermal keratinocyte colony fixed for 10 min at room temperature in 50:50 acetone:methanol [Lane, 1982; Pera and Gorman, 1984] reacted with the LP34 anti mouse keratin monoclonal antibody and stained with fluorescein-conjugated anti mouse IgG. A 3T3 cell (arrow) is not stained. The LP34 hybridoma supernatant was a generous gift of Dr. E.B. Lane, ICRF, South Mimms, UK. Bar = 20 μm. **b.** Normal human keratinocytes were fixed as in Panel a and stained by reaction with 1:10 dilution of the LP34 supernatant followed by reaction with an anti-mouse IgG alkaline phosphatase kit (Vectastain AK5002) and visualized by incubation with an alkaline phosphatase substrate kit (Vectastain SK5IOO) for 25 min in the dark. Bright-field illumination. The 3T3 feeder cells outside the colony boundary (white lines) do not stain. Bar = 500 μm. **c,d.** Keratinocytes stained with polyclonal antisera raised against desmoplakin (c) [Franke et al., 1981, 1982] and desmocollin (d) [Cowin et al., 1984] proteins of the desmosome. Bar = 20 μm. **e.** Visualization of differentiating human keratinocytes with a polyclonal rabbit antiserum to involucrin (a generous gift from Dr. F.M. Watt, ICRF, Lincoln's Inn Fields, London, UK). The micrograph shows an acetone-methanol-fixed 10-day normal human keratinocyte colony after reaction with the anti-involucrin antiserum and an anti-rabbit peroxidase kit (Vectastain PK-400l). The involucrin-positive cells were visualized by treatment for 7 min in the dark with 0.6 mg/ml diaminobenzidine and 0.6 μl hydrogen peroxide in PBSA, pH 7.4. Bright-field illumination. The colony edge is delineated by the white line, and the 3T3 feeder layer outside the colony edge does not stain. Arrow: An isolated differentiating keratinocyte. Note that the nonstratified colony edge contains few if any involucrin-positive cells but that the colony center is stained to varying intensities. Bar = 200 μm. **f.** Visualization of human nuclei with the mouse monoclonal antibody LP4N (a generous gift of Dr. E.B. Lane, ICRF, South Mimms, UK). The micrograph shows an acetone-methanol-fixed 10-day-old normal human keratinocyte colony after reaction with a 1 in 100 dilution of LP4N and visualization as with Panel b. The white line shows the border of the keratinocyte colony. The nuclei of the mouse 3T3 cells do not stain. Arrow: An isolated human keratinocyte. Bright-field illumination. Bar = 500 μm. Panels c and d from Watt et al. [1984] with permission of the Rockefeller University Press and Dr. F.M. Watt.

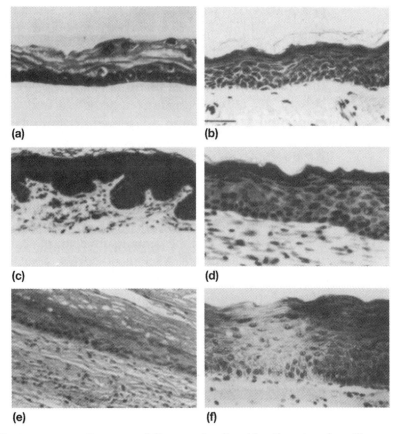

Fig 3.3. The transverse sections are as follows: **a.** A cultured keratinocyte colony. Compare with Panel b; note the absence of a granular layer and an anucleate stratum corneum. Bar = 25 μm. **b.** Human epidermis. Bar = 25 μm. **c.** Cultured human epidermis grafted onto the perniculus carnosus of a nude mouse (see Banks-Schlegel and Green [1980] for details). **d.** Cultured mouse epidermal cells seeded onto granulation tissue in a syngeneic mouse (see Fusenig et al. [1983] for details). Bar = 20 μm. **e.** Cyst derived from cultured 5V40-transformed human keratinocytes injected subcutaneously into a nude mouse (see Doran et al. [1980] for details). Bar = 50 μm. **f.** Human epidermal keratinocytes cultured on collagen rafts at an air-liquid interface (see Asselineau et al. [1985] and Kopanetal [1987] for details). Bar = 25 μm. Note the appearance in Panels c–f of an anucleate stratum corneum and a stratum granulosum and the general increase in epidermal thickness. Panels a, b, and f reproduced from Kopan et al. [1987], with permission of the Rockefeller University Press and Dr. E.V. Fuchs. Panel c reproduced from Banks-Schlegel and Green [1980], with permission of Williams and Wilkins and Dr. H. Green. Panel d reproduced from Fusenig et al. [1983], with permission of the Society of Dermatology, Inc., Cleveland, OH and Dr. N. Fusenig. Panel e is a generous gift from Dr. P.H. Gallimore of the Department of Cancer Studies, University of Birmingham.

man cultures by depleting of the fetal bovine serum that is to be used in the cultivation of the cells of vitamin A [Fuchs and Green, 1981]. It is now known that vitamin A has a strong suppressive action on many aspects of the keratinocyte differentiation program [Fuchs and Green, 1981; Kopan et al., 1987].

A more complete differentiation program than that found in vitro can be restored to the keratinocyte by grafting confluent cultures onto the perniculus carnosus connective tissue of immunosuppressed mice (Fig. 3.3c) [Banks-Schlegel and Green, 1980], seeding cell suspensions onto experimentally produced granulation tissue (Fig. 3.3d) [Fusenig et al., 1983; also see Chapter 2], or injecting cell suspensions at high cell density subcutaneously into immunosuppressed mice (Fig. 3.3e) [Doran et al., 1980].

In vitro the complete keratinocyte differentiation program can best be obtained by culturing the keratinocytes on collagen rafts until they become confluent. When confluence is reached, the collagen matrix carrying the epithelium is raised, so that the medium feeds the confluent culture with nutrients and growth factors through the collagen and the ventral surface of the epithelium. It is thought that a vitamin A gradient develops ventro-dorsally across the epidermis, and it has been demonstrated that by means of this system the complete differentiation program and all the normal epidermal layers are restored to the epithelium (Fig. 3.3f; see also Chapter 2) [Asselineau et al., 1985; Kopan et al., 1987].

ACKNOWLEDGMENTS

The authors would like to thank Dr. F.M. Watt and Dr. E.B. Lane for the gift of antisera and the following scientists for allowing the reproduction of their work in this article: Dr. F.M. Watt, Dr. E.V. Fuchs, Dr. N. Fusenig, Professor P.H. Gallimore, and Professor H. Green. The authors would also like to thank the Rockefeller University Press, Williams and Wilkins, and the Society of Dermatology, Inc. for allowing this work to be reproduced. Some of the work described in this article was supported by the Cancer Research Campaign.

REFERENCES

Alani RM, Hasskarl J, Grace M, Hernandez M-C, Israel M, Munger K (1999): Immortalisation of primary keratinocytes by the helix-loop-helix protein, Id1. Proc Natl Acad Sci USA 96: 9637–9641.

Alitalo K, Kuismanen E, Myllyla R, Kiistala U, Asko-Selgavaara S, Vaheri A (1982): Extracellular matrix proteins of human epidermal keratinocytes and feeder 3T3 cells. J Cell Biol 94: 497–505.

Allen-Hoffman BL, Rheinwald JG (1984): Polycyclic aromatic hydrocarbon mutagenesis of human epidermal keratinocytes in culture. Proc Natl Acad Sci USA 81: 7802–7806.

Appleby MW, Greenfield IM, Crook T, Parkinson EK, Stanley MA (1989): In vivo and in vitro assays for self-renewal in mouse epidermal keratinocytes expressing the v-fos and EJ-Ha-ras oncogenes. Oncogene 4: 1323–1330.

Asselineau D, Bernard B, Bailly C, Darmon M (1985): Epidermal morphogenesis and induction of the 67 kDa keratin polypeptide by culture of human keratinocytes at the liquid-air interface. Exp Cell Res 159: 536–539.

Banks-Schlegel SP, Green H (1980): Formation of epidermis by serially cultivated human epidermal cells transplanted as an epithelium to athymic mice. Transplantation 29: 308–313.

Barrandon Y, Green H (1985): Cell size as a determinant of the clone-forming ability of human keratinocytes. Proc Natl Acad Sci USA 82: 5390–5394.

Barrandon Y, Green H (1987): Cell migration is essential for sustained growth of keratinocyte colonies: The roles of transforming growth factor c and epidermal growth factor. Cell 50: 1131–1137.

Barrandon Y, Morgan JR, Mulligan RC, Green H (1989): Restoration of growth potential in paraclones of human keratinocytes by a viral oncogene. Proc Natl Acad Sci USA 86: 4102–4106.

Bodnar AG, Ouellette M, Frolkis M, Holt, SE, Chiu CP, Morin GB, Harley CB, Shay JW, Lichtsteiner S, Wright WE (1998): Extension of life-span by introduction of telomerase into normal human cells. Science 279: 349–352.

Boukamp P, Petrussevska RT, Breitkreutz D, Hornung J, Markham A, Fusenig NE (1988): Normal keratinization in a spontaneously immortalized aneuploid human keratinocyte cell line. J Cell Biol 106: 761–771.

Boukamp P, Rupnick HTR, Fusenig NE (1985): Environmental modulation of the expression of differentiation and malignancy in six human squamous cell carcinoma cell lines. Cancer Res 45: 5582–5592.

Boyce ST, Ham RG (1983): Calcium-regulated differentiation of normal human epidermal keratinocytes in chemically defined clonal culture and serum-free serial culture. J Invest Dermatol 81 (Suppl): 33s–40s.

Briggaman RA, Abele DC, Harris BA, Wheeler CE (1967): Preparation and characterization of a viable suspension of post-embryonic human epidermal cells. J Invest Dermatol 48: 159–168.

Compton CC, Gill JM, Bradford DA, Regauri S, Gallico GG, O'Connor NE (1989): Skin regenerated from cultured epithelial autografts on full-thickness burns wounds from 6 days to 5 years after grafting. A light, electron microscopic and immunocytochemical study. Lab Invest 60: 600–612.

Cowan FM, Broomfield CA, Smith WJ (1998): Sulfur mustard exposure enhances Fc receptor expression on human epidermal keratinocytes in cell culture: Implications for toxicity and medical counter measures. Cell Biol Toxicol 14: 261–266.

Cowin P, Garrod DR (1983): Antibodies to epithelial desmosomes show wide tissue and species cross-reactivity. Nature 302: 148–150.

Cowin P, Mattey D, Garrod D (1984): Identification of desmosomal surface components (desmocollins) and inhibition of desmosome formation by specific Fab^1. J Cell Sci 70: 41–60.

Clancy JMP, Shehade SA, Blight A, Young KE, Levick PL (1988): Treatment of leg ulcers with cultured epithelial grafts. J Am Acad Dermatol 18: 1356–1357.

Cruickshank CND, Cooper JR, Hooper CJ (1960): The cultivation of cells from adult epidermis. J Invest Dermatol 34: 339–342.

Dellambra E, Golisano O, Bondanza S, Siviero E, Lacal P, Molinari M, D'Atri S, De Luca M (2000): Downregulation of 14-3-3sigma prevents clonal evolution and leads to immortalization of primary human keratinocytes. J Cell Biol: 149(5): 1117–1130.

Dickson MA, Hahn WC, Ino Y, Ronfard V, Wu JY, Weinberg RA, Louis DN, Li FP, Rheinwald JG (2000): Human keratinocytes that express hTERT and also bypass a p16(INK4a)-encoded mechanism that limits lifespan become immortal yet retain normal growth: differentiation characteristics. Mol Cell Biol 20: 1436–1447.

Doran TI, Vidrich AL, Sun T-T (1980): Intrinsic and extrinsic regulation of the differentiation of skin, corneal and esophageal epithelial cells. Cell 22: 17–25.

Eisinger M, Lee JS, Hefton JM, Darzynkiewicz Z, Chiao JW, DeHarven E (1979): Human epidermal cell cultures: Growth and differentiation in the absence of dermal components or medium supplements. Proc Natl Acad Sci USA 76: 5340–5344.

Farwell DG, Shera KA, Koop JI, Bonnet GA, Matthews CP, Reuther GW, Coltrera MD, McDougall JK, Klingelhutz AJ (2000): Genetic and epigenetic changes in human epithelial cells immortalized by telomerase. Am J Pathol: 156: 1537–1547.

Fell HB (1964): The experimental study of keratinization in organ culture. In Montagna W, Lobitz WC Jr (eds): "The Epidermis." New York: Academic Press, pp 61–81.

Finch PW, Rubin JS, Mipin T, Ron D, Aaronson SA (1989): Human KGF is FGF-related with properties of a paracrine effector of epithelial cell growth. Science 245: 752–755.

Flaxman BA, Lutzner MA, Van Scott EJ (1967): Cell maturation and tissue organization in epithelial outgrowths from skin and buccal mucosa in vitro. J Invest Dermatol 49: 322–332.

Franke WW, Appelhaus B, Schmid E (1979): Identification and characterization of epithelial cells in mammalian tissues by immunofluorescence microscopy using antibodies to prekeratin. Differentiation 15: 7–25.

Franke WW, Schmidt E, Grund C, Mueller H, Engelbrecht I, Moll R, Stadler J, Jarasch E-D (1981): Antibodies to high molecular weight polypeptides of desmosomes: Specific localization of a class of junctional proteins in cells and tissues. Differentiation 20: 217–241.

Franke WW, Moll R., Schiller DL, Schmidt E, Kertenbeck J, Muller H (1982): Desmoplakins of epithelial and myocardial desmosomes are immunologically and biochemically related. Differentiation 23: 115–127.

Frost JK (1979): Gynecologic and obstetric cytopathology. In Novak ER, Woodruff JD (eds): "Obstetrics and Gynecologic Cervix Pathology." Philadelphia, London, Toronto: W.B. Saunders, pp 689–782.

Fuchs E, Green H (1981): Regulation of terminal differentiation of cultured human keratinocytes by Vitamin A. Cell 25: 617–625.

Fusenig NE (1971): Isolation and cultivation of epidermal cells from embryonic mouse skin. Naturwissenschaften 58: 421–422.

Fusenig NE, Worst PKM. (1974): Mouse epidermal cell cultures. I. Isolation and cultivation of epidermal cells from adult mouse skin. J Invest Dermatol 63: 187–193.

Fusenig NE, Breitkreutz D, Dzarlieva RT, Boukamp P, Bohnert A, Tilgen W (1983): Growth and differentiation characteristics of transformed keratinocytes from mouse and human skin in vitro and in vivo. J Invest Dermatol 81: 168s–175s.

Gilchrest BA, Marshall WL, Karassik RL, Weinstein R, Macaig T (1984): Characterization and partial purification of keratinocyte growth factor from the hypothalamus. J Cell Physiol 120: 377–383.

Gill GW, Lazar CS (1981): Increased phosphotyrosine content and inhibition of proliferation in EGF-treated A431 cells. Nature 293: 305–307.

Green H (1977): Terminal differentiation of cultured epidermal cells. Cell 11: 405–416.

Green H (1978): Cyclic AMP in relation to proliferation of the epidermal cell: A new view. Cell 15: 801–811.

Green H, Kehinde O, Thomas J (1979): Growth of cultured human epidermal cells into multiple epithelia suitable for grafting. Proc Natl Acad Sci USA 76: 5665–5668.

Green H (1980): The keratinocyte as differentiated cell type. Harvey Lect 74: 101–138.

Grimwood RE, Johnson CA, Ferris CF, Mercill DB, Mellette JR, Hull JC (1985): Transplantation of human basal cell carcinomas to athymic mice. Cancer 56: 519–523.

Halaban R, Ghosh S, Baird A (1987): bFGF is the putative natural growth factor for human melanocytes. In Vitro Cell Dev Biol 23: 47–52.

Halaban R, Langdon R, Birchall N, Cuono C, Baird A, Scott G, Moellmann G, McGuire J (1988): Paracrine stimulation of melanocytes by keratinocytes through basic fibroblast growth factor. J Cell Biol 107: 1611–1619.

Hennings M, Michael D, Cheng C, Steinert P, Holbrook K, Yuspa SH (1980): Calcium regulation of growth and differentiation of mouse epidermal cells in culture. Cell 19: 245–254.

Hernandez AD, Hibbs MS, Postlethwaite AE (1985): Establishment of basal cell carcinoma in culture: Evidence for a basal cell carcinoma-derived factor which stimulates fibroblasts to proliferate and release collagenase. J Invest Dermatol 85: 470–475.

Karasek MA, Charlton ME (1971): Growth of post-embryonic skin epithelial cells on collagen gels. J Invest Dermatol 56: 205–210.

Kiyono T, Foster SA, Koop JI, McDougall JK, Galloway DA, Klingelhutz AJ (1998): Both Rb/p16INK4a inactivation and telomerase activity are required to immortalize human epithelial cells. Nature 396: 84–88.

Kopan R, Traska G, Fuchs E (1987): Retinoids as important regulators of terminal differentiation: Examining keratin expression in individual epidermal cells at various stages of keratinization. J Cell Biol 105: 427–440.

Kubilus J, McDonald MJ, Baden HP (1979): Epidermal proteins of cultured human and bovine keratinocytes. Biochim Biophys Acta 578: 484–492.

Kulesz-Martin M, Koehler B, Hennings H, Yuspa SH (1980): Quantitative assay for carcinogen altered differentiation in mouse epidermal cells. Carcinogenesis 1: 995–1006.

Lane EB (1982): Monoclonal antibodies provide specific molecular markers for the study of epithelial tonofilament organization. J Cell Biol 92: 665–673.

Liu S-C, Karasek M (1978): Isolation and growth of adult human epidermal keratinocytes in cell culture. J Invest Dermatol 71:157–162.

Macaig T, Nemore RE, Weinstein R, Gilchrest BA (1981): An endocrine approach to the control of epidermal growth: Serum-free cultivation of human keratinocytes. Science 211: 1432–1434.

Mescon H, Grot IA (1974): The skin. In Robbins SL (ed): "Pathological Basis of Disease." Philadelphia, London, Toronto: W.B. Saunders, pp 1374–1419.

Naeyaert JM, Eller M, Gordon PR, Park H-Y, Gilchrest BA (1991): Pigment content of cultured human melanocytes does not correlate with tyrosine message level. Br J Dermatol 125: 297–303.

Paraskeva C, Buckle BG, Sheer D, Wigley CB (1984): The isolation and characterisation of colorectal epithelial cell lines at different stages in malignant transformation from familial polyposis coli patients. Int J Cancer, 34: 4956.

Park H-Y, Yaar M., Gilchrest BA (2000): Melanocytes. In Freshney, RI (ed.) "Culture of Animal Cells," 4th ed. New York: John Wiley & Sons, pp 378–381.

Parkinson EK, Newbold RF (1980): Benzo(a)pyrene metabolism and DNA adduct formation in serially cultivated strains of human epidermal keratinocytes. Int J Cancer 26: 289–299.

Parkinson EK, Grabham P, Emmerson A. (1983): A subpopulation of cultured human keratinocytes which is resistant to the induction of terminal differentiation-related changes by phorbol 1 2-myristate,13-acetate: Evidence for an increase in the resistant population following transformation. Carcinogenesis 4: 857–861.

Parkinson EK, Hume W, Potten CS (1986): The radiosensitivity of cultured human and mouse keratinocytes. Int J Radiat Biol 50: 717–726.

Parkinson EK, Al-Yaman FM, Appleby MW (1987): The effect of donor age on the proliferative response of human and mouse keratinocytes to phorbol, 12-myristate,13-acetate. Carcinogenesis 8: 907–912.

Peehl DM, Ham RG (1980a): Growth and differentiation of human keratinocytes without a feeder layer or conditioned medium. In Vitro 16: 516–525.

Peehl DM, Ham RG (1980b): Clonal growth of human keratinocytes with small amounts of dialyzed serum. In Vitro 16: 526–540.

Pera MF, Gorman PA (1984): In vitro analysis of multistage carcinogenesis: Development of indefinite renewal capacity and reduced growth factor requirements in colony forming keratinocytes precedes malignant transformation. Carcinogenesis 5: 671–682.

Phillips MA, Rice RH (1983): Convergent differentiation in cultured rat cells from non-keratinized epithelia: Keratinocyte character and intrinsic differences. J Cell Biol 97: 686–691.

Pittelkow MR, Scott RE (1986): New techniques for the in vitro culture of human skin keratinocytes and perspectives on their use for grafting of patients with extensive burns. Mayo Clin Proc 62: 777–787.

Prose PN, Friedman-Kien AE, Neistein S (1967): Ultrastructural studies of organ culture of adult human skin. Lab Invest 17: 693–716.

Rheinwald JG (1979): The role of terminal differentiation in the finite culture lifetime of the human epidermal keratinocyte. Int Rev Cytol Suppl 10: 25–33.

Rheinwald JG (1980): Serial cultivation of normal human epidermal keratinocytes. Methods Cell Biol 21A: 229–254.

Rheinwald JG, Beckett MA (1980): Defective terminal differentiation in culture as a consistent and selectable character of malignant human keratinocytes. Cell 22: 629–632.

Rheinwald JG, Beckett MA (1981): Tumorigenic keratinocyte lines requiring anchorage and fibroblast support cultured from human squamous cell carcinomas. Cancer Res 41: 1657–1663.

Rheinwald JG, Green H (1975): Serial cultivation of strains of human epidermal keratinocytes: The formation of keratinizing colonies from single cells. Cell 6: 331–344.

Rheinwald JG, Green H (1977): Epidermal growth factor and the multiplication of cultured human epidermal keratinocytes. Nature 265: 421–424.

Rice RH, Green H (1979): Presence in human epidermal cells of a soluble protein precursor of the cross-linked envelope: Activation of the cross-linking by calcium ions. Cell 18: 681–694.

Rice RH, Thacher SM (1986): Involucrin: A constituent of cross-linked envelopes and marker of squamous maturation. In Bereiter-Hahn J, Maltoltsy AG, Richard KS (eds): "Biology of the Integument 2." Berlin: Springer-Verlag, pp 752–761.

Rubin JS, Osada H, Finch PW, Taylor WG, Rudikoff S, Aaronson SA (1989): Purification and characterization of a newly identified growth factor specific for epithelial cells. Proc Natl Acad Sci USA 86: 802–806.

Shipley GD, Pittelkow MR, Willie JJ Jr, Scott RE, Moses HL (1986): Reversible inhibition of normal human prokeratinocyte proliferation by type beta transforming growth factor-growth inhibitor in serum-free medium. Cancer Res 46: 2068–2071.

Sainte-Marie I, Jumbou O, Tenaud I, Dreno B (1998): Comparative study of the in vitro inflammatory activity of three nickel salts on keratinocytes. Acta Dermato-Venereologica 78: 169–172.

Stanley MA, Parkinson EK (1979): Growth requirements of human cervical epithelial cells in culture. Int J Cancer 24: 407–414.

Steinberg ML, Defendi V (1979): Altered pattern of growth and differentiation in human keratinocytes infected by simian virus 40. Proc Natl Acad Sci USA 76: 801–805.

Sun T-T, Green H (1976): Differentiation of the epidermal keratinocyte in cell culture: Formation of the cornified envelope. Cell 9: 511–521.

Sun T-T, Green H (1977): Cultured epithelial cells of cornea, conjunctiva and skin: Absence of marked intrinsic divergence of their differentiated states. Nature 269: 489–493.

Sun T-T, Green H (1978): Keratin filaments of cultured human epidermal cells: Formation of intermolecular disulfide bonds during terminal differentiation. J Biol Chem 253: 2053–2060.

Sun T-T, Shih C, Green H (1979): Keratin cytoskeleton in epithelial cells of internal organs. Proc Natl Acad Sci USA 76: 2813–2817.

Taichman L, Reilly S, Garant PR (1979): In-vitro cultivation of human oral keratinocytes. Arch Oral Biol 24: 258–268.

Taylor-Papadimitriou J, Shearer DM, Stoker MGP (1977): Growth requirements of human mammary epithelial cells in culture. Int J Cancer 20: 903–908.

Tsau MC, Walthall BJ, Ham RG (1982): Clonal growth of normal human epidermal keratinocytes in a defined medium. J Cell Physiol 110: 219–229.

Watt FM (1983): Involucrin and other markers of keratinocyte terminal differentiation. J Invest Dermatol 81 (Suppl): 100s–103s.

Watt FM, Green H (1981): Involucrin synthesis is correlated with cell size in human epidermal cultures. J Cell Biol 90: 738–742.

Watt FM, Mattey DL, Garrod DR (1984): Calcium-induced reorganization of desmosomal components in cultured human keratinocytes. J Cell Biol 99: 2211–2215.

Wilke MS, Edens M, Scott RE (1988): Ability of normal human keratinocytes that grow in culture in serum-free medium to be derived from suprabasal cells. J Natl Cancer Inst 80: 1299–1304.

Wille JJ Jr, Pittelkow MR, Shipley GD, Scott RE (1984): Integrated control of growth and differentiation of normal human prokeratinocytes cultured in serum-free medium: Clonal analysis. J Cell Physiol 121: 31–44.

Woodcock-Mitchell J, Eichner R, Nelson WG, Sun T-T (1982): Immunolocalization of keratin polypeptides in human epidermis using monoclonal antibodies. J Cell Biol 95: 580–588.

Wu Y-J, Parker LM, Binder NE, Beckett MA, Sinard JM, Griffiths CT, Rheinwald JG (1982): The mesothelial keratins: A new family of cytoskeletal proteins identified in cultured mesothelial cells and non-keratinizing epithelia. Cell 31: 693–703.

Yaar M, Karassik RL, Schnipper LE, Gilchrest BA (1985): Effects of alpha and beta interferons on cultured human keratinocytes. J Invest Dermatol 85: 70–74.

Yuspa SH, Morgan DL, Walker RJ, Bates RR (1970): The growth of fetal mouse skin in cell culture and transplantation to F_1 mice. J Invest Dermatol 55: 379–389.

APPENDIX: SOURCES OF MATERIALS

Reagent	Catalog No.	Supplier
Adenine (hydrochloride)	A9795	Sigma
Alkaline phosphatase reaction kit (Red)	SK5100	Vector
Anti mouse IgG ABC alkaline phosphatase kit	AK5002	Vector
Anti Rabbit IgG ABC peroxidase kit	PK4001	Vector
Balb 3T3 A31 cells	CCL163	ATCC
Bovine serum (selected batch)		GIBCO BRL, ICN, Sigma, SeraLab
Cholera toxin	C3012	Sigma
Cryotubes	5000-0012	Nalge Nunc
Diaminobenzidine tablets	D5905	Sigma
DMSO	D2650	Sigma
Dulbecco's modified Eagle's medium	31885	GIBCO BRL
EDTA (sodium salt)	E8008	Sigma
Epidermal growth factor (cell culture grade)	066-53003A	GIBCO BRL
Fetal bovine serum (selected batch)	Type II	Hyclone
Glutamine ($100\times$ concentrate)	043-05030	GIBCO BRL
Glycerol	G2025	Sigma
Ham's F12 medium	21765	GIBCO BRL
HEPES, 1 M solution	15630-056	GIBCO BRL
Hydrocortisone hemisuccinate (sodium salt)	H4881	Sigma
Hydrogen peroxide (30% solution)	H1009	Sigma
Insulin	16634	Sigma
Penicillin	P3032	Sigma
Streptomycin	S9137	Sigma
Swiss 3T3 cells	CCL92	ATCC
Transferrin (bovine)	T8027	Sigma
Triiodothyronine (sodium salt)	T6397	Sigma
Trypsin (crystalline)	3703	Worthington Biochemicals

4

Culture of Human Mammary Epithelial Cells

Martha R. Stampfer[1], Paul Yaswen[1], and
Joyce Taylor-Papadimitriou[2]

[1]Lawrence Berkeley National Laboratory, Berkeley, California 94720 and
[2]Guy's Hospital, London SE1 9RT, England. mrstampfer@lbl.gov

I. BACKGROUND ISSUES IN CULTURING HUMAN MAMMARY EPITHELIAL CELLS

One of the main advantages in culturing normal human mammary epithelial cells (HMEC) is that, unlike most other human organ systems, it is easy to obtain breast tissues with normal epithelial cell content from healthy individuals. Reduction mammoplasty operations, which are commonly performed mostly on younger individuals, yield abundant quantities of HMEC. Although it is not known what is responsible for the large deposition of fat in these breasts, pathologic evaluation of these tissues generally indicates no epithelial pathology or mild to moderate fibrocystic disease. Additionally, lactation fluids provide another readily available source of smaller quantities of HMEC in a more differentiated state. The main difficulties encountered in developing culture systems for normal HMEC arise from the breast being an architecturally complex tissue containing several epithelial and nonepithelial cell types and from the fact that the breast can undergo multiple states of differentiation at different times.

Difficulties exist in distinguishing between the major epithelial cell types (luminal and basal), the interrelationship between these types, and determining which cell types are proliferating in the culture system. Furthermore, in vivo, breast epithelial cells normally interact with other cell types (e.g., fibroblast, vascular endothelial, and adipose), as well as cell matrix components, within a three-dimensional architecture. Most culture systems do not model this complexity. Basal epithelial cells line the outside of the ducts, resting upon the basement membrane. Included in the basal layer are myoepithelial cells, which contain musclelike myofilaments and which contract on appropriate hormonal stimuli to cause expulsion of milk. The luminal cells lie on top of the basal layer, although they may also have direct contact with the basement membrane. In vivo, they exhibit a polarized morphology, with microvilli at the luminal side. In the rat mammary gland, it has been suggested that a common stem cell for both myoepithelial and luminal lineages lies in the basal layer; additionally, a second type of pluripotent cell for ductal and alveolar cell types may also exist [Dulbecco et al., 1986]. It is not known for human mammary development whether both myoepithelial and luminal lineages derive from a common stem cell or whether an intermediate stem cell type exists. Other dimensions of complexity are added by topography. Cells in the large ducts show differences in structure and function compared with those found in the smaller ducts and terminal ductal lobular units (TDLU).

Unlike most other organ systems, the adult mammary gland is not always in a functionally differentiated state, as it would be during pregnancy, lactation, or involution. Other than the cells obtained from lactational fluids, human mammary tissues are not readily available from differentiated glands, making analysis of functional differentiation in culture extremely difficult. In terms of using cultured HMEC for studies of carcinogenesis, this is not a major handicap, because mammary carcinoma cells generally do not exhibit properties of functional differentiation. However, the absence of understanding of mammary epithelial cell lineages is more problematic, because cancer cells found in vivo, as well as most breast tumor cell lines in vitro, closely resemble the phenotype of the normal mature luminal cell in vivo. Yet cultured normal HMEC with this phenotype show the least proliferative potential. Thus it is difficult to compare cultured normal and tumor-derived HMEC that share the same phenotypic markers and proliferative capacity. Increased information on the mechanisms controlling HMEC development into fully mature luminal cells may shed light on the nature of malignant progression.

In an attempt to assist identification of the different epithelial cell types, considerable effort has been put into developing immunologic markers (monoclonal antibodies) against various components of HMEC. The markers have been used to define specific phenotypes in vivo (i.e., in tissue sections) and to identify phenotypes of the cultured cells. In this context, the epithelial keratins have been extremely useful, because their expression appears to be maintained in culture. In Fig. 4.1 it can be seen that all the luminal epithelial cells express keratins 8 and 18 and most express 19, whereas all the basal cells express keratins 5 and 14 and do not express keratins 8 and 18. Keratin 7 is expressed in both cell types throughout the gland, and keratins 19 and 14 are also expressed by both cell types in the large ducts but not in the TDLU. Some of the antibodies used in identifying keratins are listed in Table 4.1, which also lists antibodies directed to other phenotypes useful for HMEC identification, e.g., polymorphic epithelial mucin (PEM), expressed by luminal epithelial cells [Burchell et al., 1983; Gendler et al., 1988], and smooth muscle actin and CALLA (common leukocytic leukemia antigen), expressed by basal epithelial cells.

Cultivation of bona fide tumor cells from primary breast tumors has proven more difficult than the culture of normal HMEC. Culture of tumor tissues in media developed for normal HMEC does not lead to outgrowth of cells displaying tumor-associated phenotypes. The cells that proliferate may derive from premalignant tissue or associated benign or in situ components. In the past few years, several groups have developed specialized culture conditions that support growth of tumor-derived HMEC that display the phenotypes of the tumor cells. These methods include specialized media formulations, low calcium, oxygen, and nutrient concentrations, and specialized methods of tissue digestion. The tumor cells have generally shown limited, notably slow, growth in culture. However, because there is no one standard procedure that allows routine culture of demonstrable tumor cells from primary tumors, we do not present a method for the culture of malignant cells from the breast. The reader is referred to the several references where growth of bona fide tumor cells from primary breast cancers has been reported [Ethier, 1996; Dairkee et al., 1997; Li et al., 1998]. The development of infinite lifespan lines from primary tumor tissues has also been very difficult [Band et al., 1990; Ethier, 1996]. A recent study attempting to address this deficiency reported that 10% (18/177) of primary human breast tumors could generate continuous lines; however, these tumors had features indicative of advanced cancer with poor prognosis [Gazdar et al., 1998].

Because the culture of rodent mammary epithelial cells requires different media and another set of markers, methods for their culture are not discussed in this chapter.

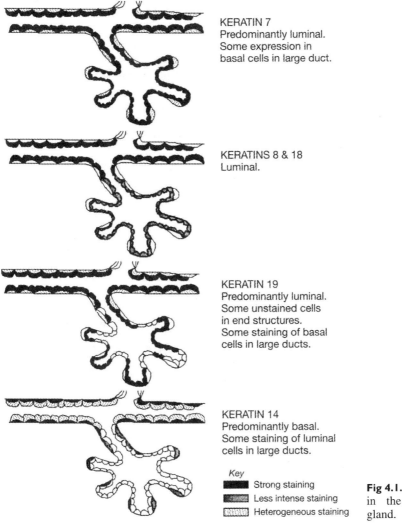

KERATIN 7
Predominantly luminal.
Some expression in
basal cells in large duct.

KERATINS 8 & 18
Luminal.

KERATIN 19
Predominantly luminal.
Some unstained cells
in end structures.
Some staining of basal
cells in large ducts.

KERATIN 14
Predominantly basal.
Some staining of luminal
cells in large ducts.

Key
■ Strong staining
▨ Less intense staining
▦ Heterogeneous staining

Fig 4.1. Keratin expression in the human mammary gland.

TABLE 4.1. Monoclonal Antibodies Useful for Characterizing Cultured Human Mammary Epithelial Cells

Antibody	Target Antigen	Reference
HMFG-1	Polymorphic	Burchell et al., 1983
HMFG-2	Epithelial mucin	Burchell et al., 1983
SM-3	(PEM)	Burchell et al., 1987
BA16	Keratin 19	Bartek et al., 1987
BA17	Keratin 19	Bartek et al., 1987
CO4	Keratin 18	Bartek et al., 1989
DA7	Keratin 18	Lauerova et al., 1988
LE61	Keratin 18	Lane, 1982
LL001	Keratin 14	Taylor-Papadimitriou et al., 1989
12C8-1	Keratin 14	Dairkee et al., 1985
M20	Keratin 8	Van Muijen et al., 1987
C-15	Keratin 8	Bartek et al., 1987
RCK 105	Keratin 7	Ramaekers et al., 1987
C-18	Keratin 7	Bartek et al., 1987
V9	Vimentin	Osborn et al., 1984
FN-3	Fibronectin	Keen et al., 1984
A12	Common acute lympho-blastic leukemia antigen (CALLA)	Gusterson et al., 1986
SM1	α-Actin	Skalli et al., 1986; Gugliotta et al., 1988

2. PREPARATION OF REAGENTS AND MEDIA

2.1. Stock Solutions, Trypsin, and Media for Milk Cell Cultures

2.1.1. Stock Solutions

1. Insulin, 1 mg/ml in 6 mM HCl
2. Hydrocortisone, 0.5 mg/ml in physiological saline
3. Cholera toxin, 50 μg/ml in physiological saline
4. Trypsin (1:250), 0.2% in Hanks' balanced salt solution (HBSS)
5. Pancreatin, 1.0% in HBSS

Serum and stock solutions of insulin, hydrocortisone, cholera toxin, pancreatin, and trypsin should be stored at −20°C.

2.1.2. Trypsinization Solution (TEGPED)
Combine:

	Final Conc.
EGTA, 0.5% (13 mM), in PBSA 10 ml	6.5 mM
EDTA, 0.02% (5 mM), in PBSA 4 ml	1.0 mM
Trypsin, 0.2% in HBSS 4 ml	0.04%
Pancreatin, 1.0% in HBSS 2 ml	0.1%

2.1.3. Growth Medium, Milk Mix (MX)

Add to RPMI 1640:

		Final Conc.
FBS		15%
Human serum		10%
Cholera toxin	50 ng/ml	0.6 nM
Hydrocortisone	0.5 μg/ml	1.4 μM
Insulin	1 μg/ml	0.2 μM

2.2. Reagents for Reduction Mammoplasty

2.2.1. Tissue Mix Medium

Add sterile solutions of the following to 1:1 DMEM:Ham's F12 medium (or equivalent) to yield the indicated final concentrations:

Insulin	10 μg/ml
Penicillin	100 U/ml
Streptomycin	100 μg/ml
Polymyxin B	50 U/ml
Fungizone	5 μg/ml

Store at 4°C.

2.2.2. Enzyme Stock Solution

(i) Dissolve collagenase in appropriate amount of tissue mix medium at 37°C to give 1500 U/ml. Filter sequentially through 0.80-μm, 0.45-μm, and 0.22-μm Nalgene filters to remove impurities and to sterilize.

(ii) Dissolve hyaluronidase (1000 U/ml) in appropriate amount of tissue mix medium at 37°C. Filter through 0.22-μm Nalgene filter.

(iii) Combine equal volumes of the sterile collagenase and hyaluronidase solutions. This is a 5× solution. Aliquot 30-ml volumes into 50-ml conical tubes. Store at $-70°C$ for up to 1 yr.

2.2.3. Tissue Digestion Medium

Add appropriate amounts of the tissue mix medium, enzyme solution, and FBS to the dissected breast tissue to yield a final concentration (including the volume of the tissue) of 150 U/ml collagenase, 100 U/ml hyaluronidase, and 10% FBS (see Protocol 4.4).

2.3. Preparation of Media for Cryopreservation

2.3.4. Cell Preservative Medium 1 (CPM1)

To make 100 ml, add 15 ml of FBS and 10 ml of DMSO to 75 ml of a 1:1 mixture of DMEM and F12. Shake gently to mix, aliquot, and store indefinitely at $-20°C$. Refrigerate after thawing. Used for freezing organoids.

2.3.5. Cell Preservation Medium 2 (CPM2)

To make 100 ml, mix 10 ml of glycerol (10%), 15 ml of FBS (15%), and 75 ml of MCDB 170 base (75%). Aliquot and store at $-20°C$. Refrigerate after thawing.

2.4. Reagents for Subculture of Primary Cultures in MCDB 170

2.4.1. STE (Saline-Trypsin-EDTA)

(i)   Solution A:

	g	mM
HEPES	7.149	30
Glucose	1.880	10
KCl	0.2238	3
NaCl	7.697	132
$Na_2HPO_4 \cdot 7H_2O$	0.268	1
Phenol red	0.010	0.028
UPW to 1 liter		

Sterilize through 0.22-μm filter and adjust pH to 7.6. Store at 4°C.

(ii) Dissolve trypsin and EDTA in solution A to yield a final concentration of 0.05% trypsin and 0.02% (0.5 mM) EDTA. Filter-sterilize and store frozen at -20°C.

NOTE ON STE: Always label trypsin solution with the date thawed; do not use trypsin more than 1 week old. Do not leave trypsin in a 37°C water bath.

2.5. Preparation of Serum-Free Medium, MCDB 170

Complete MCDB 170 medium consists of the basal MCDB 170 formula [Hammond et al., 1984] plus a set of serum-free supplements. Depending on the source of MCDB 170, some of these stocks will be supplied with the medium. Nearly complete MCDB 170 (lacking transferrin and isoproterenol) is available from Clonetics/BioWhittaker (MEGM; mammary epithelial growth medium). Medium containing fewer of the supplements is also available (MEBM; mammary epithelial basal medium). Other companies that make medium may supply basal MCDB 170. Always check to make sure which supplements come with the medium. Additionally, MCDB 170 was originally formulated to have a HEPES rather than a sodium-bicarbonate buffer base. HMEC grown in HEPES-based medium require a low-CO_2 incubator, ~0.2–1.0%. At these low settings there may be considerable variation among incubators; the best criterion for CO_2 setting is when the phenol red pH indicator is a salmon-orange. HEPES-based MCDB 170 is available from Clonetics as MEBM-SBF. We highly recommend the use of the HEPES-based medium if at all feasible, as the cells maintain their pH balance much better. Clonetics also provides a phenol red-free medium, called MEBM-PRF.

If you prefer to prepare basal MCDB 170 yourself, instructions are provided in Appendix A: Stock Solutions for MCDB 170 at the end of this chapter.

Cells growing serum-free are more sensitive to toxins in the environment. Be sure that you have not placed in the incubator, or used for cleaning, any potentially toxic compounds. Washing the incubator with distilled water and then leaving the door open for a day can alleviate some problems.

2.5.1. Stock Solutions

The following constituents are components of basal MCDB 170, but they must be added just before use to prevent precipitation or degradation. Again, you may be able to purchase these from the same supplier, but, if not, they may be made up as follows:

(i) *L-Glutamine*, 200 mM stock. Dissolve 2.92 g of L-glutamine in 100 ml of UPW. Sterilize through a 0.22-μm filter and store in 5-ml aliquots at $-20°C$.

(ii) *Stock J, 200×.* $CaCl_2 \cdot 2H_2O$, 5.88 g in 100 ml of UPW. Sterilize through a 0.22-μm filter and store at room temperature.

(iii) *Stock K_1*, 200×. $MgSO_4 \cdot 7H_2O$, 7.39 g in 100 ml of UPW. Filter, sterilize, and store at room temperature.

(iv) *Stock K_2*, 200×. $FeSO_4 \cdot 7H_2O$, 27.8 mg in 100 ml of UPW with 1 drop of 1 N HCl. Filter-sterilize and store at room temperature. Be sure to discard if solution contains a precipitate or becomes orange-colored. Best to store under nitrogen.

(v) *Stock M, 100×.* Riboflavin, 1.13 mg in 100 ml of UPW. Filter-sterilize and store at $-20°C$ in the dark. Place in aliquots so that it is not thawed more than 5 times.

2.5.2. Supplements for Serum-Free Medium

Usually, all of the following supplements will need to be added to basal MCDB 170 to make complete MCDB 170. They may be available from your media supplier, but, if not, they may be prepared as follows:

(i) *Insulin, 200× stock, 1 mg/ml.* Dissolve 1 g of insulin powder in 200 ml of 0.005 N HCl (1 ml 1 N HCl with 199 ml of UPW) by stirring on a magnetic stirrer. Add 1 N HCl dropwise if powder does not dissolve, not to exceed a final concentration of 0.005 N HCl. Bring up to 1 liter and sterilize through a 0.22-μm filter. Store aliquots at $-20°C$.

(ii) *Hydrocortisone, 2000× stock, 1 mg/ml.* Dissolve 10 mg of crystalline hydrocortisone in 10 ml of 95% ethanol. Store at $-20°C$.

(iii) *EGF (epidermal growth factor), 20,000× stock, 100 μg/ml.* Add 1 ml of sterile UPW or solution A (see Section 2.4.1 (i)) to a vial of 100 μg of sterile EGF. Mix gently. Aliquot 50-μl and 100-μl portions to Nalge Nunc ampoules and freeze at $-20°C$ for up to 3 months.

(iv) *Isoproterenol, 500 stock, 5×10^{-3} M.* Do not inhale dust. In hood, dissolve 50 mg of isoproterenol in 40 ml of 95% ethanol and store at $-20°C$. Make up fresh monthly.

(v) *Ethanolamine (2-aminoethanol), 1000× stock, 10^{-1} M.* Dissolve 61 mg of ethanolamine in 10 ml of MCDB 170 base or solution A (see Section 2.4.1, (i)). Sterilize through a 0.22-μm filter and store at 4°C.

(vi) *o-Phosphoethanolamine, 1000× stock, 10^{-1} M.* Dissolve 141 mg of phosphoethanolamine in 10 ml of MCDB 170 base or solution A (see Section 2.4.1, (i)). Sterilize through a 0.22-μm filter and store at −20°C.

(vii) *Transferrin, human, 2000× stock, 10 mg/ml.* Dissolve 50 mg of transferrin in 5 ml of sterile distilled water or solution A (see Section 2.4.1, (i)). Sterilize through a 0.22-μm filter and freeze at −20°C for up to 3 months.

(viii) *BPE (bovine pituitary extract), 200× stock, 14 mg/ml.* Centrifuge BPE at 13,000 *g* for 10 min. Sterilize by sequential filtration through 0.8-μm, 0.45-μm, and 0.22-μm Nalgene filters. Filtering proceeds slowly. Aliquot 5- to 10-ml portions into sterile screw-cap vials and store at −20°C for up to 1 year.

2.5.3. Preparation of Complete MCDB 170 from Basal MCDB 170

(i) Immediately before use, add the following filter-sterilized stocks to 967 ml of basal MCDB 170:

L-Glutamine, 200 mM	10 ml
Stocks J, K_1, and K_2	5 ml each
Stock M	10 ml

If MCDB has been supplied without trace elements, you will also need to add:

Stock L (see Appendix A: Stock Solutions for MCDB 170)	10 ml

Stir vigorously while stocks are slowly being added on magnetic stir plate with sterile stir bar.

(ii) Add the following supplements (see Section 2.5.2 for stock solutions):

Supplement	Amount	Final conc.
Insulin stock	5 ml	5 μg/ml (~1 μM)
Hydrocortisone stock	0.5 ml	0.5 μg/ml (1.4 μM)
EGF stock	100 μl	10 ng/ml (1.7 nM)
Ethanolamine stock	1 ml	6.1 μg/ml (0.1 mM)

| Transferrin stock | 1 ml | 5 μg/ml (~60 nM) |
| BPE | 5 ml | 70 μg/ml total protein |

Antibiotics are best omitted but may be added at this stage if required.

(iii) Store at 4°C for up to 2–3 weeks. Do not freeze.

3. CULTURE OF MAMMARY EPITHELIAL CELLS FROM HUMAN MILK

The earliest studies on cultured HMEC employed early lactation or postweaning milk [Buehring, 1972; Taylor-Papadimitriou et al., 1977a, 1977b, 1980], which gives the highest yield of epithelial cells, together with many macrophages. The procedure is simple and fast, the major expenditure of time being associated with the collection of the milk samples, which can be treated individually or pooled. If duplicate plates are required, it is advisable to pool the milk samples.

Media used to culture milk cells include a high-serum medium, Milk Mix (MX; see Section 2.1.3), and a lower-serum-containing medium, MM [Stampfer et al., 1980] (see Section 4.6). MX was developed for growth of the differentiated luminal cells found in milk; in this method the milk macrophages act as feeders [Taylor-Papadimitriou et al., 1977a, 1977b, 1980] and do not divide, whereas epithelial cells go through approximately 20 divisions and can be subcultured one or two times [Taylor-Papadimitriou et al., 1977b; Stoker et al., 1982]. MM was developed using HMEC from both nipple aspiration fluids and reduction mammoplasty tissues, and it also supports limited proliferation of milk-derived cells. Because milk provides keratin 19-expressing mature luminal cells, this culture method can be used to immortalize, specifically, these cells using SV40 virus [Chang et al., 1982] or SV40 DNA [Bartek et al., 1990]. Most milk-derived HMEC in the primary cultures have been characterized as belonging to the luminal cell lineage. They express keratins 7, 8, and 18 homogeneously, and 85% of the colonies express keratin 19; some keratin 14 is also expressed [Bartek et al., 1985; Taylor-Papadimitriou et al., 1989]. Additionally, they display the differentiated PEM epitopes [Taylor-Papadimitriou et al., 1989]. Those milk-derived cells that show greatest proliferative activity in culture do not express keratin 19 or PEM and may represent occasional non-luminal cells shed into the milk fluids [Bartek et al., 1985; Chang and Taylor-Papadimitriou, 1983].

Protocol 4.1. Milk Collection for Mammary Epithelial Cell Culture

Reagents and Materials

Sterile

- ❏ UPW
- ❏ Medium: RPMI 1640 (other media can be used, as appropriate)
- ❏ Universal containers

Protocol

(a) Collect milk (2–7 days postpartum) from donors at home or in hospital wards.

(b) Swab the breast with sterile H_2O.

(c) Express the milk manually into a sterile container. Usually 5–20 ml is obtained per individual. Place a maximum of 10 ml in each container.

(d) Dilute individual or pooled milks 1:1 with RPMI 1640 or other medium to facilitate centrifugation.

Protocol 4.2. Primary Culture of Mammary Epithelial Cells from Milk

Reagents and Materials

Sterile

- ❏ Universal containers of diluted milk
- ❏ Wash medium: RPMI 1640 containing 5% FBS
- ❏ Growth medium: MX (see Section 2.1.3.)
- ❏ Petri dishes, 5-cm

Protocol

(a) Spin diluted milk at 600–1000 g for 20 min.

(b) Carefully remove supernatant, leaving some liquid so as not to disturb the pellet.

(c) Wash the pelleted cells two to four times with RPMI containing 5% FBS until supernatant is not turbid, again, leaving some medium to avoid disturbing the pellet.

(d) Resuspend the packed cells in MX growth medium at the rate of 50 μl of packed cells per 6 ml of MX.

(e) Plate cell suspension in MX growth medium at 6 ml per 5-cm dish.

(f) Incubate the dishes at 37°C in 5% CO_2.

(g) Change the medium after 3–5 days and twice weekly thereafter.

(h) Colonies appear around 6–8 days and expand to push off the milk macrophages, which initially act as feeders.

When using the MX medium, it is convenient to use the macrophages that are already present in the milk as feeders; these are gradually lost as the epithelial colonies expand. However, if desired, macrophages can be removed by absorption to glass and, in that case, other feeders must be added. Irradiated or mitomycin-treated 3T6 cells show the best growth-promoting activity [Taylor-Papadimitriou et al., 1977a]. A cyclic AMP-elevating agent is crucial for growth of milk cells. However, analogs of cyclic AMP can be employed to replace the cholera toxin normally used [Taylor-Papadimitriou et al., 1980] if 3T6 cells are serving as feeders, but this is not possible with macrophage feeders, which are killed by the analogs.

Protocol 4.3. Subculture of Milk Cells

Reagents and Materials

Sterile

- ❏ TEGPED (see Section 2.1.2)
- ❏ Wash medium: RPMI 1640 containing 10% FBS
- ❏ Growth medium: MX (see Section 2.1.3)
- ❏ Petri dishes, 5-cm

Protocol

(a) Incubate colonies or resulting monolayer in TEGPED (1.5 ml per 5-cm plate) at 37°C for 5–15 min, depending on the age of the culture, to produce a single-cell suspension.

(b) Wash free of enzyme mixture by centrifuging the cells at 500 g, resuspending the pellet in 10 ml of RPMI 1640 containing 10% FBS, and recentrifuging.

(c) Resuspend the pellet in the same volume of MX medium as the original culture before trypsinization, i.e., in 6 ml for the cells from one 5-cm dish.

(d) Dilute the cell suspension 1:3 in MX medium.

(e) Replate into three 5-cm dishes.

4. CULTURE OF MAMMARY EPITHELIAL CELLS FROM REDUCTION MAMMOPLASTY

Reduction mammoplasties provide an abundant source of normal and benign HMEC. The large quantity of tissue from each operation, plus the ability to freeze the isolated HMEC, means that cells from the same individual can be used repeatedly for experimentation. Epithelial cells are isolated from the tissue using crude dissection and an enzymatic dissociation technique modified from one originally reported for rat mammary tissue [Hallowes et al., 1977]. Prolonged growth of these cells in culture was first achieved using the serum-containing MM medium [Stampfer et al., 1980; Stampfer 1982; Stampfer, 1985], and later by growth in a serum-free medium, MCDB 170 [Hammond et al., 1984]. Another technique using low-calcium medium can also provide prolonged HMEC growth [Soule and McGrath, 1986].

MM medium supports active HMEC growth for approximately 15–25 population doublings [Stampfer, 1985]. These cultures show a mixed morphology and cell composition, with both basal (keratin 5- and 14-positive, α-actin positive, keratin 19 negative) and luminal (keratin 8-, 18-, and 19-positive, PEM positive) markers initially present [Taylor-Papadimitriou et al., 1989]. As the population becomes nonproliferative, larger, flatter senescence-associated β-galactosidase (SA-β-gal)-positive cells predominate. Expression of the cyclin-dependent kinase inhibitor p16^{INK4a} increases sharply as the cell population approaches this senescence arrest [Brenner et al., 1998]. The mean terminal restriction fragment (TRF) length, a measure of telomere length, is ~6–8 kb in this senescent population.

The cells that initially maintain proliferation in MCDB 170 express a more predominantly basal phenotype. These cells also cease most growth after 15–25 population doublings and gradually become large, flatter, SA-β-gal(+), with increased levels of p16 and a mean TRF of ~6–8 kb [Stampfer, 1985; Taylor-Papadimitriou et al., 1989; Brenner et al., 1998]. However, in MCDB 170, a small subpopulation of actively proliferating cobblestone-appearing cells eventually appears. These cells no longer express p16 and show specific methylation of the p16 promoter [Brenner et al., 1998]. We have called this process associated with p16 downregulation "selection" and the p16(−) cells "postselection" HMEC [Hammond et al., 1984]. Depending on the individual specimen, postselection cells may proliferate for an additional 30–70 population doublings. The population gradually acquires a more luminal phenotype (keratins 8 and 18 and PEM, but no keratin 19), while still retaining some expression of the basal keratins 5 and 14. As this population approaches a second senescence block, cells become larger, flatter SA-β-gal($+$), with a mean TRF that has declined to ~5 kb. It is not currently known whether these postselection p16($-$) cells represent a specific epithelial population in vivo. Postselection HMEC can be generated in very large quantities, assuring a steady supply of finite-lifespan HMEC from standardized batches.

Another common method for generating populations of finite-lifespan HMEC involves using medium in which the calcium concentration has been reduced. Soule and McGrath originally demonstrated that primary cultures of HMEC grown in low (0.06 mM)-calcium medium could remain proliferative for a long time, generating approximately 50 population doublings, possibly because of inhibition of differentiation [Soule and McGrath, 1986]. Cells shed spontaneously into the medium by the primary cultures could be reestablished as secondary cultures that eventually exhibited senescence. The phenotype of these cells has not been defined in detail.

Immortal, nonmalignant cell lines that may retain wild-type p53 and RB function can be obtained from normal reduction mammoplasty-derived HMEC after exposure to chemical carcinogens [Stampfer and Bartley, 1985], the putative breast oncogene ZNF217 [Nonet et al., 2001], and ectopic expression of the catalytic subunit of the human telomerase gene, hTERT [Stampfer et al., 2001]. Growth in the low-calcium medium has also produced immortal lines from an individual subcutaneous mastectomy tissue [Soule et al., 1990]. Immortal transformation is also possible using specific viral oncogenes, e.g., the human papillomavirus E6 and E7 oncogenes [Band, 1998; Shay et al., 1993b; Wazer et al., 1995] and SV40T [Bartek et al., 1991; Shay et al., 1993a], or through loss of p53 function [Gao et al., 1996; Gollahon and Shay, 1996; Shay et al., 1995]. Further transformation of these lines to anchorage and growth factor independence, and tumorigenicity, is possible with the additional exposure to one or two specific oncogenes, e.g., oncogenic *ras* and *erb*B2 [Clark et al., 1988; Pierce et al., 1991; Russo et al., 1993; Ciardiello et al., 1992]. This chapter does not address procedures for HMEC immortalization. The reader is directed to the above references and a recent review [Stampfer and Yaswen, 2000]. Detailed information on the derivation of normal and transformed HMEC in our laboratory can be found on the web site *www.lbl.gov/~mrgs*.

4.1. Tissue Processing

The tissue digestion breaks down the stroma, freeing epithelial organoids, which can then be separated from the digested stroma by filtration. Fibroblasts from the same individual can be obtained from the filtrate. Neither the fibroblasts nor small blood vessel associated-cells pose a serious contamination problem, as they do not proliferate well in MCDB 170 medium, which was developed for the clonal growth of epithelial cells [Hammond et al., 1984].

Protocol 4.4. Processing Reduction Mammoplasty Tissue for Culture

Reagents and Materials

Sterile or Aseptically Prepared

- ❑ Human mammary tissue obtained as discarded material from reduction mammoplasty surgery
- ❑ Tissue mix medium (see Section 2.2.1) supplemented with 10% FBS
- ❑ CPM1 (see Section 2.3.4)
- ❑ Growth medium: Complete MCDB 170 (see Section 2.5)
- ❑ Enzyme solution (see Section 2.2.2)
- ❑ Petri dishes, large, e.g., 15-cm
- ❑ Petri dishes, small, 35-mm
- ❑ Sterile containers (20–30 ml) containing tissue mix medium
- ❑ Conical centrifuge tube (15 or 50 ml)
- ❑ Plastic ampoules, 1-ml capacity, (Nalge Nunc)
- ❑ Scalpels, #11
- ❑ Fine forceps
- ❑ Fine scissors
- ❑ Filter holders with 150-μm and 95-μm gauze filters: filter cloth cut and secured by clips between two metal plate holders as shown in Fig 4.2
- ❑ Container to receive filtrate

Nonsterile

- ❑ Tube rotator

Protocol

(a) Place material in sterile containers containing tissue mix medium supplemented with 10% FBS and transport to the laboratory at 4°C. Reduction mammoplasty tissue can be stored or shipped at 4°C for at least 72 h without significantly affecting subsequent cell viability.

(b) Separate the epithelial areas from the stroma using a combination of sterile scalpel, forceps, and scissors.

(c) Transfer cut pieces of tissue into a large sterile dish (e.g., 15 cm). Epithelial areas appear as white strands embedded in the more yellow stromal matrix. Dissect out these areas, scraping away grossly fatty material.

(d) Lacerate the epithelial tissue using opposing scalpels.

(e) Transfer the minced epithelium-containing tissue into a 15- or 50-ml conical centrifuge tube with the tissue making up no greater than a third of the volume of the tube. Remove fatty material remaining in the dish for disposal in the autoclave.

(f) Bring the tube up to full volume with tissue digestion medium and a final concentration of 10% FBS and 150 U/ml collagenase, 100 U/ml hyaluronidase (20% of tube volume of enzyme stock solution), leaving only a small air space to allow for gentle mixing during rotation.

(g) Place tubes on tube rotator and rotate overnight at 37°C.

(h) Centrifuge the tubes at 600 g for 5 min.

(i) Discard the supernatant fat and medium.

(j) Dilute a small aliquot of the pellet in medium to check on the microscope for degree of digestion. Digestion is complete when microscopic examination shows clumps of cells (organoids) with ductal, alveolar, or ductal-alveolar struc-

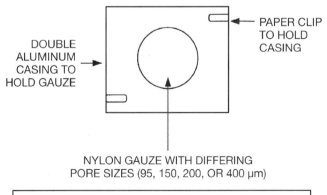

DOUBLE ALUMINUM CASING TO HOLD GAUZE

PAPER CLIP TO HOLD CASING

NYLON GAUZE WITH DIFFERING PORE SIZES (95, 150, 200, OR 400 µm)

The assembled structure is autoclaved and positioned on a beaker in order to allow the digested organoids to pass through.

Fig 4.2. Diagram of filter used for separation of organoids.

tures free from attached stroma. If the tissue is not fully digested:

  i) Resuspend pellet in fresh tissue digestion medium as previously, bringing the tube up to full volume with a final concentration of 10% FBS and enzymes. The concentration of enzymes in the tissue digestion medium can be varied according to how much more digestion is required.
  ii) Reincubate with rotation at 37°C for another 4–12 h.
  iii) Recentrifuge tubes and recheck pellet.
  iv) If digestion is still not complete, repeat above steps for an overnight digestion.

(k) When digestion is complete, centrifuge tubes at 600 g for 5 min, carefully aspirate supernatant, and resuspend pellet in tissue mix medium (approximately 15 ml/50-ml tube, 5 ml/15-ml tube).

(l) Place filter holder on top of a sterile disposable container.

(m) Wet one side of the filter cloth with about 1 ml of tissue mix medium and turn the filter over to the other side.

(n) Transfer the resuspended organoids to the top of the filter cloth a few ml at a time, letting the medium drain into the container.

(o) If there are too many organoids on the filter cloth, the medium will no longer drain through the filter. In that case, either additional filters should be used or the collected organoids should be removed (see below) and the filter reused.

(p) Carefully flip the filter cloth with the collected organoids on top of another clean container with the organoids facing down.

(q) Wash the organoids off the filter with medium. This is the 150-μm organoid pool, which contains mostly ductal structures.

(r) Take the filtrate from the 150-μm gauze filter and repeat the filtering procedure with a 95-μm filter in a holder. The organoids collected from this filter contain mostly smaller ductal and alveolar structures. The filtrate from the second container contains mostly small epithelial clumps, vascular, and stromal cells. This is the final filtrate.

(s) Transfer the pools of 150-μm and 95-μm organoids and the final filtrate to separate 50-ml tubes and centrifuge at 600 g for 5 min.

(t) Aspirate the supernatant. Resuspend the pellets in each tube in CPM1 by adding 1 ml of CPM1 per 0.1 ml of packed cell pellet.

(u) Seed a test dish for each tube by placing 0.1 ml of resuspended material into 35-mm dishes drop by drop distributed over different areas of the dish. Disperse the organoids on the dish by gently knocking the dish sideways to spread out the medium.

(v) Let the dish sit approximately 1 min, then add 1 ml of growth medium to dish.

(w) Incubate at 37°C and check for attachment and sterility the following day.

(x) Aliquot the remainder of the resuspended material into plastic ampoules (1 ml per tube).

(y) Freeze slowly at −1°C/min to −70°C and then transfer to storage in liquid nitrogen.

△ *Safety note.* Wear cryoprotective gloves, a face mask, and a closed lab coat when working with liquid nitrogen. Make sure the room is well ventilated to avoid asphyxiation from evaporated nitrogen.

4.2. Initiation and Maintenance of Primary Cultures in MCDB 170

Protocol 4.5. Primary Culture of Mammary Epithelium from Organoids

Reagents and Materials

Sterile or aseptically prepared

❑ Ampoule containing freshly digested or frozen organoids
❑ Growth medium: MCDB 170 (see Section 2.5) or MM (see Section 4.6)
❑ STE (See Section 2.4)
❑ PBSA

Protocol

(a) Quickly thaw the ampoule containing the frozen organoids in 37°C water in a container with a lid.

△ *Safety note.* An ampoule that has been stored in liquid nitrogen can inspire liquid nitrogen if not properly sealed. The ampoule will then explode violently when warmed. To protect from potential explosion of ampoules, thaw in a covered container, such as a large plastic bucket with a lid, or store in the vapor phase. Wear gloves, a face mask, and a closed lab coat.

(b) Seed 1 ampoule (1 ml) of thawed (or freshly digested) organoids into 2–10 (usually around 6) 25-cm^2 flasks or 6-cm dishes depending on visual estimation of the number of organoids in the ampoule. The thawed organoids are carefully placed, drop by drop, onto the surface of the flask or dish with a 1-ml pipette or Pasteur pipette for an even distribution of organoids. Avoid scratching the vessel surface (the cells tend not to grow past scratched surfaces).

(c) Add 2 ml of growth medium per dish slowly to avoid dislodging the organoids.

(d) Incubate at 37°C in a humidified CO$_2$ incubator (~0.2% for cells in MCDB 170, 5 % for MM). These are the primary cultures.

(e) After 1 day of incubation at 37°C, check that the organoids are attached, and add an additional 2 ml of fresh medium. Cell outgrowth should be visible by 24–48 h after seeding.

(f) Cultures should be fed every 48 h or three times a week. Cells grown in MM type media grow to near confluence within 5–8 days, whereas cells grown in MCDB 170 media may take longer (10–14 days).

(g) If fibroblastic cell growth is observed (particularly from 95-μm organoid pools), remove by differential trypsinization as follows.

　i) When epithelial patches are large, aspirate medium, and wash once with saline-trypsin-EDTA (STE).

　ii) Add 0.5 ml STE per 6-cm dish and leave STE on cells at room temperature for about 1 min, with continued observation under the microscope. Knock the dish gently. When the fibroblasts are observed to detach but the epithelial cells remain adherent, remove the STE.

　iii) For cells growing in the serum-free MCDB 170, all traces of the STE must be removed. It is therefore essential that the flask be washed an additional 2 times with PBSA before refeeding. MM grown cells can be refed with medium without additional washes.

(h) Primary cultures should not be permitted to remain at confluence, or growth potential on subculture will be diminished.

4.3. Subculture of Primary Cultures in MCDB 170

Primary cultures are subcultured when large epithelial patches are present but before they reach confluence. The density of organoid seeding and attachment will influence the time required (approximately 7–14 days) to reach subconfluence. To retain the primary culture and to generate multiple secondary cultures, spaced over time, remove only about 50% of the cells (partial trypsinization).

Protocol 4.6. Serum-Free Subculture of Mammary Epithelial Cells

Reagents and Materials

Sterile

❑ STE (see Section 2.4)
❑ PBSA
❑ Conical centrifuge tubes, 15-ml

Protocol

(a) Aspirate medium.
(b) Wash with 1–2 ml STE.
(c) Add 0.5 ml STE to dish/flask at room temperature. Observe cell detachment under the microscope at room temperature for 1–5 min, with gentle knocking of the dish to promote cell detachment. The trypsinization should be stopped when around 50% of the cells have detached. Early partial trypsinizations usually have rapid cell detachment. For later partial trypsinizations, cells can be placed at 37°C for faster detachment, but this should be carefully monitored, as all the cells may come off quickly.
(d) Add 2 ml of sterile PBSA to dish/flask; repipette to wash flask and transfer this wash to a 15-ml tube.
(e) Repeat with another 2 ml of PBSA, adding this wash to the 15-ml tube.
(f) It is essential to wash the primary flask an additional 2 times with PBSA to eliminate all traces of STE before refeeding and returning to incubator.
(g) Count an aliquot of the cells transferred to the 15-ml tubes above in a hemocytometer.
(h) Note the exact volume in the tubes, then bring the volume

Stampfer, Yaswen, and Taylor-Papadimitriou

of PBSA in the tubes up to 15 ml and centrifuge at 600 g for 5 min.

(i) Aspirate the supernatant and resuspend the cells in fresh complete MCDB 170.

(j) Seed the cells in second passage at a density of $3-5 \times 10^3$ cells/cm^2.

Partial trypsinization can be repeated, producing good growing secondary cultures, approximately 6–10 times, or until cells in the primary culture undergo "selection" (see next section). Cells removed from primary flasks can be stored frozen instead of seeding (see below).

4.4. Further Passage of Cultures in MCDB 170

4.4.1. Preselection Passages

The HMEC grow actively, with a typical epithelial cobblestone appearance for about two passages. Procedures for further subculture and appropriate seeding densities are as described below. At passage 2 or 3, most of the cell population gradually changes morphology, becoming larger, flatter, striated, and characterized by irregular edges. Fibronectin is expressed in a fibrillar pattern. These cells eventually cease proliferation. When this senescence arrest appears, maintain the cell cultures with regular feeding but without subculture. Within 1–3 wk, small pockets of actively growing cells with the typical epithelial morphology will appear. The process has been termed "selection" because only a few cells proliferate at this point and are thus selected from the background of senescing cells. The postselection cells retain the epithelial pattern of punctate, cell-associated fibronectin and express increasing levels of keratins 8 and 18 and PEM as well as keratins 5 and 14. They show no expression of p16.

An alternate method of obtaining postselection HMEC is to perform repeated (5–10) partial trypsinizations of the primary culture. The organoids will eventually no longer show widespread vigorous regrowth, rather, flat, nondividing cells predominate. Eventually, most organoid areas will give rise to postselection cells (which are more refractile looking and have active proliferation).

4.4.2. Postselection Passages

Within one or two passages, the population will consist uniformly of the morphologically epithelium-like postselection

HMEC, with 18- to 24-h doubling times. Depending on the individual specimen donor, growth will continue for an additional 20–70 population doublings after selection. At a second senescence block, cells will become larger and more vacuolated but will retain the epithelial cobblestone, smooth-edged appearance and punctate, cell-associated fibronectin pattern. When these indications of senescence appear, cell cultures are no longer used for general experimental purposes.

Some, but not all, specimen donors require the presence of a cAMP stimulator to maintain the actively growing epithelial-appearing population during selection. Isoproterenol, 1×10^{-5} M, is therefore routinely added to half of all secondary cultures for each new specimen donor. If growth during selection is enhanced in the presence of isoproterenol, it is maintained in the culture medium thereafter.

Complete MCDB 170 will support clonal growth of postselection HMEC with cloning efficiencies of 10–50%.

Protocol 4.7. Serial Subculture of Mammary Epithelium in MCDB 170

Reagents and Materials

Sterile

- ❑ STE (see Section 2.4)
- ❑ PBSA
- ❑ Growth medium: complete MCDB 170 (see Section 2.5)
- ❑ Conical centrifuge tubes, 15- or 50-ml

Protocol

(a) Aspirate medium.

(b) Wash once with STE: ~3 ml/10-cm Petri dish or 75-cm² flask; 2 ml/6-cm dish or 25-cm² flask; 1 ml/3.5-cm dish.

(c) Add just enough STE to barely cover the cells (it is important to minimize amount of STE): 1–1.2 ml/10-cm Petri dish or 75-cm² flask; ≤0.4 ml/6-cm dish or 25-cm² flask; ≤0.2 ml/3.5-cm dish.

(d) Incubate cells in 37°C incubator for 2–5 min. This time is not fixed, as cells vary. Do not leave at room temperature. The cells will not come off at room temperature.

(e) Remove cells from incubator after 2–3 min to check under microscope whether they have all "rounded up." Do not leave the STE on longer than necessary to remove most of the cells. Tap dish lightly against hand or desk if necessary to knock cells loose. Continue incubation at 37°C if cells are still attached.

(f) When most of the cells have loosened add PBSA to culture vessels. Do not wait for all the cells to come off, particularly if only small patches remain. Repipette the PBSA in the flask/dish to break up clumps, and then transfer this to 15- or 50-ml tubes (use the larger volume tube for 10-cm dishes, 75-cm^2 flasks, or more than two 6-cm dishes).

(g) Wash the flask/dish with about the same amount of PBSA one or two times and transfer to tube. The final volume in the tube should be about 6–12 ml/10-cm, 75-cm^2; 3–6 ml/6-cm, 25-cm^2; 1–3 ml/3.5 cm, depending on the cell density of the culture.

(h) Repipette to mix and to break up any cell clumps.

(i) Take a small amount in the tip of a plugged Pasteur pipette to count in a hemocytometer.

(j) Bring up volume in 15-ml or 50-ml tube to maximal with PBSA to dilute STE, and centrifuge at 600 g for 5 min.

(k) Carefully aspirate the PBS/STE away from the cell pellet.

(l) Add growth medium and dilute the cells to the desired cell concentration. Pipette a few times with 1-ml pipette to get rid of cell clumps.

(m) Seed dishes at 3–5 $\times$ 10^3 cells/cm^2 and gently swirl medium to ensure even distribution of cells in the culture vessel.

(n) Place in incubator.

4.5. Freezing of Human Mammary Epithelial Cells

Protocol 4.8. Cryopreservation of Mammary Epithelial Cells

Reagents and Materials

Sterile

❑ STE (see Section 2.4)
❑ PBSA
❑ Growth medium: Complete MCDB 170 (see Section 2.5)
❑ Conical centrifuge tubes, 15- or 50-ml
❑ CPM2 (see Section 2.3.5)

Protocol

(a) Feed cells the day before freezing.

(b) Remove the monolayer populations of HMEC in primary culture or higher passages as previously described, and count an aliquot in the hemocytometer.

(c) Centrifuge the removed cells at 600 g for 5 min.

(d) Aspirate the supernatant fraction and add CPM2 to yield a cell concentration of 1×10^6 cells/ml. Keep the cells resuspended in preservative medium on ice.

(e) Label Nunc ampoules appropriately and add 0.5–1.0 ml of resuspended cells to each ampoule.

(f) Slowly freeze the ampoules (approximately 1°C/min) to −70°C and then transfer to storage in a liquid nitrogen freezer. Do not store ampoules for more than a few days at −70°C.

Δ**Safety note.** Wear cryoprotective gloves, a face mask, and a closed lab coat when working with liquid nitrogen. Make sure the room is well ventilated to avoid asphyxiation from evaporated nitrogen.

(g) Growth is renewed by quick thawing of the frozen ampoule in water at 37°C in a covered bucket.

Δ**Safety note.** An ampoule that has been stored in liquid nitrogen can inspire liquid nitrogen if not properly sealed. The ampoule will then explode violently when warmed. To protect from potential explosion of ampoules, thaw in a covered container, such as a large plastic bucket with a lid, or store in the vapor phase. Wear gloves, a face mask, and a closed lab coat.

(h) Add the contents of 1 ampoule of 0.5 ml to a 15-ml tube containing 12 ml of the appropriate medium for seeding.

(i) Repipette gently to break up cell clumps and seed. Cells can be seeded directly into three 6-cm dishes or may first be pelleted at 600 g for 5 min in PBSA to remove the serum present in the preservative medium.

4.6. Culture of Human Mammary Epithelial Cells in Other Media

The organoids produced by digesting reduction mammoplasty tissue can be cultured in other media, such as the low-calcium medium of Soule and McGrath [1986] or variations of the medium MM, which contains conditioned medium from other cell types [Stampfer, 1982, 1985].

Stampfer, Yaswen, and Taylor-Papadimitriou

Detailed protocols for growth of HMEC in MM and making MM medium can be found on the web site *www.lbl.gov/~mrgs*. Most procedures for subculture and seeding densities are as described above for MCDB 170, except that the presence of serum in the MM allows cells removed by trypsin to be resuspended directly on MM and seeded without pelleting. It is again important to subculture the cells as soon as they reach confluence. Confluent populations of cells grown in MM can produce large quantities of lactic acid.

Cells grown in MM have a tendency to grow in multilayers when confluent, producing domes and ridges. Addition of cAMP stimulators enhances this tendency. Cholera toxin is therefore routinely omitted from MM of primary reduction mammoplasty cultures to reduce multilayering in the organoid outgrowths. MM that includes the cholera toxin is therefore used only after subculture to second passage. For freezing down cells grown in MM, use CPM1.

5. IDENTIFICATION AND MANIPULATION OF CELLS

5.1. Characterization of Cells as Epithelial

Cell phenotypes can be characterized effectively by immuno-histochemistry; Table 4.1 lists some of the antibodies that can be used. Positive staining with antibodies directed to cytokeratins identifies the cells in culture as epithelial. Fibroblasts are not present in milk and do not proliferate well in MCDB 170 medium; lack of reaction with anti-cytokeratin antibodies together with a positive reaction with an antibody to vimentin will demonstrate their presence. Also, intense fibrillar staining for cell-associated fibronectin is an easy way to detect even a single fibroblast cell in an MCDB 170-cultured population. In the epithelial cells, fibronectin is expressed in a punctate pattern [Stampfer et al., 1981]. Positive staining for PEM can also identify epithelial cells with luminal characteristics.

5.2. Distinguishing Epithelial Cell Phenotypes

As indicated above, the strong and homogeneous expression of simple epithelial keratins 8 and 18 is characteristic of the luminal epithelial cell phenotype [for review, see Taylor-Papadimitriou and Lane, 1987]. In the mammary gland, the expression of keratin 19 appears to be associated with the most mature or differentiated luminal cell in the TDLU that will secrete milk under the correct stimulus. Keratin 19 expression is found in the majority of cells cultured in MX, whether the epithelial cells derive from milk or reduction mammoplasty. Luminal cells that do not express keratin 19 have a higher proliferative potential and form large colonies in milk cell cultures [Bartek et al., 1985]. The luminal epithelial cells also express a mucin, PEM [Burchell et al., 1983; Gendler et al., 1988], that can be detected by a large number of antibodies (see Table 4.1 and Burchell and Taylor-Papadimitriou [1989] for review).

Markers for basal epithelial cells in culture include smooth muscle α-actin [Skalli et al., 1986; Gugliotta et al., 1988], the common acute lymphoblastic leukemic antigen (CALLA) [Gusterson et al., 1986], and vimentin, as well as keratins 5, 7, and 14. Definite identification of myoepithelial cells in a basal cell population would require demonstration of the presence of contractile myofibrils, or oxytocin receptors, characterizations not generally performed on cultured HMEC. Postselection cells are characterized by the absence of p16 expression [Brenner et al., 1998]. They maintain some expression of keratins 5, 7, and 14 while acquiring increasing expression of keratins 8 and 18 and PEM [Taylor-Papadimitriou et al., 1989].

5.3. Maturation and Differentiation Stages

In the culture conditions described here, none of the cultured cells have been shown to produce the functionally differentiated properties of casein or α-lactalbumin expression. Similarly, expression of a secretory component has not been detected [Bartek et al., 1990]. The expression of PEM can be considered to be a functional attribute of luminal epithelial cells, and high expression is associated with a reduced growth potential [Chang and Taylor-Papadimitriou, 1983]. Keratin 19-expressing cells most likely represent the most mature, terminally differentiated cells in the population, as they show the least proliferative potential in culture.

5.4. Cell Cycle Synchronization of Cultured HMEC

Achieving cell cycle synchrony can be useful for a variety of studies on control of cell proliferation. HMEC are easy to arrest in a G_0 state, and then release synchronously into G_1, because of their complete dependence on EGF receptor signal transduction for growth. More detailed information about this subject can be found in Stampfer et al., [1993]. Briefly, cells can be arrested in

G_0 by removal of EGF from the growth medium, coupled with the addition of 1–5 μg/ml of an anti-EGF receptor antibody, MAb225. MAb225 is isolated from a hybridoma cell line (ATCC Cat no. HB-8508), and the antibody can be obtained through standard hybridoma culture and antibody purification methods. MAb225 is added because cultured HMEC can secrete sufficient amounts of EGF receptor stimulating molecules, such as TGF-α, to sustain their own growth in the absence of exogenously added EGF. After 48 h, almost all cells are quiescent, with no DNA synthesis. The cultures can then be washed twice in PBSA and refed with complete medium containing 25 ng/ml EGF. A synchronous entry into S-phase occurs in ~12–15 h.

5.5. Introduction of Exogenous DNA

5.5.1. Transfection

We have successfully used a variety of methods (electroporation, calcium phosphate coprecipitation, lipofection) for both transient and stable transfection of exogenous DNA into HMEC. By far the easiest and most straightforward method employs cationic lipids. We use Cytofectin GSV. Transfection has been most effective into immortal HMEC and some postselection specimens.

Protocol 4.9. Transfection of Human Mammary Epithelial Cells

Reagents and Materials

Sterile or Aseptically Prepared

- ❏ Plasmid for transfection
- ❏ Growth medium: MCDB 170 (see Section 2.5)
- ❏ Cytofectin GSV stock, 2 μg/l
- ❏ Polystyrene tubes, 10 ml

Protocol

(a) Seed cells at 3.0 $\times$ 10^5 cells per 3.5-cm dish 24 h before transfection.
(b) Dilute all plasmids to 0.5 μg/μl in sterile growth medium.
(c) Dilute Cytofectin GSV to 100 ng/μl in sterile polystyrene tubes.
(d) Mix equal volumes of plasmid and Cytofectin GSV solutions together by pipetting up and down.

(e) Allow complexes to form for 10–15 min.
(f) Dilute 1:10 with growth medium.
(g) Remove medium from dishes.
(h) Add 1.0 ml of the plasmid-Cytofectin complex mixture to each plate of cells and gently rock dishes back and forth and side to side to distribute evenly.
(i) Incubate 5 h.
(j) Remove existing medium containing the plasmid-Cytofectin complex mixture, and add 2.0 ml of fresh medium. Incubate 48 h before harvesting or starting drug selection.

5.5.2. Gene transduction using retroviruses

High-efficiency transfer of genes of interest into actively replicating HMEC can be achieved using recombinant retroviruses. This method is most useful for the finite-lifespan HMEC with limited replicative potential. A variety of retroviral vectors are available that incorporate convenient cloning sites for genes of interest and selectable markers for selection of virus-expressing cells [Miller and Rosman, 1989; Morgenstern and Land, 1990]. Transcription of the inserted genes is often driven by the retroviral LTR, which we have shown has strong promoting activity in cultured HMEC. We commonly generate replication-defective retroviruses by transient cotransfection of recombinant retroviral plasmids along with a plasmid encoding packaging functions [Finer et al., 1994] into the highly transfectable 293 cell line. This packaging system allows high-titer amphotropic retrovirus to be produced without the need to generate stable producer clones. This is advantageous both in terms of time required and, more importantly, because it allows genes with possible growth-inhibiting or toxic activities to be packaged. Retrovirus-containing supernatants are harvested from transiently transfected cultures of producer cells and then applied to HMEC cultures in the presence of Polybrene, a polycation that promotes virus binding to cell surfaces. The titer of each virus stock is estimated by assaying reverse transcriptase activity and then comparing this activity to that of a β-galactosidase-encoding virus of known titer. Using this system, we have consistently obtained infection rates of greater than 60% during a single round of infection in target HMEC. Even greater infectivity can be obtained by using multiple rounds of infection.

5.6. Three-Dimensional Culture Assays

HMEC in vivo form a complex architectural arrangement that includes cell-cell and cell-matrix interactions. Additionally, the

Stampfer, Yaswen, and Taylor-Papadimitriou

polarized nature of HMEC in vivo may significantly affect their biological properties and differentiated capabilities. Culture of HMEC on plastic substrates does not support cell polarization and thus may fail to give an accurate model of in vivo behavior. Efforts to remedy this shortcoming have been attempted in a number of laboratories, using a variety of coculture and extracellular matrix extracts to model in vivo cellular microenvironments [Weaver et al., 1997]. Notably, HMEC from reduction mammoplasties and carcinomas behave very differently when cultured in the presence of reconstituted basement membrane; the former ceasing growth and forming polarized structures and the latter continuing to proliferate in a disorganized manner [Petersen et al., 1992]. We have used growth of HMEC on Matrigel, an extracellular matrix material obtained from the Engelbreth-Holm-Swarm transplantable tumor, to produce three-dimensional epithelial cell structures in culture with polarized secretion [Stampfer and Yaswen, 1992; unpublished data]. The procedure we have used for growth on Matrigel is given below [Petersen et al., 1992].

Protocol 4.10. Growth of Human Mammary Epithelial Cells in Matrigel

Reagents and Materials

❑ Reagents for subculture (see Protocols 4.6 and 4.7)
❑ PolyHEMA-coated dishes: Prepare PolyHEMA-coated dishes or wells in advance. Coat each dish or well with PolyHEMA (Sigma) dissolved at 12 mg/ml (0.8 mg/cm^2 final concentration) in 95% ethanol and air dry at 37°C overnight

Protocol

(a) Trypsinize adherent cultures, centrifuge, and count cells according to standard protocol (see Protocols 4.6 and 4.7).
(b) Aliquot cells into separate 15-ml tubes, centrifuge, aspirate supernatants, and place cell pellets on ice.
(c) Resuspend cell pellets in ice-cold Matrigel at 1.0×10^6 cells/ 1.2 ml Matrigel/35-mm dish using a cold pipette.
(d) Distribute cells in Matrigel to PolyHEMA-coated dishes or plates.
(e) Incubate 1 h at 37°C to allow the Matrigel to solidify.
(f) Add 2 ml of medium per 35-mm dish *gently* to top of solidified Matrigel.
(g) Change medium every 2–3 days.

REFERENCES

Band V (1998): The role of retinoblastoma and p53 tumor suppressor pathways in human mammary epithelial cell immortalization. Int J Oncol 12: 499–507.

Band V, Zajchowski D, Swisshelm K, Trask D, Kulesa V, Cohen C, Connolly, J, Sager R (1990): Tumor progression in four mammary epithelial cell lines derived from the same patient. Cancer Res 50: 7351–7357.

Bartek J, Durban EM, Hallowes RC, Taylor-Papadimitriou J (1985): A subclass of luminal epithelial cells in the human mammary gland, defined by antibodies to cytokeratins. J Cell Sci 75: 17–33.

Bartek J, Kovarik J, Burchell J, Taylor-Papadimitriou J, Bartkova J, Vojtesek B, Rejthar A, Schneider J, Petrek M, Staskova Z, Millis R (1987): Monoclonal antibodies to breast epithelial antigens in the study of differentiation and malignancy. In Lapis K, Eckhardt S (eds): "Molecular Biology and Differentiation of Cancer Cells," Vol. 2. Basel: Karger; Budapest: Akademiai Kiado, pp 123–130.

Bartek J, Kovarik J, Vojtesek B, Bartkova 1, Staskova Z, Rejthar A, Lauerova L (1989): Subclassification of human tumours by monoclonal antibodies to keratins. In Abelev GI (ed): "Monoclonal Antibodies to Tumour Associated Antigens and Their Clinical Application." Budapest: Akademai Kiado.

Bartek J, Bartkova 1, Lanai E-N, Brezina V. Taylor-Papadimitriou J (1990): Selective immortalisation of a phenotypically distinct epithelial cell type by microinjection of SV4O DNA into cultured human milk cells. Int J Cancer 45:1105–1112.

Bartek, J., Bartkova, J., Kyprianou, N., Lalani, E.-N., Staskova, Z., Shearer, M., Chang, S. and Taylor-Papadimitriou, J. (1991): Efficient immortalization of luminal epithelial cells from human mammary gland by introduction of simian virus 40 large tumor antigen with a recombinant retrovirus. Proc Natl Acad Sci USA 88: 3520–3524.

Brenner AJ, Stampfer MR, Aldaz CM (1998): Increased p16^{INK4a} expression with onset of senescence of human mammary epithelial cells and extended growth capacity with inactivation. Oncogene 17: 199–205.

Buehring GC (1972): Culture of human mammary epithelial cells: Keeping abreast of a new method. J Natl Cancer Inst 49: 1433–1434.

Burchell J, Taylor-Papadimitriou J (1989): Antibodies to human milk fat globule molecules. Cancer Invest 17: 53–61.

Burchell J, Durbin H, Taylor-Papadimitriou J (1983): Complexity of expression of antigenic determinants recognised by monoclonal antibodies HMFG- 1 and HMFG-2, in normal and malignant human mammary epithelial cells. J Immunol 131: 508–513.

Burchell J, Gendler S, Taylor-Papadimitriou J, Girling A, Lewis A, Millis R, Lamport D (1987): Development and characterization of breast cancer reactive monoclonal antibodies directed to the core protein of the human milk mucin. Cancer Res 47: 5476–5482.

Chang SE, Taylor-Papadimitriou J (1983): Modulation of phenotype in cultures of human milk epithelial cells and its relation to the expression of a membrane antigen. Cell Differ 12: 143–154.

Chang SE, Keen J, Lane EB, Taylor-Papadimitriou J (1982): Establishment and characterisation of SV4O-transformed human breast epithelial cell lines. Cancer Res 42: 2040–2053.

Ciardiello F, Gottardis M, Basolo F, Pepe S, Normanno N, Bianco AR, Dickson RB, Salomon DS (1992): Additive effects of c-*erb*B-2, c-Ha-*ras*, and transforming growth factor α genes on the in vitro transformation of human mammary epithelial cells. Mol Carcinogenesis 6: 43–52.

Clark R, Stampfer MR, Milley R, O'Rourke E, Walen KH, Kriegler M, Kopplin J, McCormick F (1988): Transformation of human mammary epithelial cells by oncogenic retroviruses. Cancer Res 48: 4689–4694.

Dairkee SH, Blayney CM, Asarnow D, Smith HS, Hackett AJ (1985): Monoclonal antibody that defines human myoepithelium. Proc Nail Acad Sci USA 82: 7409–7413.

Dairkee SH, Paulo EC, Traquina P, Moore DH, Ljung B-M, Smith, H (1997): Partial enzymatic degradation of stroma allows enrichment and expansion of primary breast tumor cells. Cancer Res 57: 1590–1596.

Dulbecco R, Allen RA, Bologna M, Bowman M, (1986): Marker evolution during development of the rat mammary gland: Stem cells identified by markers and the role of myoepithelial cells. Cancer Res 46: 2449–2456.

Ethier SP (1996): Human breast cancer cell lines as models of growth regulation and disease progression. J Mamm Gland Biol Neopl 1: 111–121.

Finer MH, Dull TJ, Qin L, Farson D, Roberts MR (1994): *kat*: A high-efficiency retroviral transduction system for primary human T lymphocytes. Blood 83: 43–50.

Gao Q, Hauser SH, Liu X.-L, Wazer DE, Madoc-Jones H, Band V (1996): Mutant p53-induced immortalization of primary human mammary epithelial cells. Cancer Res 56: 3129–3133.

Gazdar AF, Kurvari V, Virmani A, Gollahon L, Sakaguchi M, Westerfield M, Kodagoda D, Stasny V, Cunningham HT, Wistuba II, Tomlinson G, Tonk T, Ashfaq R, Leitch AM, Minna JD, and Shay JW (1998): Characterization of paired tumor and non-tumor cell lines established from patients with breast cancer. Int J Cancer 78:766–774.

Gendler SJ, Taylor-Papadimitriou J, Duhig T, Rothbard J, Burchell J (1988): A highly immunogenic region of a human polymorphic epithelial mucin expressed by carcinomas is made up of tandem repeats. J Biol Chem 263: 2820–2823.

Gollahon LS, Shay J (1996): Immortalization of human mammary epithelial cells transfected with mutant p53 (273[his]). Oncogene 12: 715–725.

Gugliotta F, Sapino A, Macri L, Skalli O, Gabbiani G, Bussolati G (1988): Specific demonstration of myoepithelial cells by anti-alpha smooth muscle actin antibody. J Histochem Cytochem 36: 659–663.

Gusterson BA, Monaghan P, Mahendran R, Ellis 1, O'Hare MJ (1986): Identification of myoepithelial cells in human and rat breasts by anti-common acute lymphoblastic leukemia antigen antibody A12. J Natl Cancer Inst 77: 343–349.

Hallowes RC, Rudland PS, Hawkins RA, et al. (1977): Comparison of the effects of hormones on DNA synthesis in cell cultures of non-neoplastic and neoplastic mammary epithelium from rats. Cancer Res 37: 2492–2504.

Hammond SL, Ham RG, Stampfer MR (1984): Serum-free growth of human mammary epithelial cells: Rapid clonal growth in defined medium and extended serial passage with pituitary extract. Proc Natl Acad Sci USA 81: 5435–5439.

Keen J, Chang SE, Taylor-Papadimitriou J (1984): Monoclonal antibodies that distinguish between human cellular and plasma fibronectin. Mot Biol Med 2: 15–27.

Lane EB (1982): Monoclonal antibodies provide specific intramolecular markers for the study of epithelial tonofilament organization. J Cell Biol 92: 665–673.

Lauerova L, Kovarik J, Bartek 1, Rejthar A, Vojtesek B (1988): Novel monoclonal antibodies defining epitopes of human cytokeratin 18 molecule. Hybridoma 7: 495–504.

Li Z, Bustos V, Miner J, Paulo E, Meng ZH, Zlotnikov G, Ljung B-M, Dairkee SH (1998): Propagation of genetically altered tumor cells derived from fine-needle aspirates of primary breast carcinoma. Cancer Res 58: 5271–5274.

Miller AD, Rosman GJ (1989): Improved retroviral vectors for gene transfer and expression. Biotechniques 7: 980–990.

Morgenstern JP, Land, H (1990): Advanced mammalian gene transfer: high titre retroviral vectors with multiple drug selection markers and a complementary helper-free packaging cell line. Nucl Acids Res 18: 3587–3596.

Nonet GH, Stampfer MR, Chin K, Gray JW, Collins CC, and Yaswen P (2001): The *ZNF217* gene amplified in breast cancers promotes immortalization of human mammary epithelial cells. Cancer Res, 61:1250–1254.

Osborn M, Debus E, Weber K (1984): Monoclonal antibodies specific for vimentin. Eur J Cell Biol 34: 137–143.

Petersen O, Ronnov-Jessen L, Howlett A, Bissell M (1992): Interaction with basement membrane serves to rapidly distinguish growth and differentiation patterns of normal and malignant human breast epithelial cells. Proc Natl Acad Sci USA 89: 9064–9068.

Pierce JH, Arnstein P, DiMarco E, Artrip J, Kraus MH, Lonardo F, DiFiore PP, Aaronson SA (1991): Oncogenic potential of *erb*B-2 in human mammary epithelial cells. Oncogene 6: 1189–1194.

Ramaekers FBS, Huysmans A, Schaart G, Moesker O, Vooijs P (1987): Tissue distribution of keratin 7 as monitored by a monoclonal antibody. Exp Cell Res 170: 235–249.

Russo J, Calaf G, Russo IH (1993): A critical approach to the malignant transformation of human breast epithelial cells. CRC Crit Rev Oncogenesis 4: 403–417.

Shay JW, Van Der Haegen BA, Ying Y, Wright WE (1993a): The frequency of immortalization of human fibroblasts and mammary epithelial cells transfected with SV40 Large T-antigen. Exp Cell Res 209: 45–52.

Shay JW, Wright WE, Brasiskyte D. Van Der Haegen B. (1993b): E6 of human papillomavirus type 16 can overcome the M1 stage of immortalization in human mammary epithelial cells but not in human fibroblasts. Oncogene 8: 1407–1413.

Shay JW, Tomlinson G, Piatyszek MA, Gollahon LS (1995): Spontaneous in vitro immortalization of breast epithelial cells from a patient with Li-Fraumeni syndrome. Mol Cell Biol 15: 425–432.

Skalli D, Ropraz P, Trzeciak A, Benzonana O, Gillesen D, Gabbiani G (1986): A monoclonal antibody against α-smooth muscle actin: A new probe for smooth muscle differentiation. J Cell Biol 103: 2787–2796.

Soule HD, McGrath CM (1986): A simplified method for passage and long-term growth of human mammary epithelial cells. In Vitro Cell Dev Biol 22: 6–12.

Soule HD, Maloney TM, Wolman SR, Peterson WD, Brenz R, McGrath CM, Russo J, Pauley RJ, Jones RF, Brooks SC (1990): Isolation and characterization of a spontaneously immortalized human breast epithelial cell line, MCF-10. Cancer Res 50: 6075–6086.

Stampfer MR, Hallowes R, Hackett AJ (1980): Growth of normal human mammary epithelial cells in culture. In Vitro 16: 415–425.

Stampfer MR, Vlodavsky I, Smith HS, Ford R, Becker FF, Riggs J (1981): Fibronectin production by human mammary cells. J Natl Cancer Inst 67: 253–261.

Stampfer MR (1982): Cholera toxin stimulation of human mammary epithelial cells in culture. In Vitro 18: 531–537.

Stampfer MR (1985): Isolation and growth of human mammary epithelial cells. J Tissue Cult Methods 9: 107–116.

Stampfer MR, Bartley JC (1985): Induction of transformation and continuous cell lines from normal human mammary epithelial cells after exposure to benzo(*a*)pyrene. Proc Natl Acad Sci USA 82: 2394–2398.

Stampfer MR, Pan CH, Hosoda J, Bartholomew J, Mendelsohn J, Yaswen P (1993): Blockage of EGF receptor signal transduction causes reversible arrest of normal and transformed human mammary epithelial cells with synchronous reentry into the cell cycle. Exp Cell Res 208: 175–188.

Stampfer MR, Yaswen P (1992): Factors influencing growth and differentiation of normal and transformed human mammary epithelial cells in cultures. In Milo GE, Castro BC, Shuler CF (eds): "Transformation of Human Epithelial Cells: Molecular and Oncogenetic Mechanisms." Boca Raton, FL, CRC Press, pp 117–140.

Stampfer MR., Bodnar A, Garbe J, Wong M, Pan A, Villeponteau B, Yaswen, P (1997): Gradual phenotypic conversion associated with immortalization of cultured human mammary epithelial cells. Mol Biol Cell 8: 2391–2405.

Stampfer MR, Yaswen P (2000): Culture models of human mammary epithelial cell transformation. J Mamm Gland Biol Neopl, 5:365–378.

Stampfer MR, Garbe J, Levine G, Lichtsteiner S, Vasserot AP, and Yaswen P (2001): hTERT expression can induce resistance to TGFβ growth inhibition in p16^{INK4A}($-$) human mammary epithelial cells, Proc Natl Acad Sci USA, 98:4498–4503.

Stoker M, Perryman M, Eeles R (1982): Clonal analysis of morphological phenotype in cultured mammary epithelial cells from human milk. Proc R Soc Lond B 215: 231–240.

Taylor-Papadimitriou J, Lane EB (1987): Keratin expression in the mammary gland. In Neville MC, Daniel CW (eds): "The Mammary Gland." New York: Plenum Publishing, pp 181–215.

Taylor-Papadimitriou J, Shearer M, Stoker MGP (1977a): Growth requirements of human mammary epithelial cells in culture. Int J Cancer 20: 903–908.

Taylor-Papadimitriou J, Shearer M, Tilly R (1977b): Some properties of cells cultured from early lactation human milk. J Natl Cancer Inst 58: 1563–1571.

Taylor-Papadimitriou J, Purkis P, Fentiman IS (1980): Cholera toxin and analogues of cyclic AMP stimulate the growth of cultured mammary epithelial cells. J Cell Physiol 102: 317–321.

Taylor-Papadimitriou J, Burchell J, Hurst J (1981): Production of fibronectin by normal and malignant human mammary epithelial cells. Cancer Res 41: 2491–2500.

Taylor-Papadimitriou J, Stampfer M, Bartek 1, Lewis A, Boshell M, Lane EB, Leigh IM (1989): Keratin expression in human mammary epithelial cells cultured from normal and malignant tissue: Relation to in vivo phenotypes and influence of medium. J Cell Sci 94: 403–413.

Van Muijen GNP, Warnaar SO, Ponec M (1987): Differentiation-related changes of cytokeratin expression in cultured keratinocytes and in fetal, newborn and adult epidermis. Exp Cell Res 171: 331–345.

Wazer DE, Liu X-L, Chu Q, Gao Q, Band V (1995): Immortalization of distinct human mammary epithelial cell types by human papilloma virus 16 E6 or E7. Proc Natl Acad Sci USA 92: 3687–3691.

Weaver VM, Fischer AH, Peterson OW, Bissell MJ (1997): The importance of the microenvironment in breast cancer progression: Recapitulation of mammary tumorigenesis using a unique human mammary epithelial cell model and a three-dimensional culture assay. Biochem Cell Biol 74: 833–851.

APPENDIX A: STOCK SOLUTIONS FOR MCDB 170

Preparation of Basal MCDB 170

Basal MCDB 170 medium can be purchased from Clonetics/BioWhittaker or made from stock solutions according to the following instructions. See table in this Appendix for information about stocks.

To make 1 liter of medium:

(i) Dissolve 7.149 g of HEPES (free acid) in 600 ml of UPW.

(ii) Add 1.0 ml of stock A (3.3 mM phenol red).

(iii) Adjust pH near 7.0 (yellowish orange) with stock B (4 N NaOH). This will require approximately 3.0 ml; do not overshoot 7.4 or medium will become hypertonic.

(iv) Add 10 ml each of stocks C (100× amino acids), D (100× vitamins), E (0.2 M glutamine), F (0.1 M Na pyruvate), G (7 mM cysteine), H (alanine, aspartate, glutamate, and glycine, all 10 mM), and I (bases, lipoic acid, and *myo*-inositol). (see Appendix B.)

(v) Add as solids:

Glucose	1.441 g
KCl	0.1864 g
NaCl	7.014 g
KH_2PO_4	0.06805 g

Stir until dissolved.

(vi) Adjust the volume to approximately 950 ml with UPW.

(vii) Add enough stock B to adjust the pH precisely to 7.40.

(viii) Adjust the volume to 967 ml. The osmolality should be 300 ± 5 mOsm/kg.

(ix) Store frozen at −20°C until use. The medium can be kept for up to 6 months frozen without loss of growth-promoting ability.

Just before use, add the following with continued stirring:

stock J	5 ml
stocks K_1 and K_2	5 ml each
stock L	10 ml
stock M	10 ml

(x) Sterilize by membrane filtration (0.22 μm). If stored at 4°C in the dark this medium can be used for 2–3 wk. Do not refreeze the medium after final completion with Stocks J through M or insoluble precipitates will be formed.

Composition of MCDB 170 Stock Solutions

Stock	Components	Source[1]	Molecular Weight	Concentration in Stock	
				g/L	Moles/L
A (1000×)	Phenol Red (sodium salt)	S	376.36	1.242	3.3×10^{-3}
Store indefinitely at room temperature.					
B	Sodium Hydroxide	A	40.01	160.04	4.0
Store indefinitely at room temperature in tightly closed plastic bottle.					
C (100×)	L-Arginine · HCl	S	210.7	6.321	3.0×10^{-2}
	L-Asparagine · H_2O	S	150.1	15.01	1.0×10^{-1}
	Choline chloride	S	139.6	1.396	1.0×10^{-2}
	L-Histidine · HCl · H_2O	S	209.7	2.097	1.0×10^{-2}
	L-Isoleucine (allo-free)	S	131.2	1.312	1.0×10^{-2}
	L-Leucine	S	131.2	3.936	3.0×10^{-2}
	L-Lysine · HCl	S	182.7	3.654	2.0×10^{-2}
	L-Methionine	S	149.2	0.4476	3.0×10^{-3}
	L-Phenylalanine	S	165.2	0.4956	3.0×10^{-3}
	L-Proline	S	115.1	0.5755	5.0×10^{-3}
	L-Serine	S	105.1	3.153	3.0×10^{-2}
	L-Threonine	S	119.1	3.573	3.0×10^{-2}
	L-Tryptophan	S	204.2	0.6126	3.0×10^{-3}
	L-Tyrosine	S	181.2	0.9060	5.0×10^{-3}
	L-Valine	S	117.2	3.516	3.0×10^{-2}
Stock C is prepared by dissolving the constituents in water with vigorous mechanical stirring plus mild heating as needed. Do not boil. It can be stored indefinitely in the dark at −20°C, or, if sterilized, it can be stored at 4°C for up to 2 months. Gentle heating and stirring may be required to redissolve some of its components before use.					
D (100×)	d-Biotin	S	244.3	0.0007329	3.0×10^{-6}
	Folinic acid (Ca^{2+} salt)	S	601.6	0.0006016	1.0×10^{-6}
	Niacinamide	S	122.1	0.6105	5.0×10^{-3}
	Pantothenic acid (hemi-calcium salt)	S	238.3	0.02383	1.0×10^{-4}
	Pyridoxine · HCl	S	205.6	0.006168	3.0×10^{-5}
	Thiamine · HCl	S	337.3	0.03373	1.0×10^{-4}
	Vitamin B_{12}	S	1355.4	0.01355	1.0×10^{-5}
Because of the very small amounts involved, biotin and folinic acid are normally added to Stock D from more concentrated stock solutions. Concentrations of pantothenic acid are expressed in terms of the molar concentration of the vitamin. A formula weight based on one molecule of pantothenic acid plus one half atom of calcium has been used as the molecular weight. Stock D is stored in the dark at −20°C until used.					

Appendix A continues

Composition of MCDB 170 Stock Solutions (continued)

Stock	Components	Source[1]	Molecular Weight	Concentration in Stock	
				g/L	Moles/L
E (100×)	L-Glutamine	S	146.1	29.22	2.0×10^{-1}
Stock E is stored in the dark at −20°C until used.					
F (100×)	Sodium pyruvate	S	110.0	11.0	1×10^{-1}
Stock F is stored in the dark at −20°C until used.					
G (100×)	L-Cysteine · HCl · H$_2$O	S	175.6	1.229	7×10^{-3}
Stock G is usually prepared fresh each media prep because of the lability of cysteine in solution and the extremely narrow optimal range. It can be stored at −20°C in the dark until use, but caution must be taken to ensure that there is no precipitate.					
H (100×)	L-Alanine	S	89.09	0.8909	1.0×10^{-2}
	L-Aspartic acid	S	133.1	1.331	1.0×10^{-2}
	L-Glutamic acid	S	147.1	1.471	1.0×10^{-2}
	Glycine	S	75.07	0.7507	1.0×10^{-2}
Aspartic and glutamic acids are added to slightly less than the final volume of water. One ml per liter of Stock A (phenol red) is added, and Stock B (4 N NaOH) is added with stirring just rapidly enough to keep the solution neutral (orange). When no solids remain and a stable orange color is achieved, alanine and glycine are dissolved and water is added to the final volume. If sterilized, Stock H can be stored in the dark at 4°C until use or it can be stored frozen at −20°C indefinitely.					
I (100×)	Adenine	S	135.1	0.0135	1.0×10^{-4}
	myo-Inositol	S	180.2	1.802	1.0×10^{-2}
	Lipoic acid	S	206.3	0.0002063	1.0×10^{-6}
	Thymidine	S	242.2	0.007266	3.0×10^{-5}
	Putrescine · 2HCl	S	161.1	0.00001611	1.0×10^{-7}
Adenine is dissolved in one-half the final volume with the addition of 0.3 ml of Stock B per 500 ml plus gentle warming. Lipoic acid is added from a more concentrated stock solution prepared by dissolving the solid in a few drops of Stock B followed by dilution with water. Putrescine is also added from a concentrated stock solution. myo-Inositol and thymidine are dissolved in the final solution after it has been adjusted to volume by the addition of water. The solution is left alkaline and is stored in the dark at −20°C until use.					
J (200×)	CaCl$_2$ · 2H$_2$O	A	147.02	58.81	4.0×10^{-1}
Stock J is stored at room temperature sterilized until use and added only just before the medium is to be used. The CaCl$_2$ will precipitate if frozen. When added to the medium it is added slowly dropwise to a vigorously stirred solution.					
K$_1$ (200×)	MgSO$_4$ · 7H$_2$O	A, J	246.38	73.91	3.0×10^{-1}
Stock K$_1$ is stored at room temperature sterilized until use and is added only on final completion of the medium. Do not refreeze the medium after its addition.					
K$_2$ (200×)	FeSO$_4$ · 7H$_2$O	J	278.02	0.2780	1.0×10^{-3}

Appendix A continues

Composition of MCDB 170 Stock Solutions (continued)

Stock	Components	Source[1]	Molecular Weight	Concentration in Stock	
				g/L	Moles/L

One drop of concentrated HCl is added per liter. Solution K_2 is stored sterile at room temperature. It must be discarded if it contains a precipitate or becomes orange-colored. A yellow coloration to the filter used to sterilize the medium may indicate that the solution needs to be remade.

Stock	Components	Source[1]	Molecular Weight	g/L	Moles/L
L (100×)	$CuSO_4 \cdot 5H_2O$	J	249.68	0.00002497	1.0×10^{-7}
	H_2SeO_3	J	128.98	0.0003869	3.0×10^{-6}
	$MnSO_4 \cdot 5H_2O$	J	241.08	0.00001205	5.0×10^{-8}
	$Na_2SiO_3 \cdot 9H_2O$	F	284.2	0.01421	5.0×10^{-5}
	$(NH_4)_6Mo_7O_{24}.4H_2O$	J	1235.89	0.0001236	1.0×10^{-7}
	NH_4VO_3	J	116.99	0.00005850	5.0×10^{-7}
	$NiCl_2 \cdot 6H_2O$	J	237.70	0.0000001189	5.0×10^{-10}
	$SnCl_2 \cdot 2H_2O$	J	225.63	0.0000001128	5.0×10^{-10}
	$ZnSO_4 7H_2O$	J	287.54	0.002875	5.0×10^{-5}

Because of the small amounts involved, Stock L is normally prepared from a series of more concentrated solutions, each containing one of the components at 1.0×10^{-3} M. The stock of stannous chloride is prepared at 1.0×10^4 M in 0.02 N HCl to minimize precipitation on standing. Stock L is stored at room temperature sterilized at an acidic pH (1 drop of concentrated HCl added per liter).

Stock	Components	Source	MW	g/L	mol/L
M (100×)	Riboflavin	S	376.4	0.01129	3.0×10^{-5}

Stock M is stored in the dark at $-20°C$ until use. Small aliquots are made so that the solution is not thawed more than 5×.

Components Added Directly to Medium				Concentration in Final Medium	
				g/L	mol/L
	D-Glucose	B	180.16	1.441	8.0×10^{-3}
	HEPES (free acid)	R	238.30	7.149	3.0×10^{-2}
	KCl	A, J	74.55	0.1864	2.5×10^{-3}
	NaCl	A, J	58.45	7.014	1.2×10^{-1}
	KH_2PO_4	B	136.09	0.06805	5.0×10^{-4}

[1] Sources of chemicals: [A]Alfa Inorganics, Ventron Corp., Danvers, MA (ultrapure grade), [B]Baker Chem. Co., Phillipsburg, NJ (Ultrex), [F]Fisher Scientific, Pittsburgh, PA, [G]GIBCO, Grand Island, NY, [J]Johnson Matthey Co., London, England (obtained through Jarrell Ash Division, Fisher Scientific Co., Waltham, MA), [S]Sigma Chemical Co., St. Louis, MO, [R]Research Organics Inc., Cleveland, OH

APPENDIX B: SOURCES OF MATERIALS

Materials[1]	Supplier
Bovine pituitary extract (BPE)	Hammond Cell Technology or Clonetics
Calcium chloride, dihydrate	Mallinckrodt, VWR
Cholera toxin	Sigma
Collagenase type 1	Sigma
Cytofectin GSV	Glen Research
Dimethyl sulfoxide	J.J. Baker
Dulbecco's modified Eagle's medium (DME) 50% and Ham's F12 50% (H/H)	Life Technologies (GIBCO BRL), Irvine Scientific
EDTA	Sigma
EGTA	Sigma
Epidermal growth factor (EGF)	Collaborative Research, Upstate Biotechnology
β-Estradiol	Sigma
Ethanolamine	Sigma
Ferrous sulfate	J.J. Baker
Fetal bovine (calf) serum	ICN, Life Technologies (GIBCO BRL), Hyclone
Fungizone	Squibb
Glucose	Mallinckrodt, VWR
Glycerol	Mallinckrodt, VWR
Ham's F12	Life Technologies (GIBCO BRL)
HEPES	Life Technologies (GIBCO BRL)
Human serum (HuS) Australian antigen negative)	Outdated serum from blood banks
Hyaluronidase	Sigma
Hydrochloric acid	Mallinckrodt, VWR
Hydrocortisone	Sigma
Insulin	Sigma
Isoproterenol hydrochloride	Sigma
L-Glutamine	Sigma
Magnesium sulfate	Mallinckrodt, VWR
Matrigel	Becton Dickinson
MCDB-170 and stocks	Clonetics/BioWhittaker or UCSF Cell Culture Facility

Appendix B continues

APPENDIX B: SOURCES OF MATERIALS (continued)

Materials[1]	Supplier
Pancreatin	Life Technologies (GIBCO BRL)
Penicillin-streptomycin	Life Technologies (GIBCO BRL)
Petri dishes	VWR, Corning, Nunc, GIBCO
Phenol Red	Sigma
Phosphoethanolamine	Sigma
Poly HEMA	Sigma
Polymyxin B	Life Technologies (GIBCO BRL)
Potassium chloride	Mallinckrodt, VWR
Potassium phosphate, monobasic	Mallinckrodt, VWR
Riboflavin	Sigma
RPMI 1640	Life Technologies (GIBCO BRL)
Sodium chloride	Mallinckrodt, VWR
Sodium phosphate, dibasic heptahydrate	Mallinckrodt, VWR
Sterile universals or 15 to 50-ml centrifuge tubes	VWR, Sterilin, Corning
Transferrin	Sigma
Tris base	Sigma
Trypsin, STE	Life Technologies (GIBCO BRL)
Tube rotator	New Brunswick Scientific

[1]All reagents should be highest purity or "tissue culture" grade.

5

Culture of Human Cervical Epithelial Cells

Margaret A. Stanley

Department of Pathology, University of Cambridge, Tennis Court Road, Cambridge CB2 1QP, UK. mas@mole.bio.cam.ac.uk

I. INTRODUCTION

The physiologic and pathologic conditions that affect the uterine cervix are of considerable contemporary interest. In particular, the recognition of the role of genital human papillomaviruses (HPVs) as the etiologic agent in cervical carcinoma has focused attention on the biology of cervical and vaginal epithelium. This chapter documents the protocols that have proved successful in our laboratory for monolayer and organotypic in vitro growth both of normal and neoplastic epithelium and for HPV-induced immortalization of primary cervical keratinocytes.

I.I. Anatomy and Histology of Uterine Cervix

The cervix is the lower part of the uterus that projects through the anterior wall of the vagina at the vaginal vault. The vagina is connected to the uterine cavity via the endocervical canal, which is continuous with the uterine cavity at the internal os and the vagina at the external os. The anterior and posterior lips of the ectocervix (the vaginal cervix) are covered by a stratified squamous epithelium similar to that of the vagina. The major cell

Margaret A. Stanley

component of this epithelium is the keratinocyte. Histologically this epithelium consists of five cell layers [Fluhmann, 1961]:

(i)   Basal layer of small, cylindrical cells with relatively large nuclei.
(ii) Parabasal layer of polyhedral cells with prominent nuclei and distinct intercellular bridges.
(iii) Intermediate layer of slightly flattened cells with a glycogen-rich cytoplasm and frequent vacuolation.
(iv) A layer of variable thickness with closely packed polyhedral cells with keratohyaline granules.
(v)   Superficial layer of large, flattened squames with small, dense pyknotic nuclei. This layer varies in thickness with estrogen status.
(vi) Mitotic figures are confined to the basal and first and second layers of parabasal cells. Intracellular glycogen accumulates as differentiation proceeds (Schiller, 1929].

The endocervical canal is lined by columnar epithelium composed of tall, cylindrical mucus-secreting cells with a characteristic picket fence appearance. These cells are interspersed with scattered ciliated cells. Situated between the columnar cells and the basement membrane are small, triangular subcolumnar cells. This epithelium lines both the surface and the glands of the endocervix, although the latter are in fact a complex system of clefts and pits rather than true racemose glands [Fluhmann, 1961].

The transition between the stratified ectocervical epithelium and the columnar endocervical epithelium is at the squamocolumnar junction. This junction can be abrupt but is more frequently observed as a gradual transition. The transitional area is a region of cellular instability and at certain critical periods (late fetal, menarche, and first pregnancy) cells at the junction undergo squamous metaplasia. In this process, the original simple epithelium of the endocervix is replaced by squamous epithelium. The area in which this process occurs and in which metaplastic epithelium is found is described as the transformation zone [Singer and Jordan, 1976].

The natural history of invasive cervical carcinoma has been well documented. It is preceded by histologically distinct intraepithelial lesions that form part of a spectrum of epithelial atypia. In Europe the lesions in this spectrum are described as cervical intraepithelial neoplasms (CIN) and are classified in three grades: CIN 1–mild, CIN 2–moderate, and CIN 3–severe. In the US the Bethesda classification recognizes two groups of squamous intraepithelial lesions (SIL): low grade (LGSIL) and high grade (HGSIL) [Richart and Wright, 1991]. It is clear from epidemiological studies that infection with the high-risk HPV types, 16, 18, 31, 33, 45, and their relatives, is the major risk factor for cervical cancer and the cause of SIL [Liaw et al., 1999]. Metaplasia is classified with other epithelial changes such as basal cell hyperplasia that are not regarded as having significant metaplastic potential. However, the majority of early neoplastic cervical lesions are found in or around the transformation zone at the external os, and the general view is that neoplastic change occurs as a result of persistent infection of metaplastic epithelium with high-risk genital HPVs [IARC Monographs on the Evaluation of Carcinogen Risks to Humans, 1996].

1.2. Cervical Epithelium In Vitro—Historical Review

1.2.1. Ectocervix

Culture techniques for ectocervix should result in the following:

(i)   Production of pure cultures of cervical keratinocytes without contamination with other cell types.
(ii) Serial cultivation. Cultures of normal cervical keratinocytes should have an in vitro life span comparable to that achieved for diploid fibroblasts and other cell types.
(iii) Single cell cloning.
(iv) Modulation of the differentiated phenotype in vitro.

Until 1975, when Rheinwald and Green [Rheinwald and Green, 1975] in a seminal publication demonstrated serial cultivation of neonatal foreskin keratinocytes, none of these objectives had been achieved for keratinocytes from any surface. Before this, cultures were initiated by explantation of epithelial fragments [reviewed in Wilbanks and Fink, 1976]. Sheets of epithelial cells were regularly obtained, but serial cultivation was rarely successful; passaged primary keratinocytes attached poorly and senesced rapidly in secondary culture, and the cultures rapidly became dominated by fibroblasts. The lack of success in serial culture of normal epithelium was paralleled by attempts to grow neoplastic keratinocytes from either SIL or carcinoma. Although permanent cell lines from cervical carcinomas were established, including what became probably the most widely used cell line in biology, HeLa [Gey et al., 1952], no authentic permanent line was established from SIL until the W12 line [Stanley et al., 1989] and the CIN

Margaret A. Stanley

612 line [Bedell et al., 1991], both of which were derived from LGSIL. The same technical problems encountered in the culture of normal epithelial were found with neoplastic keratinocytes plus the added complication of cellular heterogeneity in the biopsy from which the line originated. This emphasized the need for cell-specific or differentiation-specific markers other than morphology to establish the identity of cultured cells and for techniques that would allow the expression of the differentiated phenotype in vitro.

Central to the Rheinwald and Green technology was provision of connective tissue factors by an irradiated mouse feeder cell layer. In later work, the requirement for epidermal growth factor [Rheinwald and Green, 1977] and cholera toxin [Green, 1978] in deferring differentiation and enhancing colony plating efficiency was described and a rational basis for keratinocyte culture was achieved. Through this approach it was shown that ectocervical keratinocytes could be serially cultivated [Stanley and Parkinson, 1979] and that the growth requirements for these cells were similar but not identical to those of epidermal keratinocytes [Stanley and Dahlenburg, 1984].

Ham and co-workers used an alternative approach to keratinocyte culture that concentrated on the development of keratinocyte-specific defined media [Peehl and Ham, 1980; Tsao et al., 1982]. This culminated in the development of MCDB 153 [Boyce and Ham, 1986], a low-calcium defined medium supplemented with bovine-specific pituitary extract that supported the initiation of primary cultures and serial passage of human foreskin keratinocytes in the absence of serum and feeder cells.

Keratinocytes grown as monolayers do not undergo complete differentiation in vitro, although limited stratification is achieved using the feeder technique. Fusenig and his collaborators [Fusenig et al., 1978] (see Chapter 2) described a technique whereby enhanced tissue organization of stratified squamous epithelium was achieved when keratinocytes were cultivated on collagenous substrates and grown at the air-liquid interface. This technology was developed and refined by several investigators [Lillie et al., 1980; Asselineau et al., 1986; Kopan et al., 1987], and organotypic or "raft" cultures are widely used.

1.2.2. Endocervix

There are few reports detailing the successful in vitro growth of endocervical cells. Vesterinen and colleagues [Vesterinen et al., 1975] described outgrowth of cells from explants of endocervix, but these senesced within 10–12 days of culture. These cells grew as a single layer with no stratification [Kusanagi et al., 1980] and were ultrastructurally distinct from ectocervical keratinocytes [Alitalo et al., 1982]. Successful serial cultivation of endocervical cells using the feeder support system has been achieved [Dixon and Stanley, 1984].

2. PREPARATION OF REAGENTS AND MEDIA

2.1. Media and Sera

2.1.1. Transport Medium

Dulbecco's modification of Eagle's medium (DMEM) supplemented with:

Fetal bovine serum (FBS)	10%
Gentamicin sulfate	100 μg/ml
Amphotericin B	10 μg/ml

Aliquot in 10-ml lots and store at $-20°$C.

2.1.2. Keratinocyte Culture Medium (Complete Medium)

DMEM supplemented with:

FBS	10%	
Hydrocortisone	0.5 μg/ml	1.4×10^{-6} M
Cholera toxin	8.4 ng/ml	1×10^{-10} M

Store at 4°C for up to 3 wk.

2.1.3. 3T3 Culture Medium

DMEM supplemented with 10% newborn calf serum (NCS).

Store at 4°C for up to 3 wk.

2.1.4. Serum-Free Keratinocyte Growth Medium (KGM)

MCDB 153 (see supplier's instructions for preparation and storage).

2.1.5. Raft Medium

DMEM:Ham's F12 medium, 3:1, supplemented with:

FBS		10%
Cholera toxin	8.4 ng/ml	1×10^{-10} M
Insulin	5 μg/ml	9×10^{-7} M
apo-Transferrin	5 μg/ml	6.4×10^{-8} M
Hydrocortisone	0.4 μg/ml	1.1×10^{-6} M
Epidermal growth factor (EGF)	0.5 μg/ml	8.3×10^{-8} M

Store at 4°C for up to 1 week.

2.1.6. E Medium

Mix KGM and raft medium, 50:50.

Make up as required and use within 7 days.

2.1.7. Fetal Bovine Serum

Not all batches of FBS have the same capacity to support keratinocyte growth, and batches of FBS must be tested before ordering. Most suppliers will supply small aliquots (20–100 ml) of different batches for testing. When a suitable batch has been identified, at least 12 months' supply should be purchased and stored at −20°C until required.

2.2. Salt Solutions and Disaggregating Agents

2.2.1. PBSA

	g/l	mM
KCl	0.20	2.68
KH$_2$·PO$_4$	0.20	1.47
NaCl	8.00	136.89
Na$_2$HPO$_4$·7H$_2$O	2.16	8.06

Aliquot in 200-ml lots and sterilize by autoclaving.

Store at room temperature.

2.2.2. EDTA (Versene; Ethylenediamine Tetraacetic Acid-Disodium Salt)

(i) Prepared as 3.4 mM stock (0.1% w/v) in PBSA.
(ii) Filter sterilize and aliquot in 2-ml lots.
(iii) Store at room temperature.
(iv) Dilute 10× in PBSA before use.

2.2.3. EDTA (as Free Acid, Anhydrous)

Prepared as 2.7 mM stock (0.1% w/v) in sterile UPW.

Filter sterilize and aliquot in 10-ml lots.

Store at room temperature.

2.2.4. Trypsin

(i)   Prepare as stock 2.5% (25 mg/ml) in PBSA.
(ii) Check the pH, which should be 7.0.
(iii) Filter sterilize.
(iv) Aliquot in 2-ml lots.
(v)   Store at $-20°C$.
(vi) Dilute 10× before use.

2.2.5. Trypsin-EDTA

(i)   Add to sterile PBSA:
      Trypsin   0.25% (w/v)
      EDTA   0.3 mM
(ii) Adjust pH to pH 7.4
(iii) Store at 4°C for up to 1 week.

2.2.6. TE buffer pH 8.0

(i)   Tris·HCl   10 mM
(ii) EDTA   1 mM
(iii) Adjust pH to pH 8.0.
(iv) Filter sterilize.
(v)   Aliquot in 10-ml lots and store at room temperature.

2.2.7. Reconstitution Buffer for Rafts

NaHCO$_3$ 26 mM (0.22% w/v)
NaOH   0.005 N
HEPES   2 mM

2.2.8. 10× reconstitution buffer

NaHCO$_3$ 0.26 M
NaOH   0.05 N
HEPES   20 mM

2.3. Medium Additives

2.3.1. Cholera Toxin (CT; mol wt 84,000)

(i)   To make the master stock add 1.18 ml sterile UPW to 1 mg powder in the vial to give 1×10^{-5} M solution.

(ii) Store at 4°C.

(iii) As a working stock add 100 μl, 1×10^{-5} M, CT to 10 ml DMEM/10% FBS to give 1×10^{-7} M CT.

(iv) Filter sterilize and keep at 4°C.

(v) Dilute 1:17 (v/v) in medium/10% serum for use at a final concentration of 6×10^{-9} M (0.5 μg/ml).

2.3.2. Hydrocortisone

Hydrocortisone is not soluble in water but will dissolve in 50% ethanol/water (v/v).

(i) Dissolve 1 mg hydrocortisone in 1 ml sterile 50% ethanol.

(ii) Aliquot into 100-μl lots in sterile Eppendorf tubes and store at -20°C.

(iii) Use at a final concentration of 0.5 μg/ml (1.4×10^{-6} M).

2.3.3. Epidermal Growth Factor

(i) To prepare add 1 ml sterile UPW to 100 μg powder in the vial.

(ii) Aliquot in 100-μl lots and store at -20°C.

(iii) To prepare a working stock add 100 μl EGF (100 μg/ml) to 10 ml DMEM/10% FBS to give 1 μg/ml.

(iv) Store at 4°C.

(v) Dilute 1:100 (v/v) for use at a concentration of 10 ng/ml ($\sim 2 \times 10^{-9}$ M).

2.3.4. Insulin

(i) To prepare a 1000× stock solution add 20 ml sterile UPW to the 100 mg powder in the vial to give 5 mg/ml.

(ii) Incubate overnight at 4°C to allow it to go into solution.

(iii) Aliquot 1.6 ml in sterile cryovials and store at -20°C.

(iv) Dilute 1:1000 for use at a concentration of 5 μg/ml ($\sim 9 \times 10^{-7}$ M).

2.3.5. *apo*-Transferrin

(i) To prepare a 1000× stock solution dissolve 100 mg in 20 ml sterile UPW.

(ii) Aliquot in 1.6-ml lots in cryovials.

(iii) Store at -20°C.

(iv) Dilute 1:1000 for use at a final concentration of 5 μg/ml ($\sim 6 \times 10^{-8}$ M).

2.3.6. Rat Tail Collagen

Store and use according to the manufacturer's instructions.

2.4. Antibiotics

2.4.1. Geneticin Crystalline, Nonsterile (G418 sulfate)

Prepare a stock solution at 50 mg/ml in UPW, filter sterilize, and store at 4°C.

2.4.2. Gentamicin

Supplied sterile at 10 mg/ml, use at 100 μg/ml in transport medium and 50 μg/ml in PBSA wash.

2.4.3. Amphotericin B

(i)   Prepare a stock 2.5 mg/ml in sterile UPW or PBSA.
(ii) Filter sterilize, aliquot as 500-μl lots, and store at -20°C.
(iii) Use in transport medium at 10 μg/ml, 5 μg/ml in PBSA wash, and 2.5 μg/ml in culture medium.

2.4.4. Mitomycin C

(i) Dissolve contents of 2-mg vial in 5 ml UPW to give 20 stock at 400 μg/ml.
(ii) Aliquot in 0.5-ml lots and store at -20°C.

3. CELL CULTURE PROTOCOLS FOR NORMAL CERVICAL KERATINOCYTES

3.1. Culture on Fibroblast Feeder Layers

3.1.1. Ectocervix

Most ectocervical epithelium from nonneoplastic cervices is obtained from hysterectomy specimens. The cervical biopsy for culture should be taken by the pathologist and transferred immediately to transport medium. Biopsies exceeding 2 cm in diameter will remain viable in this medium for up to 3 days at 4°C. Small biopsies must be processed on the same day.

Δ*Safety note.* In the culture laboratory, biopsies are handled in a laminar flow hood (Class II microbiological safety cabinet) designated for use only with fresh human material. Laboratory personnel must wear gloves and disposable face masks. They should process the biopsy as potentially hazardous.

Protocol 5.1. Preparation of Cervical Cells

Reagents and Materials

Sterile

- ❑ Complete medium (see Section 2.1.2, above)
- ❑ Transport medium (see Section 2.1.1, above)
- ❑ PBSA containing gentamicin sulfate 50 μg/ml and amphotericin 5 μg/ml (see Sections 2.4.2 and 2.4.3, above)
- ❑ Trypsin-EDTA (see Section 2.2.5, above)
- ❑ Petri dishes, plastic, bacteriological grade, 9 cm
- ❑ Universal containers
- ❑ Forceps, fine
- ❑ Scissors, iris
- ❑ Scalpel, #22 blade
- ❑ Muslin or steel tea strainer, 0.5- to 1.0-mm mesh.

Nonsterile

- ❑ Magnetic stirrer

Protocol

(a) Remove the biopsy from the transport medium with sterile forceps and place in a 9-cm plastic Petri dish.

(b) Wash the biopsy with five applications of 5 ml of sterile PBSA containing gentamicin sulfate 50 μg/ml and amphotericin 5 μg/ml.

(c) Orient the biopsy with the epithelial surface down on the culture dish. Using a disposable scalpel fitted with a #22 blade, cut and scrape away (with a cutting direction away from the operator) as much of the stroma and muscle as possible. A thin, opaque white epithelial strip should be left after this procedure.

(d) Take this strip and mince finely with curved iris scissors. It is important that the fragments be small; the operator's wrists usually ache if this procedure is properly carried out!

(e) Add 10 ml of trypsin-EDTA preheated to 37°C to this minced tissue and transfer to a glass universal containing a sterile, plastic-coated, magnetic flea. Rinse the Petri dish with a further 10 ml of trypsin-EDTA and add to the suspension in the universal.

(f) Place the universal on a magnetic stirrer in an incubator or hot room at 37°C and stir slowly for 30–40 min.

(g) Allow the suspension to stand at room temperature for 2–3 min to allow the fragments to settle to the bottom of the universal.

(h) Using a 10-ml pipette, remove the supernatant containing single cells and filter through muslin or a stainless steel tea strainer (0.5–1.0 mm) into a sterile 50-ml centrifuge tube. Add 10 ml of complete medium to this.

(i) Add a further 10–15 ml of warm trypsin-EDTA to the fragments in the universal and repeat the above procedures, combining the trypsin supernatants in one centrifuge tube.

(j) Take the combined trypsin suspensions and spin in a bench centrifuge at 1,000 rpm (80 g) for 5 min.

(k) Remove the supernatant and add 10 ml of complete medium to the pellet. Prepare a single cell suspension by resuspending this pellet vigorously with a 10-ml pipette to which is attached a large pipette bulb.

(l) Count the cells, using a counting chamber; only count small, circular, refractile cells and ignore large squames and red blood cells. Cell viability can be assessed at this stage by trypan blue exclusion.

Protocol 5.2. Culture of Cervical Epithelium on Fibroblast Feeder Layers

Reagents and Materials

❏ Complete medium (see Section 2.1.2)
❏ Feeder layers: The feeder layers consist of lethally irradiated Swiss 3T3 cells (see Protocol 5.4) at a density of 1×10^5 cells/cm^2 (5×10^5 cells/5-cm dish, 2×10^6 cells/9-cm dish) in complete medium. The feeder layers can be prepared previously and the keratinocytes added to these layers, or feeder cells and keratinocytes can be inoculated together. In either case, it is important that the feeder cells form a continuous even layer across the dish and that there be no regions of high and low density.

Protocol

(a) Dilute the cervical cell suspension with complete medium to achieve an appropriate dilution and plate the cells out at a density of 2×10^4 cells/cm^2 (10^5 cells/5-cm Petri, 4×10^5 cells/9-cm Petri) onto preformed feeder layer or add with feeder cells (see Feeder layers in **Reagents and Materials** for this protocol).

(b) Incubate cultures at 37°C in 5% CO_2 in air.

(c) Examine the cultures by phase contrast inverted microscopy at 72 h after the initial plating to determine that the feeder layer is satisfactorily dispersed.

(d) Change the culture medium and replace with complete medium supplemented with EGF at 10 ng/ml. Further feeder cells should be added if required (i.e., if degeneration or depletion of the feeder layer is observed).

(e) The medium should be changed twice weekly, and EGF should be present in the medium, except when cells are initially plated.

(f) At 12–16 days after the initiation of the primary culture, keratinocyte colonies should be easily visible to the naked eye and should contain about 1000 cells and have a diameter of 1–3 mm (Fig. 5.1). Colonies should be subcultured at this time.

Protocol 5.3. Subculture of Keratinocytes on Fibroblast Feeder Layers

Reagents and Materials

❑ PBSA (see Section 2.2.1)
❑ EDTA, free acid, 0.3 mM (0.01%) diluted in PBSA (from stock, Section 2.2.3)
❑ Trypsin-EDTA (see Section 2.2.5)

Protocol

(a) Remove the medium from the cultures.

(b) Remove the remaining feeder cells by vigorously squirting 1–2 ml of 0.3 mM (0.01%) EDTA over the entire surface of the dish. This maneuver should not last longer than 30 s.

(c) Rinse the culture surface twice with PBSA.

(d) Add 2 ml of prewarmed 0.1% trypsin in 0.3 mM EDTA in PBSA to each 5-cm Petri dish.

(e) Leave at 37°C until the keratinocytes have detached; this should be checked microscopically. The total time in trypsin must not exceed 20 min.

(f) Remove the cell suspension from the plate and transfer to a sterile centrifuge tube.

(g) Rinse the culture surface with 5.0 ml of complete medium and add to the cell suspension.

(h) Mix gently using a 10-ml pipette.

(i) Spin at 1000 rpm (80 g) for 5 min.

(j) Remove the supernatant and resuspend the cell pellet in 10 ml of complete medium to produce a single cell suspension.

(k) Count the cells in a counting chamber. The suspension may be replated, frozen down, or subjected to chemical analysis as required by the investigator.

(l) Cells to be replated should be inoculated at 5×10^3/cm^2 or 1×10^4/cm^2 together with lethally irradiated feeder cells at 1×10^5/cm^2 and grown as described for primary cultures (see Protocol 5.2).

The colony-plating efficiency (colonies formed ÷ keratinocytes plated × 100) should be determined at each passage by staining replica plates (see Protocol 10.10 to step (e)) and recorded for each keratinocyte strain. Cytogenetic studies should be performed as soon as practicable. The number of population doublings undergone should be recorded for each strain [see Stanley, 1986]. The genital tract is susceptible to mycoplasma infection, so all cultures should be screened for mycoplasma at the time of first passage.

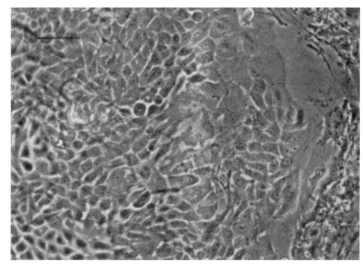

Fig 5.1. Ectocervical keratinocytes. The cells have a characteristic polygonal morphology and grow in small, tight colonies, the edge of the colony displacing the surrounding 3T3 feeder cells. Mitotic figures are evident. Bar = 10 μm.

Margaret A. Stanley

Protocol 5.4. Preparation of 3T3 Feeder Layers

The J2 clone (established by J.G. Rheinwald) of the 3T3 cell line [Todaro and Green, 1963] provides the best feeder cell support for cervical keratinocytes. The following points are some general principles for growth of 3T3 cells as feeder layers.

Reagents and Materials

Sterile or Aseptically Prepared

- ❑ 3T3 J2 cells from an authenticated distribution stock
- ❑ Medium: DMEM with 10% newborn calf serum (see Section 2.1.3)
- ❑ Flasks, 75 cm²
- ❑ Mitomycin C, 400 μg/ml (see Section 2.4.4)

Nonsterile

- ❑ Irradiation source, γ- or X-ray

Protocol

(a) Prepare a large master stock of 3T3 cells and freeze down in individual ampoules each containing 1×10^6 cells.

(b) If 3T3 cells are to remain effective feeders, the cells should not be used after passage 20. When the current stock culture reaches passage 18, thaw a new ampoule of cells from frozen stocks and reestablish new feeder stock culture.

(c) Grow cells in DMEM supplemented with 10% newborn calf serum in 75-cm² flasks. 3T3 cells grow poorly in Roller bottles.

(d) Seed cells at 1.5×10^4 cells/cm² growth area and passage just before confluence. In practice, this results in weekly passage.

(e) Maintain cells in antibiotic-free medium to avoid low-level contamination problems. Antibiotic-free cells are then used at each passage to inoculate the flasks required for that week's feeder cells.

(f) To generate feeder cells, irradiate flask cultures with 60 Gy either from an X-ray or ^{60}Co source. Irradiated cells, if kept at 4°C, retain their capacity to act as feeders for 4–5 days.

(g) If an X-ray or ^{60}Co source is not available, cells can be inactivated with mitomycin C as follows:

    i) Resuspend 3T3 cells at a concentration of 1×10^7/ml.

ii) Add 50 μl mitomycin C per ml of cell suspension to give 20 μg/ml final concentration.

iii) Resuspend carefully to ensure effective mixing of the mitomycin C.

iv) Leave at 37°C for 1 h.

v) Spin at 1000 rpm (80 g), remove the supernatant, and wash 4 times with 10 ml medium.

(h) Seed cells for feeder layers as described above in Protocol 5.2.

3.1.2. Endocervix

Biopsies are taken from the endocervical canal near the internal os. These biopsies must be selected by the pathologist to ensure that no contamination with ectocervix occurs. The tissue is processed essentially as described for ectocervix (Protocols 5.1 and 5.2) but with the following modifications.

Protocol 5.5. Culture of Cells from Endocervix

Reagents and Materials

❑ As for Protocols 5.1–5.4

Protocol

(a) Mince the epithelial sheet as described (Protocol 5.1 (d), above), but subject the minced fragments to only one cycle of disaggregation with trypsin.

(b) Wash the cell pellet once with complete medium and plate the cells at 1 $\times$ 10^4/cm^2 without filtering through a wire mesh.

(c) Maintain the cells and subculture as described in Protocols 5.2 and 5.3.

3.2. Cultures Grown with Serum-Free Keratinocyte Growth Medium (KGM)

Protocol 5.6. Culture of Cervical Epithelium in Serum-Free Medium

Reagents and Materials

❑ Serum-free keratinocyte growth medium (KGM)

Margaret A. Stanley

Protocol

(a) Dissociate the epithelium, as described in Protocol 5.1, above, to obtain a single cell suspension in complete medium.

(b) Spin this suspension at 1000 rpm (80 g) in a bench centrifuge.

(c) Remove the supernatant and resuspend in 10 ml PBSA.

(d) Spin again and wash once more with PBSA.

(e) Resuspend the cells in 10 ml KGM.

(f) Plate into culture dishes or flasks at a density of 2×10^5 cells/cm^2 (1×10^6 cells per 5-cm Petri dish, 4×10^6 cells per 9-cm dish).

(g) Primary cultures of cervical keratinocytes can be difficult to initiate with KGM alone because cell attachment can be poor. Attachment can be improved by coating the dishes with FBS as follows:

   i) Add FBS to the culture dish (2 ml/5-cm dish, 5 ml/9-cm dish).

   ii) Leave at 37°C for 1 h.

   iii) Remove the serum and plate the cells as described in (f), above.

(h) Change the medium twice weekly.

(i) Confluent monolayer cultures should be achieved after 18–21 days.

(j) Subculture the cells when they reach confluence.

Protocol 5.7. Subculture of Cervical Keratinocytes Grown in KGM

Reagents and Materials

❑ PBSA (see Section 2.2.1)
❑ Trypsin-EDTA (see Section 2.2.5)
❑ Serum-free keratinocyte growth medium (KGM; see Section 2.1.4 and supplier's instructions)

Protocol

(a) Remove the culture medium. Wash the cells once with PBSA.

(b) Add 2 ml trypsin-EDTA per 5-cm dish.

(c) Leave at 37°C until the keratinocytes detach. This should not exceed 20 min.

(d) Transfer the cell suspension to a centrifuge tube.

(e) Rinse the dish with 5.0 ml KGM; add to the trypsin suspension, mix gently, and spin at 1000 rpm for 5 min.

(f) Remove the supernatant and resuspend in 10 ml KGM.

(g) Count the cells and replate at $10^5/cm^2$.

3.3. Neoplastic Epithelium

3.3.1. Cervical Intraepithelial Neoplasms, CIN (LGSIL, HGSIL)

Biopsies are obtained either as punch biopsies taken under colposcopic direction or as epithelial strips removed from cone biopsies under the dissecting microscope. The biopsies are usually very small ($2–3$ mm^3), and disaggregation to single cells with trypsin is an inefficient procedure. The following protocol has been found to be the most effective.

Protocol 5.8 Culture of Cervical Intraepithelial Neoplasms (CIN)

Reagents and Materials

Sterile

❑ PBSA (see Section 2.2.1)
❑ FBS (see Section 2.1.7)
❑ Complete medium (see Section 2.1.2)
❑ Iris scissors, curved

Protocol

(a) Rinse the biopsy twice with 2–3 ml PBSA.
(b) Mince finely with curved iris scissors.
(c) Add 0.5–1.0 ml FBS to the minced tissue and transfer with a Pasteur pipette to the growth surface (lower surface) of a 25-cm^2 tissue culture flask.
(d) Spread the minced fragments evenly across the growth surface of the flask.
(e) Carefully turn the flask over so that the growth surface with the fragments is uppermost (Fig. 5.2).
(f) Add 4.5 ml supplemented DMEM to the surface of the flask opposite that carrying the fragments. The medium must *not* cover the fragments.
(g) Leave the flask and contents in this inverted position in the incubator for 2–3 h at 37°C.
(h) *Carefully* turn the flask to the correct position so that the medium covers the explanted fragments and leave for 72–96 h *without* touching or moving.

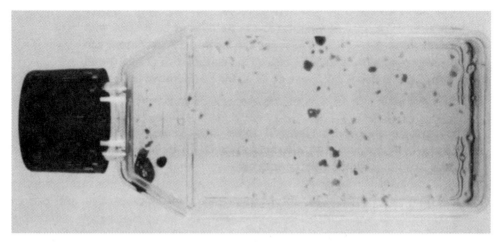

Fig 5.2. Explanted fragments of CIN or cervical carcinoma in serum attached to the growth surface. The flask is inverted and maintained in this position for 2–3 h at 37°C to promote attachment of the explanted fragments.

(i) Examine the cultures, using inverted phase microscopy to assess growth. Usually epithelial cells migrate quickly from the explants and can be passaged at 7–10 days onto feeder layers (see Protocols 5.2–5.4).

(j) Alternatively, because fibroblast contamination is a major problem in these cultures, at the first medium change replace the serum-supplemented DMEM with KGM and proceed as in Section 3.2.

3.3.2. Carcinoma

Two major problems are encountered in the culture of cervical carcinomas, microbial contamination and fibroblast contamination. Microbial contamination is caused predominantly by gram-negative bacterial species and fungal (usually *Candida*) species. Thus the growth medium for carcinomas must be supplemented initially with a broad-spectrum antibiotic (gentamicin sulfate 50 μg/ml and amphotericin 5 μg/ml). The following protocol is the most satisfactory.

Protocol 5.9. Culture of Cervical Carcinoma

Reagents and Materials

Sterile

❑ Transport medium (see Section 2.1.1)
❑ PBSA containing amphotericin, 5 μg/ml, and gentamicin, 50 μg/ml

- ❏ Complete medium (see Section 2.1.2)
- ❏ FBS
- ❏ For subculture reagents, see Protocols 5.3 and 5.4 or Protocol 5.7
- ❏ Iris scissors, curved

Protocol

(a) Carcinoma biopsies are taken in the operating room at the initial staging examination under anesthetic (EUA).

(b) Transport biopsies to the laboratory in transport medium.

(c) Malignant cervical cells are protease-sensitive, and dissociation into single cells with trypsin is not recommended; explantation is the most satisfactory initiation technique.

(d) Rinse the biopsies with PBSA containing amphotericin and gentamicin.

(e) Mince finely with curved iris scissors.

(f) Explant the minced fragments in serum as described above in Protocol 5.8 for CIN.

(g) Subsequent passage and subcultivation procedures are as described for CIN (see Protocol 5.8, (i) and (j), above). It is advisable to eliminate cholera toxin from the growth medium for carcinomas.

Fibroblast contamination is the most significant problem in the culture of cervical carcinomas. In our hands, this has been controlled effectively only by the combination of serum-free keratinocyte growth medium and physical removal of fibroblasts with a rubber cell scraper from the cultures. Cervical carcinoma lines have been established using almost every variation of culture technique including the feeder support system [Kelland et al., 1987], after transplantation in nude mice [Pal et al., 1992], and in low [Waggoner & Wang, 1994] and high [Ho et al., 1993] serum. In general, success rates are low and a cell line can be generated from about 1 in 10 biopsies.

4. IDENTIFICATION AND CHARACTERIZATION OF CERVICAL CELLS IN VITRO

4.1. Normal Ectocervical Cells

Cell cultures from ectocervical squamous epithelium consist of colonies of keratinocytes. There is a characteristic morphology of these cells at both the light and electron microscope levels. Cultures consist of small, polygonal, tightly adherent cells between that can be seen intercellular connections similar to those observed in the epithelium in the stratum spinosum (see Fig. 5.1). Cells grown on feeder support show limited stratification with 2–3 layers of cells evident in vertical section (Fig. 5.3). Ultrastructurally the cells resemble basal, parabasal, and intermediate cells in vivo [Davies and Wolfe, 1963; Shingleton and Laurence, 1976]. The apical surface is decorated with microvilli, and there are numerous junctions resembling true desmosomes between the cells that contain bundles of tonofilaments (Fig. 5.3).

Specific differentiation markers of value for the characterization of cultured cervical keratinocytes include keratin intermediate filaments, involucrin, and intracytoplasmic glycogen.

4.1.1. Keratin Expression

Monolayer cultures of cervical keratinocytes express the basal keratins of ectocervical epithelium, K5 and K19 [Moll et al.,

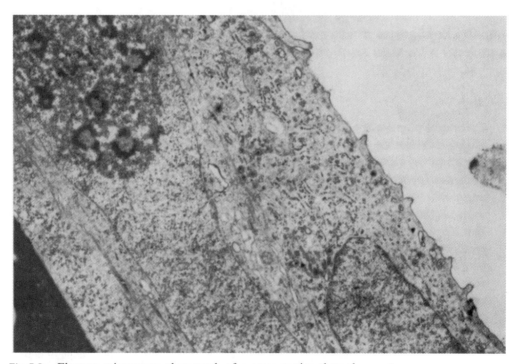

Fig 5.3. Electron microscope photograph of a cross section through an ectocervical keratinocyte colony grown with feeder cell support in serum-supplemented medium. The cells are stratified in a four-cell layer. There are numerous desmosomes and tonofilaments, and microvilli decorate the surface of the superficial cells of the colony. ×20,000.

1982], and these can be identified either biochemically by extraction and 2D gel electrophoresis or by immunostaining with monoclonal antibodies to specific keratin species. (Fig. 5.4)

4.1.2. Involucrin Expression and Glycogen Accumulation

Differentiating cells of squamous epithelium are characterized by the cornified envelope, a 12-nm band apposed to the cytoplasmic face of the plasma membrane. The cornified envelope results from the cross-linking of several proteins, one of which is the 92-kDa species involucrin [Rice and Green, 1979]. Involucrin expression is a specific marker of keratinocyte differentiation because the protein is not synthesized in significant quantity by any other cell type [Banks-Schlegel and Green, 1981]. In mucosal squamous epithelia such as the cervix, a marker of differentiation

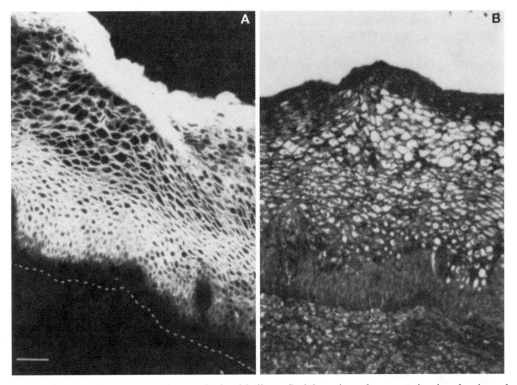

Fig 5.4. Ectocervical epithelium: Serial sections demonstrating involucrin and glycogen distribution. Bars = 10 μm. A. Immunofluorescent staining of normal ectocervix with anti-involucrin polyclonal antibody. Involucrin is synthesized in all cell layers except for the first two or three basal and parabasal layers. Dashed line: basement membrane. B. Periodic acid-Schiff (PAS) staining to demonstrate glycogen distribution. Black areas of cytoplasmic staining are PAS-positive. The distribution of glycogen parallels that of involucrin.

is the intracytoplasmic accumulation of glycogen. In the ectocervix glycogen accumulation starts in suprabasal cells with maximal expression in the superficial terminally differentiated layers. This distribution is paralleled closely by that of involucrin, which is expressed in all but the basal and parabasal layers [Walts et al., 1985; Warhol et al., 1982].

In vivo, involucrin and glycogen are coexpressed (Fig. 5.5, a and b), and this expression is related to the degree of ectocervical keratinocyte differentiation. In vitro ectocervical keratinocytes show limited stratification, usually in the center of colonies. The upper layers of these colonies consist of large squamelike cells that coexpress involucrin and glycogen (Fig. 5.5, a and b). Expression of these markers in vitro is associated with a decline in

Fig 5.5. Ectocervical keratinocytes in culture: Codistribution of involucrin and glycogen revealed by double staining. Bars = 10 μm. A. Periodic acid-Schiff (PAS) staining shows focal areas of dark cytoplasmic staining for glycogen accumulation. B. Immunofluorescent staining with an anti-involucrin polyclonal antibody reveals that the glycogen-positive and involucrin-positive areas are identical.

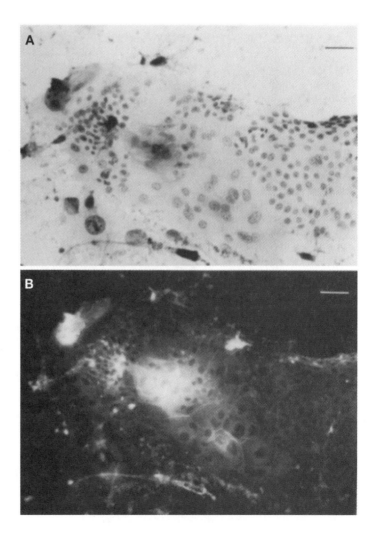

colony plating efficiency of the keratinocytes [Stanley and Dahlenburg, 1984].

4.2. Endocervix

In vitro endocervical cells grow in colonies that initially have a heterogeneous morphology (Fig. 5.6a). After approximately 14 days in culture, colony morphology changes, small polyhedral keratinocyte-like cells appear at the periphery, and these eventually come to dominate the culture (Fig. 5.6b). The endocervical origin of these cells is shown by the expression of keratin 18 (Fig. 5.7), the characteristic keratin of simple epithelia. These "endocervical keratinocytes" also express involucrin and glycogen in the center of the colonies and are the in vitro equivalent of squamous metaplasia.

Fig 5.6. Morphology of cultured endocervical epithelial cells. Bars = 10 μm. A. After 10 days in primary culture. The cells have a heterogeneous morphology and are frequently elongated with protrusions and extensions. B. After 24 days in primary culture. The cells have undergone a change in morphology and have the appearance of small keratinocytes, particularly at the edge of the colonies. Panel A reproduced from Dixon and Stanley [1984] with permission of the publisher.

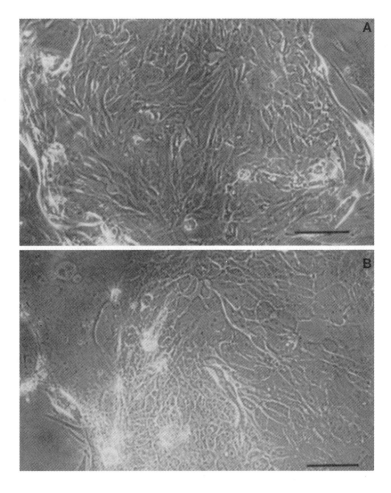

Margaret A. Stanley

5. CONDITIONS NECESSARY FOR MAXIMAL EXPRESSION OF DIFFERENTIATED PHENOTYPE IN VITRO

Submerged cultures of either ectocervical or endocervical cells consist of cells that do not completely express the differentiated phenotype either morphologically or biochemically. In vitro the differentiated phenotype of cervical cells, both morphologically and biochemically, can be induced if cultures are grown at the air-liquid interface on collagenous substrata (Fig. 5.8). The following protocol [modified from Dollard et al., 1992; Parker et al., 1997] is used in our laboratory.

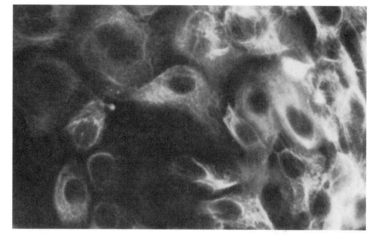

Fig 5.7. Immunofluorescent staining of "keratinocyte-like" endocervical cells (10 days after first passage) with the LE61 monoclonal antibody specific for keratin 18 [Lane, 1982]. Despite the keratinocyte-like morphology, the cells stain strongly. Reproduced from Dixon and Stanley [1984] with permission of the publisher.

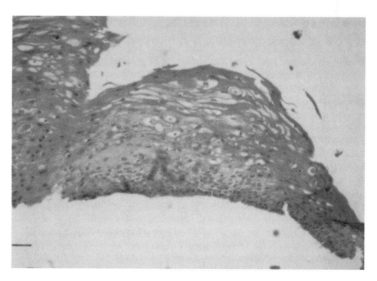

Fig 5.8. Normal ectocervical keratinocytes grown for 10 days at the air-liquid interface on a collagen matrix. The cells form a slightly hyperplastic, stratified, well-keratinized epithelium with a distinctive stratum corneum. Bar = 20 μm.

Protocol 5.10. Culture of Cervical Epithelium on Collagen Rafts

Reagents and Materials

Sterile or Aseptically Prepared

- ☐ 3T3 J2 cells
- ☐ Cervical keratinocytes (primary or subcultured)
- ☐ Reconstitution buffer, 10× (see Section 2.2.8)
- ☐ Ham's F12, 10×
- ☐ E medium (see Section 2.1.6)
- ☐ FBS
- ☐ Collagen, type A, rat tail
- ☐ Multiwell plates, 24 well
- ☐ Conical centrifuge tubes, 15 ml
- ☐ Spatula with angled tip

Protocol

(a) Seed 24-well plates with 1×10^5 3T3 J2 cells/well.

(b) Prepare a second suspension of 3T3 J2 cells at a concentration of 1.33×10^6/ml in FBS.

(c) Using disposable plastic pipettes, prepare the collagen mix. In a sterile conical 15-ml graduated, plastic tube on ice, combine:
  i) Ham's F12 medium, 10×, 0.8 ml
  ii) Reconstitution buffer, 10×, 0.8 ml

(d) Using the graduations on the side of the tube, add 8 ml 100% rat tail type A collagen.

(e) Add 5.3×10^5 J2 3T3 in 0.4 ml FBS and mix well by gently inverting the tube several times.

(f) Add 0.75 ml of this collagen/cell mix to each well of the 24-well plate from (a).

(g) Leave for 60 min, then add 1 ml E medium to each well and incubate for 4 h at 37°C.

(h) Add 1×10^5 keratinocytes in 0.5 ml KGM medium + 0.5 ml E medium to each well.

(i) Incubate overnight at 37°C.

(j) Detach the collagen raft from the sides of the well using a sterile spatula and, running the spatula around the side, gently separate the collagen from the sides of the well.

(k) Add 1 ml fresh E medium.

Margaret A. Stanley

(l) Check that the collagen raft is loose and incubate overnight at 37°C.

(m) Place sterilized stainless steel grids on stainless steel cloning rings into 6-cm plates.

(n) Transfer the rafts to grids *carefully* using a flat sterile spatula.

(o) Fill the bottom of the dish containing the grid and raft with E medium; ensure that no bubbles are caught beneath the raft. Remove any bubble so caught with a Pasteur pipette.

(p) Medium should be just below the level of the top of the grid.

(q) Medium must not flow over the top of the raft or differentiation will not occur.

(r) Incubate for 9–10 days at 37°C, changing the medium every other day.

Protocol 5.11. Harvesting Raft Cultures of Cervical Epithelium

Reagents and Materials

Nonsterile

☐ PBSA (see Section 2.2.1)
☐ Spoon forceps
☐ Nitrocellulose filter
☐ Buffered formol saline (if embedding in paraffin wax)
☐ Tissue Tek®OCT™ (if cryosectioning)

Protocol

(a) Fill the dish with PBSA.

(b) With a pair of spoon forceps, gently pull the collagen raft off the mesh and float it on the PBSA.

(c) Cut a piece of nitrocellulose just larger than the raft.

(d) Place it in the PBSA under the raft. Raise it and use it to pick up the culture, ensuring that the collagen is flat.

(e) Blot the base of the nitrocellulose on a paper towel to remove the excess PBSA.

(f) Transfer the nitrocellulose plus raft to a fixation cassette and label.

(g) Either
    i) place in 10% buffered formol saline for 4–6 h to fix and embed in paraffin wax
    or

ii) put in OCT, snap freeze in liquid nitrogen, and store at −70°C for cryosectioning.

6. HPV IMMORTALIZATION

Transfection of DNA sequences from the oncogenic HPV types 16, 18, 31, 33, and 45 immortalizes primary diploid cervical keratinocytes, generating stable, permanent cell lines in which the HPV DNA sequences are usually integrated into the cellular genome [McDougall, 1994]. In most immortalization protocols HPV DNA is cotransfected with a selectable marker, usually the neomycin resistance gene in the plasmid pSV2neo. This renders the transfected cell resistant to neomycin-mediated killing. The following protocol is used in our laboratory.

Protocol 5.12. Immortalization of Cervical Epithelium with HPV

Reagents and Materials

Sterile or Aseptically Prepared

- ❑ HPV DNA
- ❑ pSV2neo DNA
- ❑ TE buffer (see Section 2.2.6)
- ❑ LipofectACE
- ❑ E medium (see Section 2.1.6)
- ❑ Geneticin, G418 (see Section 2.4.1)
- ❑ Petri dishes, 9-cm
- ❑ Polystyrene tubes (Falcon 2054)

Protocol

Day 1

(a) Prepare the DNAs for transfection.
(b) HPV DNA resuspend at 200 ng/μl sterile TE buffer.
(c) pSV2neo DNA resuspend at 100 ng/μl sterile TE buffer.
(d) Keratinocytes should be grown on 9-cm Petri dishes in serum-free medium and be about 50% confluent.

Day 2

(e) On the morning of the transfection, change the medium on the cultures.

(f) Prepare the LipofectACE according to the manufacturer's instructions.
   - i) Use polystyrene tubes (Falcon 2054)
   - ii) Ensure that the LipofectACE is well suspended

(g) Prepare Solution A
   - i) HPV DNA (5 μg)   25 μl
   - ii) pSV2neo DNA (2 μg)   25 μl
   - iii) KGM   200 μl

(h) Prepare solution B
   - i) LipofectACE   36 μl
   - ii) KGM   214 μl

(i) Combine solution A and solution B mixing *gently* so that the DNA complex forms.

(j) Incubate at room temperature for 30 min.

(k) Remove the medium from the keratinocytes and wash the cell layer twice with 4 ml KGM.

(l) Add 0.5 ml KGM to the cell layer.

(m) Add 0.5 ml KGM to the DNA complex from (i) and add this dropwise to the cell layer.

(n) Swirl the plate gently to spread the DNA over the plate and incubate at 37°C for 5 h.
   It is wise to put the plates in a humidified container (sterile distilled water-dampened paper towel mat in a plastic lunch box) in the incubator for this operation.

(o) After incubation add 3.5 ml KGM and incubate at 37°C overnight.

(p) Plate out 2 × 10^6 irradiated 3T3 J2 into 9-cm dishes and incubate overnight

Day 3

(q) Trypsinize the transfected keratinocytes.

(r) Resuspend in 2 ml E medium.

(s) Add to the pre-prepared feeder plates from (p), above.

(t) Add a further 2 ml E medium and leave for 6 h.

(u) Add G418 at 200 μg/ml to each plate

Day 4

(v) Change the medium on the plates, replacing with 6 ml E medium + G418 at 200 μg/ml

Day 5

(w)   Change the medium and add fresh feeder cells.

(x)   Continue G418 selection for a further 10 days, changing the medium every 2 days and replacing the feeder cells every 3–4 days.

(y)   G418-resistant colonies appear within 14–28 days.

Protocol 5.13. Picking Colonies of Cervical Epithelial Cells

Reagents and Materials

Sterile

❑   PBSA (see Section 2.2.1)
❑   E medium (see Section 2.1.6)
❑   Irradiated 3T3 J2 (see Protocol 5.4)
❑   Cloning rings, stainless steel
❑   Centrifuge tubes, ~1–2 ml (e.g., Eppendorf)
❑   Melted agar, 1% in PBSA

Protocol

(a)   Remove the medium and wash the cell layer 2 with PBSA.

(b)   Take a stainless steel cloning ring and dip the base in melted agar.

(c)   Quickly place the agar-dipped ring around the colony to be picked—the agar sticks the ring to the plate, preventing cell leakage during selection.

(d)   Place 0.5 ml trypsin in each ring and leave for 15 min at 37°C.

(e)   Remove trypsin and cells and transfer to a sterile 1- to 2-ml centrifuge tube.

(f)   Wash the ring enclosed area with E medium and add the washings to the centrifuge tube.

(g)   Check microscopically that the cells have been removed and spin the centrifuge tube at 1000 rpm (80 g) for 5 min.

(h)   Resuspend the cell pellet in E medium and plate out on 6-cm Petri dishes together with 5×10^5 irradiated 3T3 J2.

REFERENCES

Alitalo K, Halila H, Vesterinen E, Vaheri A (1982): Endo- and ectocervical human uterine epithelial cells distinguished by fibronectin production and keratinization in culture. Cancer Res 42: 1142–1146.

Asselineau D, Bernard BA, Bailly C, Darmon M, Prunieras M (1986): Human epidermis reconstructed by culture: Is it "normal"? J Invest Dermatol 86: 181–186.

Banks-Schlegel S, Green H (1981): Involucrin synthesis and tissue assembly by keratinocytes in natural and cultured human epithelia. J Cell Biol 90: 732–737.

Bedell MA, Hudson JB, Golub TR, Turyk ME, Hosken M, Wilbanks GD, Laimins LA (1991): Amplification of human papillomavirus genomes in vitro is dependent on epithelial differentiation. J Virol 65: 2254–2260.

Boyce ST, Ham RG (1983) Calcium-regulated differentiation of normal human epidermal keratinocytes in chemically defined clonal culture and serum-free serial culture. J Invest Dermatol 81: 33s–40s.

Davies J, Wolfe S (1963): Histology and fine structure of the adult cervix uteri. Clin Obstet Gynecol 6: 265–304.

Dixon IS, Stanley MA (1984): Immunofluorescent studies of human cervical epithelia in vitro using antibodies against specific keratin components. Mol Biol Med 2: 37–51.

Dollard SC, Wilson JL, Demeter LM, Bonnez W, Reichman RC, Broker TR, Chow LT (1992): Production of human papillomavirus and modulation of the infectious program in epithelial raft cultures. Genes Dev 6: 1131–1142.

Fluhmann CF (1961): "The Cervix Uteri and Its Diseases." Philadelphia: W.B. Saunders, pp 30–102.

Fusenig NE, Amer SM, Boukamp P, Worst PK (1978): Characteristics of chemically transformed mouse epidermal cells in vitro and in vivo. Bull Cancer 65: 271–279.

Gey GO, Coffman WD, Kubicek MD (1952): Tissue culture studies of the proliferative capacity of cervical carcinoma and normal epithelium. Cancer Res 12: 264–265.

Green H (1978): Cyclic AMP in relation to the epidermal cell: A new view. Cell 15: 801–811.

Ho TH, Chew EC, Tam JS, Hou HJ, Yam HF, Chew-Cheng SB, Wong FW (1993): Biological characteristics of a newly established human cervical carcinoma cell line. Anticancer Res 13: 967–971.

IARC Monographs on the Evaluation of Carcinogen Risks to Humans. (1996): Vol. 64, "Human Papillomaviruses." Lyon, France: World Health Organization International Agency for Research on Cancer, 1995 (Meeting of IARC Working Group on 6–13 June 1995).

Kelland LR, Burgess L, Steel GG (1987): Characterization of four new cell lines derived from human squamous carcinomas of the uterine cervix. Cancer Res 47: 4947–4952.

Kopan R, Traska G, Fuchs E (1987): Retinoids as important regulators of terminal differentiation: Examining keratin expression in individual epidermal cells at various stages of keratinization. J Cell Biol 105: 427–439.

Kusanagi T, Matsuura M, Kudo R (1980): [Histological and histochemical observation of cultured cells derived from normal human cervical epithelium (author's translation)]. Acta Obstet Gynaecol Jpn 32: 1907–1916.

Liaw KL, Glass AG, Manos MM, Greer CE, Scott DR, Sherman M, Burk RD, Kurman RJ, Wacholder S, Rush BB, Cadell DM, Lawler P, Tabor D, Schiffman M (1999): Detection of human papillomavirus DNA in cytologically normal women and subsequent cervical squamous intraepithelial lesions. J Natl Cancer Inst 91: 954–960.

Lillie JH, MacCallum DK, Jepsen A (1980): Fine structure of subcultivated stratified squamous epithelium grown on collagen rafts. Exp Cell Res 125: 153–165.

McDougall JK (1994): Immortalization and transformation of human cells by human papillomavirus. Curr Top Microbiol Immunol 186: 101–119.

Moll R, Franke WW, Schiller DL, Geiger B, Krepler R (1982): The catalog of human cytokeratins: Patterns of expression in normal epithelia, tumors and cultured cells. Cell 31: 11–24.

Pal AK, Pratap M, Mitra AB (1992): Cervix tumour cell line established from tumour after long term passages as heterotransplant in nude mice. Indian J Exp Biol 30: 655–656.

Parker JN, Zhao W, Askins KJ, Broker TR, Chow LT (1997): Mutational analyses of differentiation-dependent human papillomavirus type 18 enhancer elements in epithelial raft cultures of neonatal foreskin keratinocytes. Cell Growth Differ 8: 751–762.

Peehl DM, Ham RG (1980): Growth and differentiation of human keratinocytes without a feeder layer or conditioned medium. In Vitro 16: 516–525.

Rheinwald JG, Green H (1975): Serial cultivation of strains of human epidermal keratinocytes: The formation of keratinizing colonies from single cells. Cell 6: 331–344.

Rheinwald JG, Green H (1977): Epidermal growth factor and the multiplication of cultured human keratinocytes. Nature 265: 421–424.

Rice RH, Green H (1979): Presence in human cells of a soluble precursor of the cross-linked envelope: Activation of crosslinking by calcium ions. Cell 18: 681–694.

Richart RM, Wright TC Jr. (1991): Pathology of the cervix. Curr Opin Obstet Gynecol 3: 561–567.

Schiller W (1929): Jodspinselung und Abschabung der Portioepithels. Zbl Gynaekol 53: 1056–1064.

Shingleton HM, Laurence WD (1976): Transmission electron microscopy of the physiological epithelium. In Jordan JA, Singer A. (eds): "The Cervix." London: W.B. Saunders, pp 36–50.

Singer A, Jordan JA (1976): The anatomy of the cervix. In Jordan JA, Singer A (eds): "The Cervix." London: W.B. Saunders, pp 89–93.

Stanley MA (1986): Human cervical epithelium. In Webber MM, Sekely LI (eds): "In Vitro Models for Cancer Research." Boca Raton, Fl: CRC Press, Vol. 3.

Stanley MA, Browne HM, Appleby M, Minson AC (1989): Properties of a non tumorigenic human cervical keratinocyte cell line. Int J Cancer 43: 672–676.

Stanley MA, Dahlenburg K (1984): Factors controlling the growth of human cervical epithelium in culture. In Vitro 20: 144–151.

Stanley MA, Parkinson EK (1979): Growth requirements of human cervical epithelial cells in culture. Int J Cancer 24: 407–414.

Todaro JG, Green H (1963): Quantitative studies of the growth of mouse embryo cells in culture and their development into established cell lines. J Cell Biol 17: 199–213.

Tsao MC, Walthall BJ, Ham RG (1982): Clonal growth of normal human epidermal keratinocytes in a defined medium. J Cell Physiol 110: 219–229.

Vesterinen E, Leinikki P, Saksela E (1975): Cytopathogenicity of cytomegalovirus to human ecto- and endocervical epithelial cells in vitro. Acta Cytol 19: 473–481.

Waggoner SE, Wang X (1994): Effect of nicotine on proliferation of normal, malignant, and human papillomavirus transformed human cervical cells. Gynecol Oncol 55: 91–95.

Walts AE, Said JW, Siegel MB, Banks-Schlegel S (1985): Involucrin, a marker of squamous and urothelial differentiation. An immunohistochemical study on its distribution in normal and neoplastic tissues. J Pathol 145: 329–340.

Warhol MJ, Antonioli DA, Pinkus GS, Burke L, Rice RH (1982): Immuno-peroxidase staining for involucrin: A potential diagnostic aid in cervico-vaginal pathology. Hum Pathol 13: 1095–1099.

Wilbanks GD, Fink CG (1976): Tissue and organ culture of cervical epithelium. In Jordan JA, Singer A. (eds): "The Cervix." London: W.B. Saunders, pp 429–441.

APPENDIX: SOURCES OF MATERIALS

Item	Catalog No.	Supplier
Amphotericin B	A2411 15290	Sigma GIBCO
Cholera toxin (mol wt 84,000)	C3012	Sigma
DMEM (Dulbecco's modification of Eagle's medium)	31885	GIBCO

EDTA:
  Ethylenediamine tetraacetic
    acid disodium salt
  Free acid, anhydrous
	E1644
	
	E66758
		Sigma
		
		Sigma

Epidermal growth factor	E4127	Sigma
Formol saline, buffered	HT50	Sigma
Geneticin crystalline nonsterile (G418 sulfate)	11811	GIBCO
Gentamicin sulfate solution	G1264	Sigma
Ham's F12	21765	GIBCO
Hydrocortisone	H-4251	Sigma
Insulin	I-1882	Sigma
Tissue Tek®OCT™	4583	Sakura (Raymond Lamb in UK)
Rat tail collagen	354236	Becton Dickinson

Serum-free defined keratinocyte growth medium:
  KGM
  Keratinocyte SFM
  Epi-Life™ serum-free
    medium plus keratinocyte
    medium supplement
	
	BW3194
	17005-034
	E 0151
	K 2007
		
		BioWhittaker
		GIBCO
		Sigma
		Sigma

apo-Transferrin	T-1147	Sigma
Trypsin	T-4665	Sigma

6

Human Prostatic Epithelial Cells

Donna M. Peehl

Department of Urology, Stanford University School of Medicine, Stanford, CA 94305, USA dpeehl@leland.stanford.edu

Culture of Epithelial Cells, pages 171–194

I. BACKGROUND

The prostate is a small gland of the male genitourinary tract. Maturing at puberty in response to androgen, the prostate's major function in the adult is to provide approximately 30% of the components of seminal fluid [Cunha et al., 1987]. This seemingly innocuous gland becomes conspicuous because of its propensity for developing disease. The prostate has the highest frequency of any organ for manifesting a benign proliferative disorder called *benign prostatic hyperplasia* or BPH [McNeal, 1984]. Prostate cancer is ubiquitous worldwide and is the second leading cause of cancer deaths among men in the United States [Landis et al., 1999].

The human prostate differs considerably from that of rodents with regard to embryological development, adult anatomy, and etiology of disease. Nevertheless, the rat has been used extensively as an animal model to study normal prostatic development and physiology and hormonal initiation and promotion of cancer [Lucia et al., 1998]. Transgenic mice are now available with genes targeted specifically to the prostate (for reviews, see [Green et al., 1998; Sharma and Schreiber-Agus, 1999]. Similarly, the canine prostate develops hyperplasia, dysplasia, and cancer in aged animals and has been used as an animal model for BPH and neoplasia [Waters et al., 1998].

The development of in vitro culture systems has permitted many studies aimed at defining the biological properties of prostatic epithelial cells, a primary goal being the identification of the molecular changes in prostate cells that lead to the development of cancer and proliferative disease. From early studies with explant cultures in relatively undefined conditions, techniques have been refined to permit monolayer culture of epithelial as well as stromal cells in serum-free media and in sophisticated three-dimensional histocultures. Optimized culture methods are now available for human prostatic epithelial cells as well as prostatic cells derived from rat, mouse, and dog. Great strides have been made toward a better understanding of the biology of the normal adult prostate and the development of benign and malignant diseases. The availability of optimal culture systems beckons to those who would participate in efforts toward control of these diseases through research.

2. PREPARATION OF SOLUTIONS AND MEDIA

2.1. Media and Salt Solutions

2.1.1. HEPES-Buffered Saline (HBS)

(i)   Dissolve HEPES, free acid, (11.915 g) in 900 ml of UPW (to give final concentration of 50 mM).
(ii) Bring pH to 7.6 with NaOH.
(iii) Add:

	g	mM
Glucose	0.721	4
KCl	0.224	3
NaCl	7.597	130
$Na_2HPO_4 \cdot 7H_2O$	0.268	1
Phenol red-Na salt	0.001	0.003

(iv) Stir to dissolve, then bring to final volume of 1 liter with UPW.
(v)   Sterilize by vacuum-filtration through a 0.22-μm filter unit.
(vi) Store at 4°C for up to 1 month or freeze at -20°C for up to 1 yr.

2.1.2. Medium PFMR-4A

(i)   Prepare stock solutions listed in Appendix A: PFMR-4A Stocks.
(ii) To prepare 1 liter of PFMR-4A, add to 700 ml of UPW while stirring (note, there is no stock 6a):

Stock 1a	20 ml
Stock 1b	20 ml
Stock 1c	20 ml
Stock 2	10 ml
Stock 3	10 ml
Stock 5	1 ml

Stock 6b	10 ml
Stock 6c	10 ml
Stock 7	10 ml
Stock 8	10 ml
Stock 9	10 ml
Stock 10	10 ml
L-glutamine	2.922 g
D(+)-glucose	1.261 g
NaCl	5.845 g
KH_2PO_4	0.0585 g
HEPES	7.149 g

(iii)   Bring pH to 7.4 with 4 N NaOH and add:

$NaHCO_3$	1.176 g

(iv)   Bring to volume of 989 ml with UPW.

(v)   The medium can now be frozen, minus stocks 4 and 11, at −20°C for up to 1 yr.

(vi)   Before use, add while stirring:

Stock 4	10 ml
Stock 11	1 ml

(vii)   Sterilize by vacuum filtration through a 0.22-μm filter unit.

(viii)   Store at 4°C for up to 1 month.

2.1.3. Complete PFMR-4A

(i)   Prepare PFMR-4A as listed in Section 2.1.2.

(ii)   To 1 liter of sterile PFMR-4A, add the following amounts of sterile stock solutions:

	ml
Epidermal growth factor, 100 μg/ml stock	0.1
Cholera toxin, 100 μg/ml stock	0.1
Bovine pituitary extract (BPE), 14 mg/ml stock	2.8
Insulin, 4 mg/ml stock	1.0
Gentamicin sulfate, 40 mg/ml stock	2.5
Hydrocortisone, 10 mg/ml stock in 100% EtOH	0.1
Phosphoethanolamine, 0.1 M stock	1.0
Selenous acid, 3×10^{-4} M stock	0.1
α-Tocopherol, 2.3×10^{-2} M stock in DMSO	0.1
Retinoic acid, 3×10^{-7} M stock in DMSO	0.1

(iii)   Store at 4°C for up to 2 wk

2.1.4. Complete MCDB 105

Prepare MCDB 105 according to manufacturer's instructions. To 1 liter of sterile MCDB 105, add the supplements indicated for the preparation of complete PFMR-4A (see Section 2.1.3), except add 0.7 ml instead of 2.8 ml of BPE. Store at 4°C for up to 2 wk.

2.2. Disaggregation Solutions

2.2.1. Trypsin/EDTA solution (T/E)

(i) Dissolve:

Trypsin	0.2 g	
EDTA·Na$_2$·2H$_2$O	0.2 g	6.8 mM
in HBS	100 ml	

(ii) Sterilize by vacuum-filtration through a 0.22-μm filter unit.
(iii) Transfer 5-ml aliquots to tubes and freeze at -20°C for up to 1 yr.
(iv) Each aliquot should be thawed just before use, and remaining solution should be refrozen. Each aliquot may be freeze-thawed several times before trypsin loses adequate potency.

2.2.2. Trypsin Inhibitor (TI)

Dissolve 0.5 g of type 1 soybean trypsin inhibitor in 500 ml of HBS. Sterilize by vacuum-filtration through a 0.22-μm filter unit. Store at 4°C

2.2.3. Collagenase-Digestion Medium

To 10 ml of complete PFMR-4A, add 100 units/ml of collagenase. Stir to dissolve; then filter-sterilize through a 0.22-μm filter. Use fresh.

2.3. Collagen-Coated Dishes

(i) Add 1 ml of cold Vitrogen-100 collagen to 4 ml of sterile 0.013 N HCl at room temperature.
(ii) Distribute aliquots to plastic tissue culture dishes (0.2 ml per 35-mm dish, 0.3 ml per 6-cm dish, 0.5 ml per 10-cm dish).
(iii) Swirl and knock to disperse collagen solution evenly over bottom of dish.
(iv) Store at room temperature for several days to dry thoroughly. In humid climates, it may be necessary to dry by

placing dishes with lids ajar in a laminar flow hood overnight. It is essential that the collagen film is absolutely dry
before use or the collagen film may peel off on the addition
of medium and cells. Once dry, collagen-coated dishes can
be stored indefinitely at room temperature.

3. PROTOCOLS FOR PRIMARY CULTURE OF HUMAN PROSTATIC EPITHELIAL CELLS

3.1. Acquisition of Tissue

Adult human prostatic tissues can be procured from specimens
obtained by autopsy, cystoprostatectomy, radical prostatectomy,
open prostatectomy, transurethral resection of the prostate, and
needle biopsy or aspiration. Each source provides various advantages and disadvantages. The intact prostate is removed by radical
prostatectomy, and dissection of normal (undiseased) tissues, as
well as BPH and cancer, is often feasible. Cystoprostatectomies,
which are performed to treat bladder cancer, also provide an intact
prostate and a source of normal tissues. However, careful histologic analysis is essential to ensure that the putative normal tissue
obtained for culture is not contaminated by transitional carcinoma
of the bladder, BPH, or cancer of the prostate. Open prostatectomies are performed to remove large volumes of BPH and should
provide pure BPH tissue. Transurethral resections of the prostate
are becoming infrequent as alternate treatments for BPH become
more popular and probably will not provide much material for
culture in the future. We have no personal experience with autopsy material, but such tissue, if secured in a timely manner,
should present no unusual problems. Cell cultures can be derived
from needle biopsies, but the small size of the biopsy makes histologic verification of the tissue problematic.

3.2. Histologic Classification of Tissue

The prostate is a heterogeneous gland and therefore does not
present an easy subject for the biologist who is not a pathologist.
It is essential that a person familiar with the morphology and
histology of the prostate be available for tissue acquisition and
subsequent histologic analysis. A detailed description of the prostate cannot be provided here, but the publications of McNeal
[McNeal, 1984, 1988a, b] are excellent. Briefly, the adult human
prostate is composed of the central, peripheral, and transition

zones, each with distinguishing morphologic features. Cancer of the prostate occurs most frequently in the peripheral zone, whereas BPH is predominantly a disease of the transition zone. The central zone appears to be relatively immune to the development of cancer and BPH.

The protocol used in our laboratory to obtain and evaluate tissues is described in Schmid and McNeal [1992]. Small wedges of tissue (~ 10 mm^3) are dissected from prostate specimens using sterile technique. Colored inks are used to mark the cut edges within the prostate where wedges were removed, and then the prostate is fixed and serially sectioned. In this way, it is possible to map the origin of the dissected material precisely and to characterize, histologically, the tissue adjacent to and surrounding the wedges removed for culture.

It must be emphasized that in the absence of in vitro markers to distinguish, definitively, normal from BPH or cancer cells (see Section 6), it is of the utmost importance that a detailed histologic analysis be provided for each sample from which a cultured cell strain is derived. It is not sufficient to presume the nature of a sample on the basis of the type of procedure used to procure the tissue. Thus, although patients whose prostates are removed by cystoprostatectomy often have no clinical symptoms of BPH or prostate cancer, it is quite probable that BPH and/or cancer is present because of the high incidence of these diseases in the older male population.

3.3. Isolation of Cells

Protocol 6.1. Collection and Disaggregation of Prostate Tissue

Reagents and Materials

Sterile

- ❑ HBS, 4°C (see Section 2.1.1)
- ❑ Collagenase digestion medium (see Section 2.2.3)
- ❑ Complete PFMR-4A (see Section 2.1.3)
- ❑ Petri dishes, 6 cm
- ❑ Forceps
- ❑ Scissors

Protocol

(a) Collect tissue sample in sterile vessel containing cold HBS. Store at 4°C for processing within a few hours.

(b) Transfer sample from collection vessel to a 6-cm dish containing 5 ml of HBS.

(c) Rinse tissue three times with 5 ml of HBS each time.

(d) Using sterile forceps and scissors, mince to pieces of approximately 1 mm^3.

(e) With a wide-bore pipette, transfer pieces to a centrifuge tube.

(f) Spin in a clinical centrifuge at 250 g for 5 min.

(g) Discard supernatant and resuspend tissue in 10 ml of collagenase digestion medium.

(h) Rock tissue gently at 37°C for 12–18 h.

(i) Vigorously pipette fragments to break up clumps.

(j) Spin for 20 s in a clinical centrifuge at 250 g.

(k) Discard supernatant. Resuspend pellet in 5 ml of HBS and vigorously pipette.

(l) Repeat steps (j) and (k) two more times.

(m) After the final spin, discard supernatant and resuspend pellet in 5 ml of complete PFMR-4A.

3.4. Primary Culture

Protocol 6.2. Primary Culture of Prostatic Epithelium

Reagents and Materials

Sterile

❑ Complete PFMR-4A (see Section 2.1.3)
❑ Collagen-coated dishes, 6 cm (see Section 2.3)

Protocol

(a) Transfer cell suspension in 5 ml of complete PFMR-4A (see Protocol 6.1) to one 6-cm, collagen-coated dish.

(b) Incubate at 37°C in a 95% air-5% CO_2 humidified incubator.

(c) After 3–4 days, clumps of epithelial cells should have attached. Remove medium and replace with fresh complete PFMR-4A.

(d) Feed with complete PFMR-4A every 3–4 days until cells are semiconfluent (approximately 1×10^6 cells per 6-cm dish).

Typically, cells reach this stage at about 1 wk after initiation of the culture. At this time, subculture or freeze the cells.

3.5. Subculture

Protocol 6.3. Subculture of Prostatic Epithelial Cultures

Reagents and Materials

- ❏ Complete MCDB 105 (see Section 2.1.4)
- ❏ Complete PFMR-4A (see Section 2.1.3) if confluent cultures required
- ❏ HBS (see Section 2.1.1)
- ❏ T/E: Trypsin/EDTA (see Section 2.2.1)
- ❏ TI: HBS containing 0.1% soybean trypsin inhibitor (see Section 2.2.2)
- ❏ Hemocytometer or electronic cell counter (Beckman Coulter, Schärfe)

Protocol

(a) Remove medium.
(b) Rinse once with HBS.
(c) Add T/E, 1 ml per 6-cm dish.
(d) Incubate at 37°C for approximately 3 min or until cells round up.
(e) Resuspend cells by adding TI, 5 ml per 6-cm dish, and pipetting vigorously.
(f) Transfer suspended cells to a centrifuge tube. Rinse dish with 5 ml of HBS and add rinse to centrifuge tube.
(g) Remove small aliquot of cell suspension to determine cell number with a hemocytometer or electronic cell counter.
(h) Spin cells in clinical centrifuge at 250 g for 5 min.
(i) Discard supernatant and resuspend cells in complete MCDB 105.
(j) Distribute up to 5×10^4 cells per dish into 10-cm collagen-coated dishes (final volume of medium = 10 ml). It is important that the cells be seeded sparsely for optimal growth.
(k) Incubate at 37°C and feed with complete MCDB 105 every 3–4 days until cultures become semiconfluent (generally 7–10 days, depending on initial inoculum). It is important to subculture when cells are still subconfluent and actively dividing. If confluent cultures are desired, then switch to complete PFMR-4A and feed every 3–4 days until confluence is achieved.

Colony-forming efficiencies average 30% for secondary cultures and decrease with serial culture. Cell lines generally undergo 30 population doublings (~3–5 passages, depending on the cell densities of serial cultures) before becoming senescent.

3.6. Freezing and Thawing Cells

Because of the limited life span and relatively low plating efficiency of prostatic epithelial cells in vitro, it is wise to freeze numerous ampoules containing small numbers of cells from primary cultures. This offers the investigator the opportunity to study an individual cell line over a long period of time without losing the line.

Protocol 6.4. Cryopreservation of Prostatic Epithelial Cultures

Reagents and Materials

Sterile

- ❏ Freezing medium: Complete MCDB 105 with 10% DMSO and 10% fetal bovine serum
- ❏ HBS (see Section 2.1.1)
- ❏ Complete MCDB 105 (see Section 2.1.4)
- ❏ Complete PFMR-4A if cells to be grown to confluence (see Section 2.1.3)
- ❏ Cryotubes (Nalge Nunc)
- ❏ Collagen-coated dish, 10-cm

Protocol

(a) Resuspend cells as in Protocol 6.3, steps (a) through (h).
(b) Resuspend pellet in freezing medium to yield a concentration of 1×10^4 cells/ml.
(c) Transfer 1 ml of cell suspension in freezing medium to each sterile cryotube.
(d) Place cryotubes at 4°C for 3 h. Do not place in any sort of holder (such as Styrofoam), which would impede cooling.
(e) Transfer cryotubes to −70°C overnight.
(f) Transfer vials to a liquid nitrogen cryogenic refrigerator for long-term storage.

△*Safety note*. A transparent face mask, cryoprotective gloves, and a fastened lab coat must be worn when placing any material into or removing from liquid nitrogen.

(g) To thaw cells, remove cryotube from liquid nitrogen storage and immediately place in 37°C water in a covered bucket to thaw. After the risk of explosion has passed (~30 s) you may agitate by hand to hasten thawing.

Δ *Safety note.* Ampoules stored in liquid nitrogen can explode when warmed if they have inspired any liquid nitrogen during storage. They are, therefore, best thawed in a covered container. Alternatively, ampoules may be stored in the vapor phase, eliminating the risk of explosion and allowing ampoules to be thawed in an open vessel.

(h) Wash cryotube with 95% ethanol. Dry for a few seconds.
(i) Transfer cells from cryotube to a centrifuge tube containing 5 ml of HBS.
(j) Spin in clinical centrifuge at 250 g for 5 min.
(k) Discard supernatant and resuspend cells in 10 ml of complete MCDB 105.
(l) Transfer cells to one 10-cm collagen-coated dish.
(m) Incubate at 37°C and feed with complete MCDB 105 every 3–4 days until semiconfluent. At this time, either serially passage or feed with complete PFMR-4A every 3–4 days until confluent.

3.7. General Comments

No additional techniques are required to select against the growth of fibroblasts or other nonepithelial cells because of several elements of this culture system. First, collagenase is somewhat toxic to fibroblasts. Second, collagenase digests prostatic tissue into clumps of epithelial cells and predominantly single stromal cells. The brief 20-s spins in the isolation protocol separate the heavier clumps of epithelial cells from the single fibroblasts. Finally, the growth medium, used during primary culture, was optimized specifically for the growth of epithelial cells, and fibroblasts do not proliferate in this medium. The resulting cultures are composed of 100% epithelial cells, as determined by techniques described in Section 6, Cell Identification.

Questions may arise concerning the use of complete MCDB 105 for subcultures of prostatic epithelial cells. After comparing the ability of numerous basal media to support very low-density or clonal growth, we determined that MCDB 105 was superior to PFMR-4A in this regard. Similarly, we found that PFMR-4A supported better high-density cell growth than MCDB 105. Therefore, we use complete MCDB 105 for low-density conditions (clonal growth assays or subcultures at <50% confluence) and complete PFMR-4A for high-cell-density conditions (primary cultures or subcultures at >50% confluence).

Similarly, no special techniques are required to culture tumor cells. Normal, BPH, and malignant tissues all yield finite cell lines with similar efficiencies (approaching 90% in our laboratory with tissues derived from radical prostatectomies). However, it may be important to reduce the length of collagenase digestion for tissues derived from very high-grade cancers, which lack an acinar structure. We have had little experience with such tumors and are unable to make firm recommendations. Cells derived from needle biopsies can be cultured by slight modifications of the techniques described above [Peehl et al., 1991]. Stromal cells can also be cultured from the same specimens from which epithelial cells are derived [Peehl and Sellers, 1997].

The population doubling time of prostatic epithelial cells cultured according to these protocols is approximately 24 h during exponential growth. A number of peptide growth factors that regulate proliferation of prostatic epithelial cells have been identified [for reviews, see Culig et al., 1996; Djakiew, 2000; Lee et al., 1997; Peehl, 1996]. Among the extensive list of factors with growth-stimulatory properties are keratinocyte growth factor (KGF), hepatocyte growth factor (HGF), and insulin-like growth factor (IGF). Growth-inhibitory factors include retinoic acid, 1,25-dihydroxyvitamin D_3, and transforming growth factor (TGF)-β. Androgen responsiveness is not typically exhibited by primary cultures of prostatic epithelial cells [Berthon et al., 1997].

4. VARIATIONS

Other formulations of media and different techniques for establishment and propagation of human prostatic epithelial cells have been described [Bologna et al., 1993; Chaproniere and Mc-Keehan, 1986; Chopra et al., 1997; Cronauer et al., 1997; Cussenot et al., 1994; Delos et al., 1995; Gilad et al., 1996; Krill et al., 1997; Mitchen et al., 1997; Pantel et al., 1995; Robinson et al., 1998; Zwergel et al., 1998]. Prostatic epithelial cells from rodents have also been cultured by a variety of methods [Danielpour et al., 1994; Lipschutz et al., 1997; McKeehan et al., 1984; Ravindranath and Dym, 1999; Taketa et al., 1990]. Most of these protocols are similar in principle but involve diverse mixtures of enzymes for tissue dissociation, the use of Percoll gradients to separate epithelial from stromal cells, a variety of basal media, and serum or supplements of hormones and growth factors. Three-dimensional cultures of prostatic epithelial cells have been created, with or without the inclusion of stromal cells, in supports such as sponges, Matrigel, or collagen [Geller et al., 1992; O'Connor, 1999; Perrapato et al., 1990]. Improved methods for organ culture of human and rodent prostatic tissues have also been described [Lopes et al., 1996; Nevalainen et al., 1993; Sharma and Schreiber-Agus, 1999].

5. CONTINUOUS CELL LINES

Spontaneously immortalized cell lines are not easily derived from prostatic tissues. The most widely used human prostatic cell lines are LNCaP, DU 145, and PC-3, all derived from metastases [for review, see Peehl, 1994]. Other commonly used cell lines include TSU-Pr1, JCA, and ALVA-31 [for review, see Bosland et al., 1996]. New lines with characteristics particularly relevant to prostate cancer include the LuCaP, LACP, and CWR series of xenografts and derived cell cultures [Sramkoski et al., 1999; Stearns et al., 1998] and MDA PCa 2a and 2b, isolated from a metastasis to the bone [Navone et al., 1997]. Cell lines are generally grown in standard, serum-supplemented media such as RPMI 1640 with 10% fetal bovine serum. Serum-free media for some of the cell lines have been described [Pretlow et al., 1993]. Characteristics of each of the cell lines have been compiled [Liu et al., 1999; Mitchell et al., 2000].

Immortal and/or tumorigenic prostatic cell lines that represent the spectrum of prostate cancer progression have been developed from primary cultures by the introduction of oncogenes or exposure to chemicals or radiation [for reviews, see Rhim et al., 1996; Webber et al., 1996, 1997]. These transformed cell lines are often grown in keratinocyte serum-free medium (KSFM) supplemented with bovine pituitary extract and epidermal growth factor.

6. CELL IDENTIFICATION

Normal prostatic tissue contains glandular epithelia surrounded by a fibromuscular stroma [Cunha et al., 1987]. The epithelium in the mature male is typically a bilayer of basal cells and columnar secretory cells that line the lumen. Keratins, classic markers of epithelial cells, are differentially expressed in the basal and luminal cells. Keratins 5 and 14 are markers of basal cells, whereas keratins 8 and 18 are expressed by luminal cells [Brawer et al., 1985; Feitz et al., 1986; Nagle et al., 1987]. Stem cells (pluripotent cells that are capable of regenerating all elements of prostatic glandular structures) are believed to comprise a subset of basal cells, but definitive markers are still sought [De Marzo et al., 1998b; Reiter et al., 1998].

Two tissue-specific proteins that are made by the epithelial element of the gland have been described for the human prostate. The first is prostatic acid phosphatase (PAP) [Vihko et al., 1988], which is secreted in large amounts by the prostate. The other tissue marker is prostate-specific antigen (PSA), a protein with structural and functional similarity to kallikreins [Riegman et al., 1989; Watt et al., 1986].

Morphologic and immunocytochemical analyses can be used to characterize the phenotype of cell lines cultured from prostatic tissues.

6.1. Morphology

Epithelial cells cultured from normal, BPH, or malignant tissues retain their epithelial morphology in vitro. Typically, cultures contain small cuboidal cells that arrange themselves in a cobblestone pattern. Depending on the culture conditions, the cells may adhere tightly to each other and form cohesive colonies (such as when grown in medium containing keratinocyte growth factor) or they may be very migratory and form loose colonies (such as when grown in medium containing epidermal growth factor) [Peehl et al., 1996]. No morphologic features have been noted that distinguish cultures derived from normal, BPH, or malignant tissues.

6.2. Keratin Expression

The demonstration of keratin in a cell is positive proof of epithelial origin and can be accomplished by immunocytochemical labeling. The use of pan-keratin antibodies, which recognize epitopes of many keratins, would be appropriate for this purpose, or antibodies with more stringent specificity can be employed. Antibodies specific for keratin 5 or 14 stain all prostatic epithelial cells in culture, regardless of morphologic or histologic origin [Brawer et al., 1986]. Antibodies specific for keratin 8 or 18 label only a subset of cells. The simultaneous expression of basal and luminal cell-associated keratins by cultured prostatic cells resembles that described for the regenerating epithelium of the rat prostate on administration of androgen after castration [Bonkhoff et al., 1994].

6.3. Expression of Tissue-Specific Markers

PAP and PSA are not typically expressed in significant amounts by monolayer cultures of prostatic epithelial cell strains [Berthon et al., 1997]. Methods purported to promote expression of PSA include culture on Matrigel [Fong et al., 1991] and coculture with prostatic stromal cells [Bayne et al., 1998].

6.4. Cancer-Specific Markers

No marker has yet been identified that definitively distinguishes normal or BPH from cancer cells in culture. In the absence of distinctive biochemical markers for prostatic cancer cells in vitro, behavioral properties have been sought to identify cancer populations. Like cell lines from normal and BPH tissues, cell lines from cancer are mortal in culture. Tumorigenicity assays in *nude* mice do not provide a good index of the malignant potential of cultured prostatic epithelial cells. As has been noted for certain other types of human cancers, the formation of tumors by prostate cancer tissue in *nude* mice is very infrequent [Schroeder et al., 1976], apparently because of rejection by natural killer cells and macrophages [Reid et al., 1980]. Cancer-derived cells also do not generally differ from normal or BPH cells in their responses to stimulatory factors (such as epidermal growth factor or pituitary factors) or to inhibitory factors (including TGF-β or high levels of retinoic acid) [Peehl et al., 1989]. Karyotypic abnormalities have been noted in some finite cancer cell lines [Arps et al., 1993; Brothman et al., 1992; Chopra et al., 1997; Konig et al., 1998; Webb et al., 1996], but no consistent markers have been found and some investigators suggest that diploid cancer cells selectively grow in vitro [Ketter et al., 1996].

7. DIFFERENTIATION

Two alternative pathways of differentiation are believed to lead to the development of secretory luminal epithelial cells or neuroendocrine cells from precursor basal, or stem cells, in the prostate [Bonkhoff and Remberger, 1996]. An extensive list of markers of each of these cell lineages is becoming available to assess the differentiated phenotype of cultured prostatic epithelial cells. Genes that are expressed by basal cells in tissue as well as by cultured epithelial cells include telomerase [Belair et al., 1997], epidermal growth factor receptor [Cohen et al., 1994], CD44 [De Marzo et al., 1998a], and cytokeratins 5 and 14 [Peehl et al., 1994]. Certain markers of secretory luminal cells are also expressed by cultured epithelial cells, including cytokeratins 8 and 18 [Cussenot et al., 1994; Peehl et al., 1994; Pretlow et al., 1995; Robinson et al., 1998]. The simultaneous expression in a single cell of both basal and secretory cell markers is typical of so-called transit or amplifying cells that are seen in prostatic tissues [Bonkhoff et al., 1994; English et al., 1987; Evans and Chandler, 1987; Verhagen et al., 1992]. Further information regarding cell-specific gene expression and biological properties will come as protocols to isolate and culture pure populations of basal and secretory luminal cells are optimized [Liu et al., 1997, 1999; Ravindranath and Dym, 1999].

REFERENCES

Arps S, Rodewald A, Schmalenberger B, Carl P, Bressel M, Kastendieck H (1993): Cytogenetic survey of 32 cancers of the prostate. Cancer Genet Cytogenet 66: 93–99.

Bayne CW, Donnelly F, Chapman K, Bollina P, Buck C, Habib F (1998): A novel coculture model for benign prostatic hyperplasia expressing both isoforms of 5 alpha-reductase [published erratum appears in J Clin Endocrinol Metab 1998 Mar;83(3): 910]. J Clin Endocrinol Metab 83: 206–213.

Belair CD, Yeager TR, Lopez PM, Reznikoff CA (1997): Telomerase activity: a biomarker of cell proliferation, not malignant transformation. Proc Natl Acad Sci USA 94: 13677–13682.

Berthon P, Waller AS, Villette JM, Loridon L, Cussenot O, Maitland NJ (1997): Androgens are not a direct requirement for the proliferation of human prostatic epithelium in vitro. Int J Cancer 73: 910–916.

Bologna M, Vicentini C, Corrao G, Festuccia C, Muzi P, Tubaro A, Biordi L, Miano L (1993): Early diagnosis of prostatic carcinoma may be achieved through in vitro culture of tumor cells harvested by prostatic massage. Eur Urol 24: 148–155.

Bonkhoff H, Remberger K (1996): Differentiation pathways and histogenetic aspects of normal and abnormal prostatic growth: A stem cell model. Prostate 28: 98–106.

Bonkhoff H, Stein U, Remberger K (1994): Multidirectional differentiation in the normal, hyperplastic, and neoplastic human prostate: Simultaneous demonstration of cell-specific epithelial markers. Hum Pathol 25: 42–46.

Bosland MC, Chung LWK, Greenberg NM, Ho S, Isaacs JT, Lane K, Peehl DM, Thompson TC, van Steenbrugge GJ, van Weerden WM (1996): Recent advances in the development of animal and cell culture models for prostatic cancer research. Urol Oncol 2: 99–128.

Brawer MK, Bostwick DG, Peehl DM, Stamey TA (1986): Keratin protein in human prostatic tissue and cell culture. Ann NY Acad Sci 455: 729–731.

Brawer MK, Peehl DM, Stamey TA, Bostwick DG (1985): Keratin immuno-reactivity in the benign and neoplastic human prostate. Cancer Res 45: 3663–3667.

Brothman AR, Patel AM, Peehl DM, Schellhammer PF (1992): Analysis of prostatic tumor cultures using fluorescence in-situ hybridization (FISH). Cancer Genet Cytogenet 62: 180–185.

Chaproniere DM, McKeehan WL (1986): Serial culture of single adult human prostatic epithelial cells in serum-free medium containing low calcium and a new growth factor from bovine brain. Cancer Res 46: 819–824.

Chopra DP, Sarkar FH, Grignon DJ, Sakr WA, Mohamed A, Waghray A (1997): Growth of human nondiploid primary prostate tumor epithelial cells in vitro. Cancer Res 57: 3688–3692.

Cohen DW, Simak R, Fair WR, Melamed J, Scher HI, Cordon-Cardo C (1994): Expression of transforming growth factor-alpha and the epidermal growth factor receptor in human prostate tissues. J Urol 152: 2120–2124.

Cronauer MV, Eder IE, Hittmair A, Sierek G, Hobisch A, Culig Z, Thurnher M, Bartsch G, Klocker H (1997): A reliable system for the culture of human prostatic cells [letter]. In Vitro Cell Dev Biol Anim 33: 742–744.

Culig Z, Hobisch A, Cronauer MV, Radmayr C, Hittmair A, Zhang J, Thurnher M, Bartsch G, Klocker H (1996): Regulation of prostatic growth and function by peptide growth factors. Prostate 28: 392–405.

Cunha GR, Donjacour AA, Cooke PS, Mee S, Bigsby RM, Higgins SJ, Sugimura Y (1987): The endocrinology and developmental biology of the prostate. Endocr Rev 8: 338–362.

Cussenot O, Berthon P, Cochand-Priollet B, Maitland NJ, Le Duc A (1994): Immunocytochemical comparison of cultured normal epithelial prostatic cells with prostatic tissue sections. Exp Cell Res 214: 83–92.

Danielpour D, Kadomatsu K, Anzano MA, Smith JM, Sporn MB (1994): Development and characterization of nontumorigenic and tumorigenic epithelial cell lines from rat dorsal-lateral prostate. Cancer Res 54: 3413–3421.

De Marzo AM, Bradshaw C, Sauvageot J, Epstein JI, Miller GJ (1998a): CD44 and CD44v6 downregulation in clinical prostatic carcinoma: relation to Gleason grade and cytoarchitecture. Prostate 34: 162–168.

De Marzo AM, Meeker AK, Epstein JI, Coffey DS (1998b): Prostate stem cell compartments: Expression of the cell cycle inhibitor p27Kip1 in normal, hyperplastic, and neoplastic cells. Am J Pathol 153: 911–919.

Delos S, Carsol JL, Ghazarossian E, Raynaud JP, Martin PM (1995): Testosterone metabolism in primary cultures of human prostate epithelial cells and fibroblasts. J Steroid Biochem Mol Biol 55: 375–383.

Djakiew D (2000): Dysregulated expression of growth factors and their receptors in the development of prostate cancer. Prostate 42: 150–160.

English HF, Santen RJ, Isaacs JT (1987): Response of glandular versus basal rat ventral prostatic epithelial cells to androgen withdrawal and replacement. Prostate 11: 229–242.

Evans GS, Chandler JA (1987): Cell proliferation studies in rat prostate. I. The proliferative role of basal and secretory epithelial cells during normal growth. Prostate 10: 163–178.

Feitz WF, Debruyne FM, Vooijs GP, Herman CJ, Ramaekers FC (1986): Intermediate filament proteins as tissue specific markers in normal and malignant urological tissues. J Urol 136: 922–931.

Fong CJ, Sherwood ER, Sutkowski DM, Abu-Jawdeh GM, Yokoo H, Bauer KD, Kozlowski JM, Lee C (1991): Reconstituted basement membrane promotes morphological and functional differentiation of primary human prostatic epithelial cells. Prostate 19: 221–235.

Geller J, Sionit LR, Connors K, Hoffman RM (1992): Measurement of androgen sensitivity in the human prostate in in vitro three-dimensional histoculture. Prostate 21: 269–278.

Gilad E, Laudon M, Matzkin H, Pick E, Sofer M, Braf Z, Zisapel N (1996): Functional melatonin receptors in human prostate epithelial cells. Endocrinology 137: 1412–1417.

Green JE, Greenberg NM, Ashendel CL, Barrett JC, Boone C, Getzenberg RH, Henkin J, Matusik R, Janus TJ, Scher HI (1998): Workgroup 3: transgenic and reconstitution models of prostate cancer. Prostate 36: 59–63.

Ketter R, Zwergel T, Romanakis K, Unteregger G, Ziegler M, Zang KD, Wullich B (1996): Selection toward diploid cells in prostatic carcinoma derived cell cultures. Prostate 28: 364–371.

Konig JJ, Teubel W, Kamst E, Romijn JC, Schroder FH, Hagemeijer A (1998): Cytogenetic analysis of 39 prostate carcinomas and evaluation of short-term tissue culture techniques. Cancer Genet Cytogenet 101: 116–122.

Krill D, Shuman M, Thompson MT, Becich MJ, Strom SC (1997): A simple method for the isolation and culture of epithelial and stromal cells from benign and neoplastic prostates. Urology 49: 981–988.

Landis SH, Murray T, Bolden S, Wingo PA (1999): Cancer statistics. CA Cancer J Clin 49: 8–31.

Lee C, Kozlowski JM, Grayhack JT (1997): Intrinsic and extrinsic factors controlling benign prostatic growth. Prostate 31: 131–138.

Lipschutz JH, Foster BA, Cunha GR (1997): Differentiation of rat neonatal ventral prostates grown in a serum-free organ culture system. Prostate 32: 35–42.

Liu AY, True LD, LaTray L, Ellis WJ, Vessella RL, Lange PH, Higano CS, Hood L, van den Engh G (1999): Analysis and sorting of prostate cancer cell types by flow cytometry. Prostate 40: 192–199.

Liu AY, True LD, LaTray L, Nelson PS, Ellis WJ, Vessella RL, Lange PH, Hood L, van den Engh G (1997): Cell-cell interaction in prostate gene regulation and cytodifferentiation. Proc Natl Acad Sci USA 94: 10705–10710.

Lopes ES, Foster BA, Donjacour AA, Cunha GR (1996): Initiation of secretory activity of rat prostatic epithelium in organ culture. Endocrinology 137: 4225–4234.

Lucia MS, Bostwick DG, Bosland M, Cockett AT, Knapp DW, Leav I, Pollard M, Rinker-Schaeffer C, Shirai T, Watkins BA (1998): Workgroup I: Rodent models of prostate cancer. Prostate 36: 49–55.

McKeehan WL, Adams PS, Rosser MP (1984): Direct mitogenic effects of insulin, epidermal growth factor, glucocorticoid, cholera toxin, unknown pituitary factors and possibly prolactin, but not androgen, on normal rat prostate epithelial cells in serum-free, primary cell culture. Cancer Res 44: 1998–2010.

McNeal JE (1984): Anatomy of the prostate and morphogenesis of BPH. In Kimball FA, Buhl AE, Carter DB (eds): "New Approaches to the Study of Benign Prostatic Hyperplasia." New York: Alan R. Liss, pp 17–53.

McNeal JE (1988a): Normal histology of the prostate. Am J Surg Pathol 12: 619–633.

McNeal JE (1988b): The prostate gland: Morphology and pathobiology. Monogr Urol 9: 36–54.

Mitchell S, Abel P, Ware M, Stamp G, Lalani E (2000): Phenotypic and genotypic characterization of commonly used human prostatic cell lines. BJU Int 85: 932–944.

Mitchen J, Oberley T, Wilding G (1997): Extended culturing of androgen-responsive human primary epithelial prostate cell isolates by continuous treatment with interstitial collagenase. Prostate 30: 7–19.

Nagle RB, Ahmann FR, McDaniel KM, Paquin ML, Clark VA, Celniker A (1987): Cytokeratin characterization of human prostatic carcinoma and its derived cell lines. Cancer Res 47: 281–286.

Navone NM, Olive M, Ozen M, Davis R, Troncoso P, Tu SM, Johnston D, Pollack A, Pathak S, von Eschenbach AC, Logothetis CJ (1997): Establishment of two human prostate cancer cell lines derived from a single bone metastasis. Clin Cancer Res 3: 2493–2500.

Nevalainen MT, Harkonen PL, Valve EM, Ping W, Nurmi M, Martikainen PM (1993): Hormone regulation of human prostate in organ culture. Cancer Res 53: 5199–5207.

O'Connor KC (1999): Three-dimensional cultures of prostatic cells: Tissue models for the development of novel anti-cancer therapies. Pharm Res 16: 486–493.

Pantel K, Dickmanns A, Zippelius A, Klein C, Shi J, Hoechtlen-Vollmar W, Schlimok G, Weckermann D, Oberneder R, Fanning E, et al. (1995): Establishment of micrometastatic carcinoma cell lines: a novel source of tumor cell vaccines. J Natl Cancer Inst 87: 1162–1168.

Peehl DM (1994): The male reproductive system: Prostatic cell lines. In Hay RJ, Park J-G, Gazdar A (eds): "Atlas of Human Tumor Cell Lines." San Diego: Academic Press, pp 387–411.

Peehl DM (1996): Cellular biology of prostatic growth factors. Prostate Suppl 6: 74–78.

Peehl DM, Leung GK, Wong ST (1994): Keratin expression: a measure of phenotypic modulation of human prostatic epithelial cells by growth inhibitory factors. Cell Tissue Res 277: 11–18.

Peehl DM, Sellers RG (1997): Induction of smooth muscle cell phenotype in cultured human prostatic stromal cells. Exp Cell Res 232: 208–215.

Peehl DM, Wong ST, Bazinet M, Stamey TA (1989): In vitro studies of human prostatic epithelial cells: Attempts to identify distinguishing features of malignant cells. Growth Factors 1: 237–250.

Peehl DM, Wong ST, Rubin JS (1996): KGF and EGF differentially regulate the phenotype of prostatic epithelial cells. Growth Regul 6: 22–31.

Peehl DM, Wong ST, Terris MK, Stamey TA (1991): Culture of prostatic epithelial cells from ultrasound-guided needle biopsies. Prostate 19: 141–147.

Perrapato SD, Slocum HK, Huben RP, Ghosh R, Rustum Y (1990): Assessment of human genitourinary tumors and chemosensitivity testing in 3-dimensional collagen gel culture. J Urol 143: 1041–1045.

Pretlow TG, Ogrinc GS, Amini SB, Delmoro CM, Molkentin KF, Willson JK, Pretlow TP (1993): A better defined medium for human prostate cancer cells [letter]. In Vitro Cell Dev Biol Anim 29A: 528–530.

Pretlow TG, Yang B, Pretlow TP (1995): Organ culture of benign, aging, and hyperplastic human prostate. Microsc Res Tech 30: 271–281.

Ravindranath N, Dym M (1999): Isolation of rat ventral prostate basal and luminal epithelial cells by the STAPUT technique. Prostate 41: 173–180.

Reid LCM, Minato N, Rojkind M (1980): Human prostatic cells in culture and in conditioned animals. In Spring-Mills E, Hafez ESE (eds): "Male Accessory Sex Glands." Vol 4. New York: Elsevier/North-Holland Biomedical Press, pp 617–640.

Reiter RE, Gu Z, Watabe T, Thomas G, Szigeti K, Davis E, Wahl M, Nisitani S, Yamashiro J, Le Beau MM, Loda M, Witte ON (1998): Prostate stem cell antigen: A cell surface marker overexpressed in prostate cancer. Proc Natl Acad Sci USA 95: 1735–1740.

Rhim JS, Peehl DM, Webber MM, Jay G, Dritschilo A (1996): In vitro multistep human prostate epithelial cell models for studying prostate carcinogenesis. Rad Oncol Invest 3: 326–329.

Riegman PH, Vlietstra RJ, van der Korput JA, Romijn JC, Trapman J (1989): Characterization of the prostate-specific antigen gene: a novel human kallikrein-like gene. Biochem Biophys Res Commun 159: 95–102.

Robinson EJ, Neal DE, Collins AT (1998): Basal cells are progenitors of luminal cells in primary cultures of differentiating human prostatic epithelium. Prostate 37: 149–160.

Schmid HP, McNeal JE (1992): An abbreviated standard procedure for accurate tumor volume estimation in prostate cancer. Am J Surg Pathol 16: 184–191.

Schroeder FH, Okada K, Jellinghaus W, Wullstein HK, Heinemeyer HM (1976): Human prostatic adenoma and carcinoma. Transplantation of cultured cells and primary tissue fragments in "nude" mice. Invest Urol 13: 395–403.

Sharma P, Schreiber-Agus N (1999): Mouse models of prostate cancer. Oncogene 18: 5349–5355.

Sramkoski RM, Pretlow TG 2d, Giaconia JM, Pretlow TP, Schwartz S, Sy MS, Marengo SR, Rhim JS, Zhang D, Jacobberger JW (1999): A new human prostate carcinoma cell line, 22Rv1. In Vitro Cell Dev Biol Anim 35: 403–409.

Stearns ME, Ware JL, Agus DB, Chang CJ, Fidler IJ, Fife RS, Goode R, Holmes E, Kinch MS, Peehl DM, Pretlow TG 2d, Thalmann GN (1998): Workgroup 2: Human xenograft models of prostate cancer. Prostate 36: 56–58.

Taketa S, Nishi N, Takasuga H, Okutani T, Takenaka I, Wada F (1990): Differences in growth requirements between epithelial and stromal cells derived from rat ventral prostate in serum-free primary culture. Prostate 17: 207–218.

Verhagen AP, Ramaekers FC, Aalders TW, Schaafsma HE, Debruyne FM, Schalken JA (1992): Colocalization of basal and luminal cell-type cytokeratins in human prostate cancer. Cancer Res 52: 6182–6187.

Vihko P, Virkkunen P, Henttu P, Roiko K, Solin T, Huhtala ML (1988): Molecular cloning and sequence analysis of cDNA encoding human prostatic acid phosphatase. FEBS Lett 236: 275–281.

Waters DJ, Sakr WA, Hayden DW, Lang CM, McKinney L, Murphy GP, Radinsky R, Ramoner R, Richardson RC, Tindall DJ (1998): Workgroup 4: Spontaneous prostate carcinoma in dogs and nonhuman primates. Prostate 36: 64–67.

Watt KW, Lee PJ, M'Timkulu T, Chan WP, Loor R (1986): Human prostate-specific antigen: structural and functional similarity with serine proteases. Proc Natl Acad Sci USA 83: 3166–3170.

Webb HD, Hawkins AL, Griffin CA (1996): Cytogenetic abnormalities are frequent in uncultured prostate cancer cells. Cancer Genet Cytogenet 88: 126–132.

Webber MM, Bello D, Quader S (1996): Immortalized and tumorigenic adult human prostatic epithelial cell lines: Characteristics and applications. Part I. Cell markers and immortalized nontumorigenic cell lines. Prostate 29: 386–394.

Webber MM, Bello D, Quader S (1997): Immortalized and tumorigenic adult human prostatic epithelial cell lines: Characteristics and applications. Part 3. Oncogenes, suppressor genes, and applications. Prostate 30: 136–142.

Zwergel T, Kakirman H, Schorr H, Wullich B, Unteregger G (1998): A new serial transfer explant cell culture system for human prostatic cancer tissues preventing selection toward diploid cells. Cancer Genet Cytogenet 101: 16–23.

APPENDIX A: PFMR-4A STOCKS

(Note: there is no Stock 6a)

	Component	Concentration in Stock Solution (g/liter)
Stock 1a (50×)[a]	L-Arginine HCl	21.070
	Choline chloride	0.698
	L-Histidine HCl·H_2O	2.096
	L-Isoleucine	3.936
	L-Leucine	13.120
	L-Lysine HCl	3.654
	L-Methionine	4.476
Stock 1b (50×)[b]	L-Phenylalanine	0.496
	L-Serine	1.051
	L-Threonine	11.910
	L-Tryptophan	0.204
	L-Valine	1.172
Stock 1c (50×)[c]	L-Tyrosine	0.544
Stock 2 (100×)[d]	Biotin	0.00733
	Ca pantothenate	0.02383
	Niacinamide	0.00366
	Pyridoxine HCl	0.00617
	Thiamine HCl	0.03375
	KCl	28.348
Stock 3 (100×)[e]	$Na_2HPO_4·7H_2O$	21.7161
	Folic acid	0.1324
Stock 4 (100×)[f]	$FeSO_4·7H_2O$	0.0834
	$MgCl_2·6H_2O$	10.5716
	$MgSO_4·7H_2O$	3.9440
	$CaCl_2·2H_2O$	13.5240
Stock 5 (1000×)[g]	Phenol red-sodium salt	2.221
Stock 6b (100×)	Sodium pyruvate	22.00
Stock 6c (100×)[i]	Riboflavin	0.00376
Stock 7 (100×)[j]	L-Cystine	3.605
Stock 8 (100×)[k]	L-Asparagine	3.002
	L-Proline	6.906
	Putrescine 2HCl	0.032

Appendix A continues

(Note: there is no Stock 6a)

	Component	Concentration in Stock Solution (g/liter)
Stock 8 (100×)[k]	Vitamin B_{12}	0.136
Stock 9 (100×)[l]	L-Aspartate	2.662
	L-Glutamate	2.942
	L-Alanine	1.782
	Glycine	1.502
Stock 10 (100×)[m]	Hypoxanthine	0.4083
	6,8-Thioctic acid	0.0206
	myo-Inositol	18.0200
	Thymidine	0.7270
	$CuSO_4 \cdot 5H_2O$	0.00025
Stock 11 (1,000×)[n]	$ZnSO_4 \cdot 7H_2O$	0.1438

[a] Gently heat while stirring to dissolve. Store aliquots at −20°C for up to 1 yr. After thawing, gently warm to dissolve precipitate.

[b] Stir to dissolve. Store aliquots in dark at −20°C for up to 1 yr. After thawing, gently warm to dissolve precipitate.

[c] Dissolve solid in 50 ml of 4 N NaOH; then dilute to 1 liter with UPW. Store aliquots at −20°C for up to 1 yr.

[d] Stir to dissolve. Store aliquots in dark at −20°C for up to 1 yr.

[e] Completely dissolve sodium phosphate; then add folic acid. Be sure that folic acid completely dissolves. Store aliquots in dark at −20°C for up to 1 yr.

[f] Stir to dissolve. After preparation of stock, add 1 drop of concentrated HCl per 100 ml of stock to prevent precipitation. Store sterile at room temperature for up to 1 yr.

[s] Stir to dissolve. Store sterile at room temperature indefinitely.

[h] Stir to dissolve. Store in aliquots at −20°C for up to 1 yr.

[i] Riboflavin is difficult to dissolve and requires extensive stirring; cover with foil while stirring because riboflavin is light-sensitive. Store aliquots in dark at −20°C for up to 1 yr.

[j] Add concentrated HCl dropwise while stirring until all of solid dissolves. Make fresh immediately before use.

[k] Stir to dissolve. Store in dark in aliquots at −20°C for up to 1 yr.

[l] To prepare one liter of stock solution, add aspartic acid and glutamic acid to 900 ml of UPW containing 1 ml of Stock 5. While stirring, add 4 N NaOH dropwise to maintain neutrality (orange-pink color) as the acids dissolve. Then add alanine and glycine, stir to dissolve, and bring to final volume with UPW. Store in aliquots at −20°C for up to 1 yr.

[m] To prepare 1 liter of stock solution, dissolve hypoxanthine in 100 ml of boiling UPW; cool. Dissolve thioctic acid in a few drops of 1 N NaOH, dilute with 10 ml of UPW. Add hypoxanthine and thioctic acid solutions to 850 ml of UPW in which the remaining components have been dissolved; then bring to final volume with UPW. $CuSO_4 \cdot 5H_2O$ is prepared by dissolving 0.025 g in 1 liter of UPW; 10 ml of this is added to stock. Store in aliquots in dark at −20°C for up to 1 yr.

[n] Stir to dissolve. Store sterile at room temperature indefinitely.

APPENDIX B: MATERIALS AND SUPPLIERS

Material	Supplier
L-Alanine	Sigma-Aldrich[a]
L-Arginine HCl	Sigma-Aldrich
L-Asparagine	Sigma-Aldrich
L-Aspartic acid	Sigma-Aldrich
d-Biotin	Sigma-Aldrich
Bovine pituitary extract	Hammond Cell/Tech
$CaCl_2 \cdot 2H_2O$	Sigma-Aldrich
Cholera toxin	List Biological Laboratories
Choline chloride	Sigma-Aldrich
Collagenase, type I	Sigma-Aldrich
$CuSO_4 \cdot 5H_2O$	Sigma-Aldrich
L-Cystine	Sigma-Aldrich
DMSO	Sigma-Aldrich
$EDTA \cdot Na_2 \cdot 2H_2O$	Sigma-Aldrich
Epidermal growth factor	Becton Dickinson Labware
$Fe_2SO_4 \cdot 7H_2O$	Sigma-Aldrich
Folic acid	Sigma-Aldrich
$D(+)$-glucose	Sigma-Aldrich
Gentamicin sulfate	Gemini Bioproducts
L-Glutamic acid	Sigma-Aldrich
L-Glutamine	Sigma-Aldrich
Glycine	Sigma-Aldrich
HCl	Sigma-Aldrich
HEPES	Sigma-Aldrich
L-Histidine $HCl \cdot H_2O$	Sigma-Aldrich
Hydrocortisone	Sigma-Aldrich
Hypoxanthine	Sigma-Aldrich
myo-Inositol	Sigma-Aldrich
Insulin	Sigma-Aldrich
L-Isoleucine	Sigma-Aldrich
KCl	Sigma-Aldrich
KH_2PO_4	Sigma-Aldrich
KSFM	GIBCO-BRL
L-Leucine	Sigma-Aldrich

Appendix B continues

Material	Supplier
L-Lysine HCl	Sigma-Aldrich
MCDB 105	Sigma-Aldrich
$MgCl_2 \cdot 6H_2O$	Sigma-Aldrich
$MgSO_4 \cdot 7H_2O$	Sigma-Aldrich
L-Methionine	Sigma-Aldrich
NaCl	Sigma-Aldrich
$NaHCO_3$	Sigma-Aldrich
$Na_2HPO_4 7H_2O$	Sigma-Aldrich
NaOH	Sigma-Aldrich
Niacinamide	Sigma-Aldrich
D-Pantothenic acid $\cdot$ hemi-Ca-salt	Sigma-Aldrich
Phenol red-Na salt	Sigma-Aldrich
L-Phenylalanine	Sigma-Aldrich
Phosphoethanolamine	Sigma-Aldrich
L-Proline	Sigma-Aldrich
Putrescine 2HCl	Sigma-Aldrich
Pyridoxine HCl	Sigma-Aldrich
Retinoic acid-all *trans*	Sigma-Aldrich
Riboflavin	Sigma-Aldrich
Selenous acid	Sigma-Aldrich
L-Serine	Sigma-Aldrich
Sodium pyruvate	Sigma-Aldrich
Soybean trypsin inhibitor	Sigma-Aldrich
Thiamine-HCl	Sigma-Aldrich
DL-6,8-Thioctic acid	Sigma-Aldrich
L-Threonine	Sigma-Aldrich
Thymidine	Sigma-Aldrich
$(+)$-α-Tocopherol	Sigma-Aldrich
Trypsin, crystalline, type I	Sigma-Aldrich
L-Tryptophan	Sigma-Aldrich
L-Tyrosine	Sigma-Aldrich
L-Valine	Sigma-Aldrich
Vitamin B_{12}	Sigma-Aldrich
Vitrogen-100 collagen	Cohesion Technology
$ZnSO_4 \cdot 7H_2O$	Sigma-Aldrich

[a] Cell culture-tested reagents

7

Human Oral Epithelium

Roland C. Grafström

Experimental Carcinogenesis, Institute of Environmental Medicine,
Karolinska Institutet, Stockholm, Sweden. roland.grafstrom@imm.ki.se

Culture of Epithelial Cells, pages 195–255

I. GENERAL INTRODUCTION

1.1. Aim of Chapter

The main purpose of this chapter is to provide the basic and necessary methodology required for growth of human oral keratinocytes in both monolayer and organotypic culture. After a brief introduction of the epithelial structures found in the oral mucosa, a review of the methods utilized by various investigators for culture of nonmalignant oral epithelium is presented including a tabulated presentation of the respective research areas and results. Technical aspects applicable to monolayer, multilayer, explant, and organotypic culture are summarized. Subsequently, detailed protocols for serum-free culture of oral epithelium are shown based on the experiences derived from specimens obtained from more than 800 individuals over the last two decades. Step-by-step protocols for media fabrication include information on commercial source, preparation, and storage for each of the components. The basic protocols for deriving, handling, and storage of cells include primary and transfer culture at low (clonal) and high density. The overall information presented demonstrates that basic laboratory resources are sufficient to reproducibly generate reagents and conditions for oral keratinocyte culture from single chemicals and bovine pituitaries without the necessity of purchasing buffers and media from commercial sources. Notably, the conditions developed for normal oral keratinocytes are also applicable to at least some immortalized (nonmalignant) and malignant variants in both monolayer and organotypic culture.

1.2. Structure of Oral Mucosa

Related to its many functions, the oral cavity contains several different types of stratified squamous epithelia, including those classified as nonkeratinized, parakeratinized, and orthokeratinized [Burkhardt and Maerker, 1981]. Regional variation and heterogeneity within each type of epithelium also include glandular epithelium (salivary glands) and taste buds, the latter on the dorsal and lateral tongue. Primarily nonkeratinized epithelium provides a lining in the cheeks, lips, floor of mouth, ventral aspect of the tongue, soft palate, and upper and lower vestibular sulci. Parakeratinized and orthokeratinized epithelium lines the hard palate and the mucosa that surrounds the teeth (attached gingiva). Transitions, abrupt or gradual, take place in several regions of the oral cavity, often making it difficult to define clearly the type of epithelium present in specimens used for derivation of cell cultures. The dorsal tongue and gingival margin are such zones. The basement membrane zone, the papilla and reticular zones of the lamina propria, and, beneath these, the submucosa, typically support the various oral epithelia. The very similar structure of the oral epithelium and the epidermis, including the squamous nature of both and the generation of a surface barrier, naturally implies that many of the research results with epidermal keratinocytes are also applicable to the oral epithelium. The fact that relatively similar culture conditions can be applied for culture of a variety of human epithelia also implies that many aspects of the specific nature of keratinocytes may be the same in different tissues [Grafström, 1990]. Subtle differences in culture conditions among epithelia, or differences in the biological properties expressed between different epithelia in vitro, sometimes in one standardized condition, argue for the existence of many unique epithelial phenotypes, even within the oral cavity. Notably, the oral epithelia in common laboratory animals, i.e., rodents, are primarily of the squamous keratinized type, and, thus, the morphology and biochemistry often differ from the human equivalent.

1.3. Overview of Methods for Monolayer Culture

1.3.1. Tissue Sites–Explant Outgrowth, or Enzymatic Digestion

Epithelial cells from normal oral mucosa have been grown from several functionally and histologically differing sites (Tables 7.1 and 7.2). Several general conclusions can be drawn from side-by-side comparisons of methodological reports dating primarily from 1987 to 2000 [see MacCallum et al., 1987, for an excellent review of earlier studies]. Oral surgery including removal of wisdom teeth, tonsillectomy, and maxillo-facial reconstructive surgery has

TABLE 7.1. Examples of Methodological Reports on Monolayer Culture of Human Oral Epithelium[a]

State/Origin[b]	Method/Culture Conditions[c]	Longevity/Type of Culture[d]	Studies/Characteristics of Cell Line	References[e]
Normal Tissue				
Buccal mucosa	Explant outgrowth; MEM + 10% FBS; Chick plasma and extracts; 34°C; 0.5% dimethyl sulfoxide	2 passages	Evidence of senescence at 5 wk; some functionality up to 14 wk; expression of keratinocyte markers by microscopic analysis	Arenholt-Bindslev et al., 1987
Buccal mucosa	Explant outgrowth; BEG medium, fibronectin/collagen coating	~2 months 5 passages	≤6%CFE (≥16 cells/colony); CG, 0.8 PD/D; expression of keratins and involucrin; GI by TGF-β; TD by Ca^{2+} and FBS; toxicity of areca nut alkaloids and N-nitrosamines	Sundqvist et al., 1989, 1991b
Buccal mucosa	Trypsin-digested tissue and mechanical scraping; EMHA, fibronectin/collagen coating or no coating	~7 months 10 passages	≤40% CFE (≥16 cells/colony); CG, ≤1.2 PD/D; GI by TGF-β; TD by FBS; medium suitable also for growth of an oral carcinoma cell line	Sundqvist, 1991a
Buccal mucosa and uvula	Trypsin-digested tissue and mechanical scraping; DMEM:F12 (3:1) + 20% FBS; Swiss 3T3 cells as feeder layer	Primary culture	Assessment of different protocols for primary culture, morphology, yield of cells, colony formation and time of stratification; generation of grafts suitable for surgical application; comparisons to epidermal cells	Tomson et al., 1994
Gingiva	Explant outgrowth on non-coated dishes or collagen, F12:DMEM (1:1) and modified MCDB 153	4–5 passages	≤10% CFE (≥4 cells/colony); CG; 0.8 PD/D; analysis of growth factor requirement and keratin expression; TD induced by suspension culture; expression of keratinocyte markers by microscopic analysis; Ca^{2+}-induced generation of grafts suitable for surgical application	Wille et al., 1990

TABLE 7.1. Examples of Methodological Reports on Monolayer Culture of Human Oral Epithelium[a] (continued)

State/Origin[b]	Method/Culture Conditions[c]	Longevity/Type of Culture[d]	Studies/Characteristics of Cell Line	References[e]
Normal Tissue (continued)				
Gingiva	Dispase/trypsin-digested tissue; KGM	~3 months 7 passages	Expression of keratins; TD by Ca^{2+}; expression of keratinocyte markers by microscopic analysis	Oda and Watson, 1990
Gingiva	Explant outgrowth; DMEM:F12 (3:1) + 10% FBS	4–6 weeks	Generation of graft (4–6 cell layers) suitable for surgical application	Lauer, 1991, 1994
Gingiva/buccal mucosa	Dispase/trypsin-digested tissue; PFM-7 and K-SFM	3–4 passages	Expression of mRNA for various growth factors and their receptors; medium suitable also for growth of an oral carcinoma cell line	Kamata et al., 1999
Oral tissue (several sites)	Trypsin-digested tissue; DMEM:F12 (3:1) + 5% FBS; Swiss 3T3-J2 cells as feeder layer	3–10 passages; 30–80 cell generations	Expression of keratins and involucrin; conditions applicable to fetal oral tissue and leukoplakia; confluent sheets xenografted in nude mice	Lindberg and Rheinwald, 1990
Oral tissue (several sites)	Trypsin-digested tissue; modified MCDB 153	Not reported	≥90% CFE (≥4 cells/colony); GI by TGF-β and ethionine; TD by FBS	Kasperbauer et al., 1990
Oral keratinizing tissue	Collagenase/dispase for separation of epithelium from connective tissue; trypsin digestion; KGM; collagen coating	~20–25 PD	Culture of basal epithelial cells; assessment of replication, senescence, and terminal differentiation	Kang et al., 1998, 2000
Oral tissue (not specified)	Dispase/trypsin-digested tissue; DMEM: F12 (3:1) + 5% FBS; Swiss 3T3 feeder layer	Primary culture, sheets graftable after 20 days	Structural changes and viability of cultured grafts after freezing; peri-implant soft tissue management with mucosal grafts	Ueda et al., 1995; Hibino et al., 1996; Ueda et al., 1998
Oral tissue (from wisdom teeth removal)	Explant outgrowth; RPMI:DMEM (1:1) with variable serum and factor supplementation	~3 months 5–6 passages	Assessment of growth factor requirement and keratin expression; expression of keratinocyte markers by microscopic analysis	Southgate et al., 1987

TABLE 7.1. **Examples of Methodological Reports on Monolayer Culture of Human Oral Epithelium[a] (continued)**

State/Origin[b]	Method/Culture Conditions[c]	Longevity/Type of Culture[d]	Studies/Characteristics of Cell Line	References[e]
Normal Tissue (continued)				
Oral tissue (from third molar removal)	Dispase/trypsin-digested tissue; KBM + modified BEGM	7–9 passages	Epithelial morphology; keratin expression; conditions also applicable to esophageal cells	Oda et al., 1998
Palate	Explant outgrowth; PF86-1	2 months, primary culture	Epithelial morphology; medium suitable also for growth of oral carcinoma cell lines	Rikimaru et al., 1990
Palate	Trypsin-digested tissue; DMEM:F12 (3:1) + 10% FBS; Swiss 3T3-J2 cells as feeder layer	Variable and age-dependent	Histologic evaluation; expression of keratin; generation of graft surgically applied onto patient gingiva	De Luca et al., 1990
Parotid gland	Explant outgrowth; KBM	35 passages; 120–140 PD	Expression of keratinocyte markers by microscopic analysis and keratins; β-adrenergic receptor function	Chopra and Xue-Hu, 1993
Peritonsilar mucosa	Collagenase-digested tissue; DMEM + 10% FBS	Short-term culture (5 days)	Various conditions promoted growth	Formanek et al., 1996
Peritonsilar mucosa (TE1177)	Modified alpha medium + 10% FBS	45 PD	Epithelial morphology; expression of retinoic acid receptor-β, mucin and keratin	D'Ambrosio et al., 2000
Peritonsilar mucosa	Trypsin-digested tissue; DMEM:F12 (3:1) + 10% FBS; Swiss 3T3-J2 cells as feeder layer	0.22 PD/D	Epithelial morphology; assessment of feeder cell dependence, growth, and keratin expression	Neugebauer et al., 1996
Peritonsilar mucosa and other sites	Explant outgrowth or dispase-dissociated epithelium, Amniomax-C100; KGM	3–5 passages	Assessment of yield and TD with different methodological approaches; epithelial morphology; expression of keratins; GI by TGF-β	Xu et al., 1996

TABLE 7.1. Examples of Methodological Reports on Monolayer Culture of Human Oral Epithelium[a] (continued)

State/Origin[b]	Method/Culture Conditions[c]	Longevity/Type of Culture[d]	Studies/Characteristics of Cell Line	References[e]
Normal Tissue (continued)				
Salivary gland	Explant outgrowth; modified MCDB153-LB	Primary culture	Epithelial morphology	Rhim et al., 1988
Tongue	Trypsin-digested tissue; DMEM + 20% FBS, Swiss 3T3 feeder layer	Not reported	Epithelial morphology	Chang et al., 1992
Uvula and other sites	Thermolysin/protease followed by trypsin digestion; KGM	6–7 passages	Storage of tissue in medium with antibiotics for 3–4 days before derivation of primary cultures decreases risk of infection	Reid et al., 1997
Premalignant Tissue/Immortalized Cells				
Buccal mucosa and gingiva	Transfection of normal keratinocytes with HPV16 genes; RM[+] + 10% FBS	>18 months; 35 passages	Expression of HPV16 E7 protein and keratins; correlative assessment of transfection and immortalization; lack of HPV11 immortalization; nontumorigenic in immunodeprived host	Sexton et al., 1993
Buccal mucosa (SVpgC2a)	Transfection of normal keratinocytes with SV40 T; EMHA	>2 yr; >700 PD	Genomic integration of SV40T; aneuploid; expression of keratins; partial resistance to GI and TD by TGF-β and FBS	Kulkarni et al., 1995
Buccal mucosa (H157) and tongue (H103) squamous cell carcinomas	Explant outgrowth, DMEM + 20% FCS; Swiss 3T3 feeder layer initially	~3 yr; >30 passages, 200 PD	Expression of keratins; feeder layer independent; anchorage-independent; nontumorigenic in immunodeprived host; conditions suitable also to tumorigenic carcinoma lines	Prime et al., 1990

TABLE 7.1. Examples of Methodological Reports on Monolayer Culture of Human Oral Epithelium[a] (continued)

State/Origin[b]	Method/Culture Conditions[c]	Longevity/Type of Culture[d]	Studies/Characteristics of Cell Line	References[e]
Premalignant Tissue/Immortalized Cells (continued)				
Gingiva (S-G); apparently normal mucosa	Explant outgrowth; Alpha-modified Eagle's medium + 15 % FBS;	41 passages	80–90% plating efficiency; ~1 PD/D; focus formation and loss of contact inhibition; nontumorigenic in hamster cheek pouch assay; biocompatibility of dental materials	Smulow and Glickman, 1966; Kasten et al., 1989
Gingiva (IHGK)	Retroviral infection of E6/E7 from HPV16; KGM initially; K-SFM	>4 yr; >350 passages	Expression of keratins and vascular endothelial growth factor, progressive chromosomal abnormalities; malignant transformation from chemical exposure; cell cycle phase analysis	Oda et al., 1996a,b; Yoo et al., 2000
Gingiva (HOK16A, HOK16B)	Transfection of normal keratinocytes with HPV16 genes; KGM	>8 months; 40 passages	Genomic integration of HPV16; overexpression of c-myc; malignant transformation from chemical exposure	Park et al., 1991; Kim et al., 1993
Gingiva (HOK18)	Transfection of normal keratinocytes with HPV18 genes; KGM	>2 yr; 90 passages	Genomic integration of HPV18; resistance to GI by Ca^{2+}; increased expression of TGF-α and c-myc; malignant transformation from chemical exposure	Shin et al., 1994
Larynx papillomas and erythroplakia (BICR P1-6 & E1-5)	Explant outgrowth (papillomas) and trypsin digestion (erythroplakia); DMEM + 20% FBS; Swiss 3T3 feeder cells initially	Not specified	Abnormal TD but not immortal; normal coding region of the p53 gene; papilloma cell lines contain HPV 6 or HPV11 DNA	Burns et al., 1994
Dysplastic leukoplakia (Leuk1 and Leuk2)	KGM	>100 PD	Abnormal TD (resistance to Ca^{2+} and serum)	Sacks, 1996

TABLE 7.1. Examples of Methodological Reports on Monolayer Culture of Human Oral Epithelium[a] (continued)

State/Origin[b]	Method/Culture Conditions[c]	Longevity/Type of Culture[d]	Studies/Characteristics of Cell Line	References[e]
Premalignant Tissue/Immortalized Cells (continued)				
Labial vestibule, fetal (GMSM-K)	Transfection of normal keratinocytes with SV40 T; KSFM	0.27 PD/D	Epithelial morphology; T antigen-negative; hypotetraploid; anchorage-independent growth; lack of tumorigenicity in immunodeprived host	Gilchrist et al., 2000
Oral (HPV16 oral EPI)	Retroviral infection of E6/E7 from HPV16; KGM	>90 passages	Expression of cytochrome P450s and microsomal epoxide hydrolase	Farin et al., 1995
Tongue (DOK) Dysplastic tissue, i.e., erythroleukoplakia	Trypsin-digested tissue; DMEM + 10% or 20% FBS; Swiss 3T3 feeder cells initially	≥150 PD; 1 yr	Analysis of growth factor requirement and keratin expression; aneuploidy; tumor suppressor p53 is mutated	Chang et al., 1992
Tongue SCC (SCC-83-01-82)	Soft agar cloning of minced tumor tissue, Eagle's MEM + 10% FBS	Not reported	Anchorage-independent growth; lack of tumorigenicity in immunodeprived host; malignant transformation by chemical exposure; the genes encoding for p53 and H-ras are mutated	Shuler et al., 1990; Lee et al., 1997

[a]The listing of these references is an effort to provide an indication of methodology and research area, and the reader is referred to the original articles for details. The information provided also reflects the variable depth of details provided by different authors. [b]Listing of the reports is based on site in oral cavity in alphabetical order and year of publication in succession. Priority has been given to articles from 1987 onward because of existing reviews of reports older than 1987 (see text). [c]A brief description of the culture method is followed by type of medium with specification of complex components, e.g., serum supplementation (if used). Media abbreviations are used, and the reader is referred to the original articles for details. [d]The time stated indicates longevity as provided by the authors or what could be deduced from results in the text. [e]On occasion, parts of the information were retrieved from reports other than those listed, e.g., application of the identical technique for epidermal keratinocytes at earlier date.

Abbreviations: CFE, colony forming efficiency; CG, clonal growth; EMHA, see Appendix A; FBS, fetal bovine serum; GI, growth inhibition; HPV, human papillomavirus; PD, population doublings; PD/D, population doublings per day; SV40T, simian virus 40 T antigen; TD, terminal differentiation of the squamous type; TGF-α, human transforming growth factor α; TGF-β, human transforming growth factor β1.

TABLE 7.2. Methodological Reports on Organotypic Culture of Human Oral Epithelium[a]

State/Origin/ Cell Line[b]	Method/Culture Conditions[c]	Longevity of Study/ Longevity[d]	Studies/Characteristics of Cell Line	Reference[e]
Buccal mucosa and gingiva	De-epidermalized human dermis; RM[+] medium including 10% FBS; submerged or air-liquid interface	15 days or 1 + 14 days	Submerged cells showed superior TD than air-liquid interface cells; HPV16-immortalized expressed an undifferentiated phenotype	Sexton et al., 1993
Buccal mucosa	Explant culture on tissue culture plastic or gelatin sponge; BEX medium	2–5 days longevity	Histology comparable to noncultured tissue; N-nitrosamine metabolism and tissue binding of reactive intermediates	Liu et al., 1993
Buccal mucosa and gingiva	Contracted collagen lattice + oral or dermal fibroblasts; DMEM + 10% FBS; submerged followed by air-liquid interface	1 + 2 weeks	Assessment of morphology; keratinizing vs. nonkeratinizing epithelia; normal vs. delipidized serum; influences of retinoic acid on TD and keratin expression	Kautsky et al., 1995
Buccal mucosa	De-epidermized human buccal mucosa or collagen lattice + buccal fibroblasts; F12:DMEM (3:1) + 10% FBS; submerged followed by air-liquid interface	2 + 7 or 7 + 7 days	Assessment of morphology; expression of keratins, growth, basement membrane, and TD markers; influences of retinoic acid and calcipotriol; comparisons to epidermal cells	Chung et al., 1997
Buccal mucosa	Collagen lattice + buccal fibroblasts; supplemented KGM w/o pituitary extract; submerged followed by air-liquid interface	1 + 10 days	Expression of keratins, basal membrane components, integrins, cell-surface carbohydrates, and wound healing markers; comparisons to epidermal cells	Grøn et al., 1999

State/Origin/ Cell Line[b]	Method/Culture Conditions[c]	Longevity of Study/ Longevity[d]	Studies/Characteristics of Cell Line	Reference[e]
Buccal mucosa	Collagen lattice + buccal fibroblasts; EMA; submerged followed by air-liquid interface	2 + 10 days	Assessment of morphology and invasiveness; expression of keratins; conditions applicable to SV40T-immortalized and carcinoma cells; multistage model of carcinogenesis	Hansson et al., 2001
Gingiva (junctional epithelium)	Outgrowth between explant and high-protein-binding membrane; EMEM + 10% FBS; submerged culture	4, 6 and 8 days	Epibolus of 5–8 cell layers formed between connective tissue of explant and substratum; assessment of morphology, migration, and keratins; comparisons to the in vivo situation	Salonen et al., 1989
Gingiva	Collagen lattice + embryonic dermal fibroblasts; DMEM:F12 (3:1) + 5% FBS; submerged culture	17 days	Assessment of morphology and keratin expression; comparison to grafts generated on 3T3-feeder layers	Gosselin et al., 1989, 1990
Gingiva	Explant culture on decalcified dentin matrix + or w/o filter separation; EMEM + 10% FBS	10 days	Expression of cell migration, DNA synthesis, keratins, and collagenolytic enzyme activity	Salonen et al., 1991
Gingiva	Stroma of gingival fibroblasts on nylon mesh; DMEM + 5% FBS, moist nonsubmerged culture	3 weeks; 35-day longevity	Assessment of morphology, viability and proliferation; expression of fibronectin, keratin, basement membrane and stromal markers	Odioso et al., 1995
Gingiva	Collagen lattice + NIH-3T3 fibroblasts; E-medium; submerged followed by air-liquid interface	7 + 10 days	Assessment of morphology and filaggrin expression; normal vs. HPV16-immortalized and carcinogen-transformed cells; multistage model of carcinogenesis	Park et al., 1995

TABLE 7.2. Methodological Reports on Organotypic Culture of Human Oral Epithelium[a] **(continued)**

State/Origin/Cell Line[b]	Method/Culture Conditions[c]	Longevity of Study/Longevity[d]	Studies/Characteristics of Cell Line	Reference[e]
Gingiva and other sites	Contracted collagen lattice + foreskin dermal fibroblasts; DMEM:F12 (3:1) + 5% FBS; submerged followed by air-liquid interface	4 + 10 days	Influences of retinoic acid on differentiation; assessment of keratin and filaggrin expression; retroviral transfection and expression of retinoic acid receptors; comparison to epidermal cells	Schön and Rheinwald, 1996
Gingiva	Collagen lattice + foreskin dermal fibroblasts; DMEM + 10% FBS; submerged followed by air-liquid interface	4–6 + 7 days	Assessment of morphology; expression of keratins and filaggrin; conditions applicable to HPV16-immortalized cells; model of carcinogenesis	Oda et al., 1996b
Gingiva	Contracted collagen lattice + dermal foreskin fibroblasts; transfer to second collagen lattice; DMEM + 10% FBS; submerged followed by air-liquid interface	6 + 4 days	Model of re-epithelialization and wound healing; assessment of proliferation, migration and expression of TGF-β and matrix metalloproteinase	Garlick et al., 1996
Gingiva	Polycarbonate filter + 3T3 feeder layer; epithelium generated separately from fibroblast support (antipodal culture); submerged followed by air-liquid interface	5 + 11–14 days	Assessment of morphology and keratin expression; nonsubmerged culture promotes differentiation; comparisons to other supports, i.e., collagen lattice and 3T3 feeder layer	Delcourt-Huard et al., 1997
Gingiva	Collagen lattice + gingival fibroblasts; KGM; submerged followed by air-liquid interface	2 days +1, 2 or 3 weeks	Assessment of morphology, proliferation, keratins, and basement membrane components; tissuelike differentiation at later time points	Tomakidi et al., 1997, 1998, 1999

TABLE 7.2. Methodological Reports on Organotypic Culture of Human Oral Epithelium[a] (continued)

State/Origin/ Cell Line[b]	Method/Culture Conditions[c]	Longevity of Study/ Longevity[d]	Studies/Characteristics of Cell Line	Reference[e]
Gingiva (peri-odontal pocket)	Polyester or collagen membrane; KSFM ± elevated Ca^{2+} and 10% FBS; submerged culture	1 week + 1, 2 or 3 weeks	Assessment of mor-phology and keratin expression; junc-tional-like or sulcular-like epithelium was induced dependent on conditions	Papaioannou et al., 1999
Gingiva/buccal mucosa (non-keratinizing epithelia)	Culture on de-epidermal-ized human dermis soaked in collagen; MCDB153 medium + or w/o 10% FBS; sub-merged followed by air-liquid interface	4 + 4, 11 or 18 days; 4 days + 1 or 2 weeks	Assessment of mor-phology, proliferation, keratins, and fatty acids; organotypic ep-ithelium appeared to be more active and proliferative than na-tive keratinized mucosa	Izumi et al., 1999; 2000
Gingiva	Collagen lattice + NIH-3T3 fibroblasts; 1:1 mixture of DK-SFM: DMEM/F12 (1:3) +10% FBS; submerged followed by air-liquid interface	1 + 10–14 days	Assessment of mor-phology and invasive-ness; normal vs. HPV16-immortalized, carcinogen-trans-formed, and carci-noma cells; multi-stage modeling of carcinogenesis	Yoo et al., 2000
Gingiva	Keratinocytes grown on polyethylene membrane with agar overlay; fibro-blasts grown on lower surface; FAD with 5% FBS; submerged culture	3 weeks	Assay standardized by application of keratin-ocytes immortalized by HPV-E6 and E7. Assessment of surface integrity, proliferation and keratin expres-sion after exposure to dental materials	Tomakidi et al., 2000
Palate (hard)	Culture on de-epider-mized human dermis of human skin; DMEM: F12 (3:1) + 10% FBS; submerged followed by air-liquid interface, the latter + delipidized FBS	2 + 14 days	Assessment of mor-phology and keratin expression; conditions with normal serum preferable to buccal cells	Cho et al., 2000

TABLE 7.2. Methodological Reports on Organotypic Culture of Human Oral Epithelium[a] (continued)

State/Origin/ Cell Line[b]	Method/Culture Conditions[c]	Longevity of Study/ Longevity[d]	Studies/Characteristics of Cell Line	Reference[e]
Peritonsilar mucosa and other sites	Explant culture; EMEM + 10% decalcified FBS	3–4 days	Assessment of histology; differentiation regulated by Ca^{2+}; a destratified explant with a dorsal layer of basal keratinocytes can be redifferentiated	Sacks et al., 1985

[a]The listing of these references indicates methodology and research areas, and the reader is referred to the original articles for details. The information provided also reflects the variable depth of details provided by the respective authors. [b]Listing of the reports is based on site in oral cavity in alphabetical order and year of publication in succession. Priority has been given to articles from 1987 onward because of existing reviews of reports older than 1987 (see text). [c]A brief description of the culture method is followed by type of medium with specification of serum supplementation (if used). Media abbreviations were used as reported. [d]The information on length of study often involves separation of the time in submerged culture (first) and air-liquid interface culture (second); time indicating longevity is stated. [e]On occasion, parts of the information were retrieved from reports other than those listed, e.g., application of the identical technique for epidermal keratinocytes at earlier date.

Abbreviations: FBS, fetal bovine serum; HPV, human papillomavirus; TD, terminal differentiation of the squamous type; SV40T, simian virus 40 T antigen; TGF-β, human transforming growth factor-β.

been the primary source for obtaining oral epithelium but some studies also included autopsy specimens. Primary cultures were obtained as outgrowths from explanted tissue or, alternatively, by initial dissociation of tissue using trypsin, collagenase, dispase, or other digestive enzymes singly or in combination. In the latter case, proteolytic treatment, often combined with mechanical dissociation of the cells of the epithelium, was followed by subsequent culture of the resulting suspension of tissue fragments, clumps of cells, and individual cells. A clear trend toward the latter approach is noted in the more recent studies.

About half of the listed reports utilized conditions with serum and feeder layers for monolayer culture (if serum is present in the culture medium, the percentage is specified in Table 7.1). Many of these utilize variations of the method for epidermal keratinocytes described by Rheinwald and Green [1975] and later modified by Allen and Rheinwald [1984]. The 3T3 fibroblast line from the Swiss albino mouse (sometimes specifying the J2 strain), exposed to ionizing radiation or radiomimetic drugs, serves as a feeder layer in this protocol. Furthermore, application of 5–20% FBS to a mixture of media, often DMEM:Ham's F12 in ratios of 1:1 or 3:1 plus additional factors, has been part of this protocol.

The majority of the other reports employed media that are serum-free but supplemented with small amounts of pituitary extract. In this case, the amount of protein added is around 2 orders of magnitude lower compared with that of a medium with 10% serum. These methods are often variations of the protocol for epidermal keratinocytes described by Boyce and Ham [1983 and 1986]. Conditions without either serum or pituitary extract were developed for explant culture and subsequently refined for monolayer culture, involving the possibility of short-term culture of oral keratinocytes at chemically defined conditions [Rikimaru et al., 1990; Kamata et al., 1999]. Most serum-free methods are based on the MCDB 153 medium [Boyce and Ham, 1986] including various supplements. The fabrication of a variant of this medium, termed EMHA (epithelial medium with high levels of amino acids) [Sundqvist et al., 1991a], for the purpose of oral keratinocyte culture is described in detail in this chapter. This medium was previously known as EMA but has been altered to EMHA to avoid confusion with "epithelial membrane antigen," abbreviated as EMA elsewhere in this book.

Several points can be made in comparisons of culture conditions with or without serum. Serum exposure of keratinocytes may, to some extent, mimic the state of wound healing, although the regular diffusion of serum factors from vessels in the underlying connective tissue would probably involve exposure to lower amounts than those used in cell culture. Although the defined approach without serum offers several advantages, including less experimental variability, the possibility of identifying factors that directly regulate proliferation and differentiation, ease of isolation of cellular products, and utilization of selective growth conditions for different cell types, conditions with serum may produce cultures with higher cloning efficiency and longevity than serum-free conditions.

1.3.2. Substrates and Longevity

Most studies of oral keratinocytes have relied on regular tissue culture plastic as substrate (culture surface) although some utilized dishes coated with proteins typically found in the extracellular environment of keratinocytes, including those in the proximity of the basement membrane. With EMHA as culture medium, coating with fibronectin and collagen markedly improved colony-forming efficiency, growth rate, and harvests of primary cultures more than other combinations of medium and culture surfaces [Sundqvist et al., 1991a]. However, transfer of oral keratinocytes in EMHA after primary culture is equally effective with or without this coating mixture in terms of net generation of cells per passage [Grafström, unpublished observation].

Oral keratinocyte cultures derived from normal, nonpathologic tissue express many features of normality including finite life spans. The longevity of normal oral keratinocyte cultures has been variably described as length of time in culture or number of passages and population doublings. In the more recent reports, from 4 to 10 passages seem to be possible, with or without serum, over periods of up to 3 months. One study reported even longer culture periods approximating those commonly shown for immortal cell lines [Chopra and Xue-Hu, 1993]. In EMHA, buccal keratinocytes commonly undergo 60 population doublings resulting in yields of $1 \times 10^8 - 1 \times 10^{11}$ cells per cm^2 of mucosal specimen [Sundqvist et al., 1991a]. This longevity and harvest appear to be among the highest reported for serum-free culture of human epithelial cells, including tissues other than oral mucosa [Grafström et al., 1997]. In practical terms, for the purpose of expanding cultures, oral keratinocytes are rarely cultured beyond the third or fourth passage because the number of new cells generated decreases to approximate the number of cells dying. Confirming the reduction in the growth fraction, the cloning efficiency decreases from 40–90% at passages 1–3 to usually 1–2% at later passages, i.e., within about 1 month from initiation of the primary culture. Furthermore, the clonal growth rates reported are typically between 0.8 to 1.2 population doublings per day (PD/D) in early passages, whereas in later passages cells divide at around 0.5 PD/D [Sundqvist et al., 1991a].

1.3.3. Characteristics of Monolayer Cultures

Typical characteristics of oral keratinocytes in monolayer culture have been reviewed [Dale et al., 1990; Sacks, 1996; Grafström et al., 1997]. Such cultures in early passage are reminiscent of normal basal epithelium, that is, the cells exhibit a diploid karyotype, high proliferative ability, a relatively small cell size, low expression of markers associated with terminal differentiation (TD) of the squamous type, and the expression of basal cell keratins. Furthermore, the cells respond positively and negatively to growth factors, for example, epidermal growth factor and transforming growth factor-β, respectively. The cells retain the ability to undergo TD from a number of stimuli, for example, Ca^{2+} and serum as well as tumor promoting and cytotoxic agents. The typical criteria of TD include those observed by microscopy, like tonofilaments and desmosomes, or proteins detected from immunochemical assessment like involucrin, filaggrin, and differentiation-related keratins. The reports listed in Table 7.1 variably describe such data along with methodological advances in the culture of oral keratinocytes. Notably, most of the authors listed have characterized oral keratinocytes in additional studies, and the readers are referred to those and other literature for further information on the characteristics of cultured oral epithelium.

1.3.4. Fabrication of Grafts

A number of methodological studies focused on the fabrication of epithelial grafts for surgical application; they are listed in Table 7.1 on the basis that the epithelia were generated without the involvement of a cultured dermal equivalent in the initial phase of the experiments. Grafts are organotypic to some degree in that they contain both proliferative basal-like cells as well as those committed to TD. Confluent monolayers of keratinocytes were derived primarily from application of serum and feeder cell-dependent methods. Continued growth in serum-supplemented media results in multilayering of the cultures, typically involving from 3 to 10 cell layers. Such cultured grafts were successfully applied by surgical procedures in the oral cavity as well as in other body sites as the inner ear. Procedures for preservation and storage of intact grafts in liquid nitrogen were also developed (see Table 7.1).

1.3.5. Establishment of Immortalized Cell Lines by Experimental Approaches

Reports on the generation of immortal, nonmalignant oral keratinocyte lines by experimental means or from culture of tumor material are listed in the second part of Table 7.1; the generation of mostly malignant cell lines from oral tumor tissue was extensively reviewed by Sacks [1996]. The longevity of so-called "immortalized" lines exceeds considerably that of normal keratinocytes with finite life span, involving culture periods of commonly 1–4 yr (sometimes without interruption), 30–350 passages, or an estimated number of population doublings that vary from 100 to more than 700. By way of transfection of DNA tumor virus oncogenes, that is, E6/E7 genes from HPV 16 or HPV 18 and the T antigen gene from simian virus 40 (SV40T), various immortal, permanent cell lines were generated (see Table 7.1). The E6 and E7 proteins form complexes with the tumor suppressor p53 and Rb proteins, respectively, leading to inactivation of the latter

[Levine et al., 1991; Weinberg, 1991]. Because the HPV E6 protein, unlike SV40T, which complexes with both the p53 and Rb proteins, also catalyzes degradation of the p53 protein, cell lines transfected with SV40T or HPV E6/E7 offer complementary systems of transformation.

Immortal keratinocyte lines often develop through an extension of their normal life spans followed by one or two crises. A rare immortalizing event likely occurs in one cell from which a permanent line develops. The cell lines generally exhibit a nontumorigenic phenotype in the immune-deprived host, at least in the early passages, and they can be grown rapidly to high cell numbers. Other typical characteristics include partial to complete loss of features associated with TD, including responsiveness to agents that induce growth inhibition or TD in normal cells. Increased expression of growth-promoting genes related to cell cycle regulation or oncogenic transformation is common. The cell lines are aneuploid and generally show chromosomal instability, although the degree of this instability has not been thoroughly investigated. Full transformation to a malignant phenotype can sometimes be accomplished by continued culture, or with good success after supertransfection with an oncogene or treatment with chemical carcinogens [Grafström, 1990].

The reports in Table 7.1 include several examples of immortal cell lines that exhibit the above criteria and which undergo transformation to a fully malignant phenotype after exposure to carcinogens, including those typically found in tobacco and tobacco smoke. Among many interesting results, these studies naturally imply that malignant transformation of oral epithelium may be caused by sequential or combined effects of infection with high-risk HPVs and exposure to tobacco-related carcinogens.

1.3.6. Establishment of Immortal Cell Lines from Tumor Tissue

Immortal, nontumorigenic oral keratinocyte lines were also derived from apparently normal tissue (one study) as well as tumor material (see Table 7.1). The listed reports indicate that the cell lines were unable to form tumors in the immune-deprived host, and as such they may represent premalignant cells. The majority of studies involve culture of the cells in serum-supplemented conditions. Accumulating evidence indicates that the process of transformation involves development of resistance to the TD-promoting effect of serum and even dependence on certain serum factors for growth, unlike the preferences or requirements of normal cells.

However, information is lacking as to what extent serum-free conditions were applied to these cell lines. Typical premalignant characteristics of these cell lines involve loss of dependence of feeder cells, focus formation, loss of contact inhibition, anchorage-independent growth, aneuploidy, and genetic alterations in genes controlling growth (see Table 7.1).

1.3.7. Applications of Immortalized Cell Lines

Immortalized lines are likely to be valuable tools for future investigations relating to intermediate stages of the multistep process of carcinogenesis. However, immortalized lines may preserve many features of normal cells, and as such they may be reproducible and easily grown models for exploitation of normal oral epithelial functions. Cell lines from normal or dysplastic tissue should be tested for the preservation of normal tissue functions because cells immortalized by DNA tumor virus oncogenes often exhibit at least some characteristics of severe epithelial dysplasia [Park et al., 1995; Hansson et al., 2001]. Recent studies showed marked persistence of normal or even activated drug metabolism activity in HPV- or SV40T-immortalized oral keratinocytes [Farin et al., 1995; Vondracek et al., 2001; Hedberg et al., 2000, 2001].

A number of general points can be made as to the potential usefulness of human oral keratinocytes in transformation studies.

1. Commonly, both quantitative and qualitative differences are generally found in the metabolism of carcinogens between human and animal cells [Harris et al., 1984; Boyd and Reade, 1988].
2. Rodent cells undergo immortalization and malignant transformation more frequently than human cells [DiPaolo et al., 1986; Grafström, 1990; Chang, 1991].
3. Human keratinocytes generally show a higher capability for metabolism of carcinogens than fibroblasts from the same tissue [Autrup and Grafström, 1982], whereas phenotypic changes associated to transformation were previously demonstrated primarily in mesenchymal cells.

Thus further studies are needed to demonstrate the degrees of normality or abnormality exhibited in transformed keratinocytes, including those of oral origin.

I.4. Overview of Methods for Organotypic Culture

1.4.1. Explant Culture and Regeneration of Epithelia from Monolayer Cultures

Oral keratinocytes can be cultured in organized tissuelike states in vitro using various supports (Table 7.2). Also listed in Table 7.2 are attempts of organ culture of oral epithelium (maintenance of a tissue specimen in explant culture is naturally an alternative to organotypic culture of cells initially derived in monolayer culture). Some general conclusions can be made from a comparison of the listed reports. Explant culture only permits the maintenance of normal tissue architecture and function for at most a few days, whereas substantially longer periods are possible with epithelia regenerated from monolayer cultures. The latter approach variably includes using a lattice of collagen, de-epidermized oral mucosa or skin, artificial membranes or matrices, often involving the application of methods established for epidermal keratinocytes. Interestingly, comparisons in some reports showed that oral keratinocytes were more easily grown than epidermal keratinocytes, involving both the monolayer and organotypic culture stage.

Fibroblasts are commonly incorporated in the collagen matrices or added as feeder layers on membranes. These support cells have included different types of oral or epidermal fibroblast cell lines as well as the Swiss mouse 3T3 fibroblasts. The most commonly used principle initially involves the growth of a submerged culture of the keratinocytes to a confluent monolayer on a fibroblast-enriched collagen matrix, after which the keratinocytes are allowed to stratify into an organotypic epithelium at the air-liquid interface. Notably, the efficiency of this general protocol may vary with the type of oral epithelium. Nonkeratinized or parakeratinized epithelia may develop equally well or even better in continuously submerged conditions, whereas the generation of keratinized epithelia may be more easily promoted by the utilization of the air-liquid interface during the final phase of the experiment. Several studies, in fact, report this as a means of directing the pattern of differentiation to a particular type of oral epithelium.

The conditions for monolayer culture may often be applied also to organotypic culture. The majority of methods employ serum supplementation. However, several reports, some recent, describe the successful generation of organotypic epithelia in serum-free conditions. Notably, the serum-free period is limited to the generation of the epithelium. Fibroblasts, if used, are still derived in conditions with serum, and future application of methods for low-serum or serum-free culture of oral fibroblasts [Liu et al., 1991] may aid efforts to develop further refined conditions also for organotypic cultures. The conditions optimal for normal keratinocytes were occasionally shown to be applicable also to immortalized and tumor-derived cells or both. Multistage modeling of oral cancer development in vitro is therefore an option with some culture conditions.

The selected methodological reports have involved extensive characterizations of the cultures in efforts to investigate their usefulness as a tissue equivalent, some involving comparison with the respective monolayer culture. Organotypic culture of oral epithelium clearly involves larger efforts and longer time than monolayer culture. However, the unanimous conclusion is that the behavior of keratinocytes resembles the in vivo state more closely in organotypic models, particularly when epithelial-mesenchymal interactions are permitted. Normalization of morphogenesis, improved differentiation, and downregulation of proliferation at certain thickness is typically reported in matured organotypic epithelia, suggesting that the keratinocytes may be under a lower burden of "stress" compared with traditional monolayer culture. A number of research areas are presented in the listing of the methodological reports in Table 7.2, implying that the general methodology of organotypic culture is increasingly used in both basic and applied research on the oral epithelium. Notably, other published literature has applied these methods for studies of oral epithelium in an organotypic state.

2. REAGENTS AND MATERIALS

2.1. Preparation of EMHA, a Medium for Serum-Free Culture of Oral Keratinocytes

The medium EMHA (an epithelial medium with high amino acid supplementation) is based on MCDB 153 enriched with various growth supplements, including a stock of several amino acids · in high concentration. EMHA, initially termed EMA, was developed for serum-free culture of oral keratinocytes [Sundqvist et al., 1991a], but it is also applicable to keratinocytes from other squamous epithelia, including epidermis. The medium is similar or possibly identical to the commercially available medium KGM. However, the protocol for preparation and mixing of the individual stocks and components is different from the original protocol provided by Boyce and Ham [1983, 1986]. Almost 20 years of efforts to optimize cell yields and reproducibility of cultures derived from more than 800 oral mucosal specimens in our laboratory has generated a cost-saving protocol in which a solution termed pre-MCDB 153 is supplemented with selected stocks and individual growth supplements when preparing the final growth medium (EMHA). For example, 20 rather than 35 μg/ml of bovine pituitary extract (PEX) is required for optimal growth in EMHA compared with KGM.

As the instructions for preparation and the lists of constituents of EMHA are quite extensive, they have been listed in a series of appendixes at the end of this chapter. Preparation of complete EMHA from the appropriate stocks is tabulated in Appendix A. A protocol for the preparation of a solution named pre-MCDB 153 is tabulated in Appendix B. This pre-MCDB 153 is more stable than MCDB 153 when made without the five different stocks indicated. Instructions for preparation of each of the stocks in EMHA and pre-MCDB 153 are tabulated in Appendix C based on the original denominations (numbers and letters) given to these stocks by Ham and Boyce [1986]. This Appendix also includes instructions for preparation of a high-amino acid stock developed by Pittelkow and Scott [1986] and the various single supplements in EMHA and pre-MCDB 153. Appendix D contains the instructions for the single solutions used to make up the trace element stock (Stock L in Appendix C). Finally, Appendix E completes the instructions for preparation of EMHA by providing the stepwise protocol used to make up an extract from bovine pituitaries. This Appendix also contains a typical testing protocol that can be used for evaluation of new batches. As can be seen, the Appendixes for media fabrication are presented in a reversed order with the intent of indicating where the individual solutions, stocks, or supplements should be ultimately used. Each Appendix contains a heading describing the logistics underlying the procedure and a subheading with pertinent details on preparation, storage, and longevity.

All but one of the chemicals are obtained from Sigma and marked according to their product catalog for the year 2000; only selenious acid is from Kebo. As these constituents are so numerous, and almost all are from Sigma, they are not listed in the Sources of Materials at the end of this chapter. Suppliers' names and addresses are provided at the end of the book. Information on handling and storage of purchased individual chemicals is provided in the product catalogs and should be followed. However, the current protocols contain the information needed with regard to source, handling, and storage/longevity of stocks made from individual components or mixtures of components that are included in EMHA and pre-MCDB 153.

Note that:

(i) Chemicals are repurchased on at least an annual basis provided that the company has a new batch of the chemical (this should be checked before ordering!).

(ii) A "pre-MCDB 153" is fabricated based on efforts to improve longevity and reproducibility of the cultures. Therefore, some of the stocks originally designed for MCDB 153 are added just before use to make EMHA.

(iii) New MCBD stocks (and those used for making EMHA) are routinely made on a 3-month basis, and the old stocks are discarded after the new ones have been tested, i.e., after proof that the new stocks support growth in EMHA at least as well as the previous ones.

(iv) After thawing of "frozen stocks" they are generally never refrozen. If not used at once, they are only used on a short-term basis for preparation of additional medium within a week or two.

2.2. Preparation of Stocks/Solutions (Other Than for Growth Medium) for Serum-Free Culture of Oral Keratinocytes

Six solutions are necessary for monolayer and organotypic serum-free culture of oral keratinocytes. In order, these include: the solution used for transport of donor tissue from the clinic, the buffer used in all protocols except for media preparation (PBSA: Dulbecco's phosphate-buffered saline lacking Ca^{2+} and Mg^{2+}), the trypsin solutions used for digestive treatment of tissue for the purpose of generating primary cultures and for passage of primary and transfer cultures, the coating solution consisting of fibronectin, collagen, and bovine serum albumin that is used in the establishment of primary cultures, the serum-free medium used for long-term frozen storage of the cells in liquid nitrogen, and finally, the collagen stock (type I collagen isolated from rat tail) used in the establishment of a dermal equivalent applicable to organotypic culture of the cells. The subheadings provide additional information on preparation, procedure, and applicability of the respective solution. Sources of the various reagents and chemicals are provided in Appendix F at the end of this chapter.

2.2.1. Medium for Transport of Oral Tissue Specimens

Component	Stock Concentration	Amount (ml)
For surgical specimens:		
Leibovitz 15 medium[a]		500
Gentamicin[b]	50 mg/ml	1.0
Glutamine	200 mM	7.5
For autopsy specimens also include:		
Gentamicin[b]	50 mg/ml	1.0 (i.e., additional 1 ml; total amount is 2.0 ml)
Penicillin-streptomycin[c]	10,000 U/ml, 10 mg/ml	5.0
Fungizone[d]	250 μg/ml	2.0

[a]Without glutamine. [b]Gentamicin sulfate; active against *Mycoplasma* and gram (+) and (−) bacteria (See Appendix C). [c]Penicillin-streptomycin combined (See Sources of Materials); active against gram (+) and (−) bacteria; 10,000 units penicillin and 10 mg streptomycin per ml; store refrigerated. [d]Fungizone (amphotericin B), 250 μg/ml (See Sources of Materials); active against yeasts and molds; store frozen.

2.2.2. Ca^{2+}-Mg^{2+}-Free Phosphate-Buffered Saline (PBSA)

Component	Amount per 1 L (10×)	Amount per 3 L (1×)
NaCl	80 g	24 g
KCl	2.0 g	0.6 g
KH_2PO_4	2.0 g	0.6 g
$Na_2HPO_4 \cdot 2H_2O$	14.4 g	4.32 g

For preparation of a 10× stock, mix the components, adjust to pH 7.4 with HCl and subsequently add UPW to make up to final volume. Dilute 1:10 with sterile UPW for use.

2.2.3. Trypsin Solution for Digestion of Oral Tissue

Component	Stock Concentration	Amount (ml)	Final Concentration
Trypsin	2.5%	6.8	0.17%
PBSA		93.2	

Make aliquots and freeze at −20°C until use. Discard thawed solutions after use.

2.2.4. Trypsin Solutions for Passaging Oral Cell Cultures

Component	Stock Concentration, % w/v	Amount (ml)	Final Concentration, % w/v
PET[a]:			
Polyvinylpyrrolidone, 40,000 Da	10	10	1
EGTA	0.2	10	0.02
Trypsin	2.5	1.0	0.025
PBSA		79	

2.2.4. Trypsin Solutions for Passaging Oral Cell Cultures (continued)

Component	Stock Concentration, % w/v	Amount (ml)	Final Concentration, % w/v
PET, 3 × T[b]:			
Polyvinylpyrrolidone, 40,000 Da	10	10	1
EGTA	0.2	10	0.02
Trypsin	2.5	3.0	0.075
PBSA		77	
E-PET, 3 × T[c]:			
Polyvinylpyrrolidone, 40,000 Da	10	10	1
EGTA	0.2	10	0.02
EDTA	2.0	1.0	0.02
Trypsin	2.5	3.0	0.075
PBSA		76	

[a]PET is suitable for most cells, e.g., oral keratinocytes and fibroblasts. [b]PET 3 × T is suitable if the cells detach slowly in PET. [c]E-PET is used for confluent cultures of oral carcinoma cells (SqCC/Y1); this solution also decreases aggregation of detached cells.

2.2.5. Fibronectin/Collagen (FN/C/BSA) Coating of Plastic Culture Vessels

Component	Stock Concentration, mg/ml	Amount (ml)	Final Concentration, μg/ml
Fibronectin[a]	1.0	1.0 ml	10
Vitrogen[b]	~3	1.0 ml	~30
BSA[c]	1.0	1.0 ml	10
PBSA		97 ml	

[a]Use the lyophilized preparation; store at −20°C. [b]Vitrogen is a sterile solution of purified, pepsin-solubilized bovine dermal collagen dissolved in 0.012 N HCl; store refrigerated. [c]Make sterile stocks of 1.0 and 10 mg/ml in PBSA; store refrigerated.

Coat dishes with the solution for between 1 and 6 h at 37°C; the surface area of the dish should be covered, for example, add 1 ml per 60-mm dish. The FN/C/BSA solution can be collected and reused at least twice if maintained sterile. Store refrigerated.

2.2.6. Serum-Free Freezing Medium for Oral Keratinocytes

(From Boyce and Ham [1986]).

Component	Stock Concentration	Amount (ml)	Final Concentration
MCDB 153		84.66	
PEX	5 mg/ml	5.0	250 μg/ml
Ca^{2+}	100 mM	0.1	100 μM

2.2.6. Serum-Free Freezing Medium for Oral Keratinocytes (continued)

(From Boyce and Ham [1986]).

Component	Stock Concentration	Amount (ml)	Final Concentration
EGF	10 μg/ml	0.1	10 ng/ml
HC	0.36 mg/ml (1.0 mM)	0.14	0.5 μg/ml (1.4 μM)
DMSO		10	10% v/v

Abbreviations: PEX, pituitary extract; EGF; epidermal growth factor; HC, hydrocortisone; DMSO, dimethyl sulfoxide.

2.2.7. Preparation of Collagen Stock for Organotypic Culture of Oral Epithelium

Store rat tails at $-70°C$. Perform the preparation in a sterile hood.

(i)   Thaw in 70% alcohol and rinse twice in UPW.

(ii) Cut off the upper thick end (~1 cm) of each tail and discard.

(iii) Incise full length of skin on remaining tail and strip off.

(iv) Fracture tails into smaller segments with two clamps, pull out the tendons, clip, and collect them in a Petri dish containing PBSA.

(v)   Pluck tendons into pieces and spread out, remove blood vessels and peritendineum carefully using tweezers.

(vi) Blot tendons dry on preweighed sterile blotting paper.

(vii) Weigh tendons under sterile conditions.

(viii) Add to the moist weight an amount of 0.1% (sterile) acetic acid to achieve a final concentration of 4 mg per ml.

(ix) Stir at 4°C using a magnetic stir plate for 24 h (a homogeneous gel that can be poured is achieved).

(x)   After extraction, clear the supernatant by centrifugation (30 min at 10,000 g; repeat if necessary).

(xi) Divide the collagen solution in aliquots, e.g., in 100-ml flasks, and store at 4°C.

3. PROTOCOLS FOR MONOLAYER AND ORGANOTYPIC CULTURE OF HUMAN ORAL EPITHELIUM

Six basic protocols are presented for serum-free growth of oral keratinocytes in monolayer and organotypic culture. In order, these include instructions for tissue processing and initiation of primary cultures, sequential passage of monolayer cultures, freezing of cells for storage, thawing of cells from frozen storage for reinitiation of cultures, determination of colony forming efficiency (this is a highly useful assay for assessment of clonal growth; it is recommended for assessment of pituitary extract to standardize the growth-promoting effect of different preparations), and, finally, preparation of organotypic cultures.

Protocol 7.1. Tissue Processing for Initiation of Primary Cultures of Oral Keratinocytes

Reagents and Materials

Sterile

- ❏ Transport medium: Leibowitz L-15 (see Section 2.2.1)
- ❏ Growth medium (see Section 2.1 and Appendix A)
- ❏ Antibiotic-supplemented growth medium: growth medium supplemented with gentamicin 100 μg/ml, penicillin-streptomycin 100 U/ml, and Fungizone, 1 μg/ml
- ❏ PBSA: Dulbecco's PBS lacking Ca^{2+} and Mg^{2+} (see Section 2.2.2)
- ❏ Trypsin, 0.17% in PBSA (see Section 2.2.3)
- ❏ Scalpels, #11 blade
- ❏ Scissors, fine
- ❏ Forceps, fine, 2 pairs
- ❏ Petri dishes, non-tissue culture grade for dissection, 3.5 cm, 10 cm
- ❏ Centrifuge tubes, 15 ml, conical
- ❏ Micropipette, e.g., Gilson, 100 μl
- ❏ FN/C/BSA-coated culture dishes, 5 cm (see Section 2.2.5)

Protocol

(a) Obtain the tissue from surgery or early autopsy, place in cold L-15 medium ("transport medium") and transfer to the laboratory as soon as possible.

(b) Transfer the tissue to a 10-cm dish and rinse with phosphate-buffered saline (PBSA).

(c) Remove as much connective tissue as possible, including parts containing blood. If the tissue specimen(s) have a surface area of ≥ 1 cm^2, divide them into smaller pieces.

(d) Place the specimens in a 3.5-cm dish and add enough 0.17%

trypsin solution for coverage (1–2 ml) and incubate overnight at 4°C.

(e) Hold each specimen, using forceps, for example, then peel and scrape away the epithelium with another pair of forceps into the trypsin solution.

(f) Triturate the suspension carefully a few times, to further disaggregate the cells, and transfer the cell suspension to a centrifuge tube.

(g) Rinse the dish with PBSA and subsequently add this rinsing solution to the cell suspension. Use the same volume for rinsing as of the trypsin solution used for tissue digestion.

(h) Remove an aliquot by micropipette for determination of cell yield. (Another approach is to determine yield of the cells after centrifugation and resuspension in fresh medium as described below).

(i) Pellet the cells at 125 g at 4°C, preferably using a refrigerated centrifuge, and resuspend the cells in growth medium. (Determine the number of cells, if not done while cells are being collected by centrifugation as above).

(j) Dilute with additional growth medium as required and then seed the cells at $5 \times 10^3/cm^2$ on FN/C/BSA-coated culture dishes. If cells are derived from autopsy material use antibiotic-supplemented growth medium for the initial 3–4 days in culture.

(k) Feed the cells with fresh medium after 24 h to remove possible cell debris and erythrocytes and, from then on, feed the cells every second day.

Protocol 7.2. Passage of Oral Keratinocytes

Reagents and Materials

Sterile

❏ PBSA
❏ PET solution (see Section 2.2.4)
❏ Growth medium (see Section 2.1 and Appendix A)
❏ Petri dishes, tissue culture grade, 5 or 10 cm

Nonsterile

❏ Neubauer hemocytometer counting chamber

Protocol

(a) Rinse the cells once with PBSA.

(b) Add PET solution, covering the cells completely with the solution, e.g., use 3 ml/10-cm dish.

(c) Incubate at room temperature until the cells begin to round up and/or detach from the dish. Follow the cell detachment under the microscope (the procedure generally takes 5–10 min). The rate of detachment can be enhanced by addition of trypsin at higher concentrations (see Section 2.2.4) or by increasing the temperature to 37°C.

(d) When most cells have detached, carefully tap on the side of dish and pipette the trypsin solution gently over the growth surface to mechanically enhance detachment.

(e) When the cells have detached, add 5–10 ml of PBSA to the dish to inactivate the action of trypsin by dilution.

(f) Transfer the cell suspension to centrifuge tubes and triturate gently to obtain an even distribution of the cells in the suspension.

(g) Using a 1-ml pipette, take out a sample for a cell count and transfer to a Neubauer chamber, taking care to fill but not overfill the counting chamber.

(h) Determine the number of cells.

(i) Pellet the cells by centrifugation for 5 min at 125 g at 4°C. Follow the manual for the centrifuge for a correct formula to convert g to rpm.

(j) Remove the supernatant and tap the tube gently against the fingers until the pellet disperses.

(k) Add growth medium as desired and triturate the cell suspension gently with a pipette. To avoid variation in number of cells seeded per vessel (when many vessels are seeded), make up a cell suspension of the total volume required for all the dishes instead of filling the vessels with most of the medium and subsequently inoculating a small volume of concentrated cell suspension.

(l) Add the cell suspension to each vessel. A variation in the volume of ±0.1 ml per vessel is acceptable.

(m) Place all the vessels on a tray. Agitate the vessels gently by holding and moving the tray in your hands alternating between different directions, to ensure even density of the cells in each vessel (simply swirling the dishes will focus the cells in the center of the dish). It is also important that the shelves are evenly fixed in the incubator where the vessels are placed, and that the incubator is free of vibration, to avoid an uneven distribution of cells during attachment.

(n) Incubate the cells undisturbed for 4–24 h before changing the medium.

Protocol 7.3. Freezing of Oral Keratinocytes for Storage in Liquid Nitrogen

Reagents and Materials

Sterile

❑ Freezing medium, serum-free (see Section 2.2.6)
❑ PET (see Protocol 7.2 and Section 2.2.4)
❑ Vials for freezing (i.e., vials that are suited for storage at $-170°$); 1–5 ml

Protocol

(a) Detach cells by trypsin treatment (see Protocol 7.2), determine total number of cells, and pellet by centrifugation.

(b) Resuspend the cells in freezing medium at a final concentration of $1-10 \times 10^6$ cells/ml.

(c) Aliquot the cell suspension into freezing vials.

(d) Follow the directions for freezing supplied by the manufacturer of the liquid nitrogen container or as published elsewhere [e.g., Freshney, 2000].

Cells can generally be stored for at least a year, maintaining a high growth potential, but the success of the storage of frozen cells will depend on the storage temperature and how much it fluctuates.

Protocol 7.4. Thawing of Oral Keratinocytes for Culture

Reagents and Materials

Sterile

❑ Growth medium (see Section 2.1 and Appendix A)
❑ Flasks or dishes for thawed cells

Protocol

(a) Prepare cell culture dishes or flasks with growth medium. To minimize the possible toxicity by dimethyl sulfoxide (DMSO, a component of the "freezing medium"), the cell suspension should be diluted at least 10-fold with growth medium. (When used as solvent, DMSO is usually considered nontoxic at $\leq 0.1\%$ v/v).

(b) Thaw the frozen cells by placing the ampoule briefly in a water bath at 37° or by gently shaking it in the water.

$\triangle$ **Safety note.** Take care when thawing vials that have been submerged in liquid nitrogen as they can explode violently if they have inspired liquid nitrogen. Thaw in a covered container and do not handle the vial until 20–30 s after placing in the container. Alternatively, store vials in the vapor phase of the liquid nitrogen freezer.

(c) As soon as the cell suspension has thawed, transfer the suspension to a 15-ml tube and gently dilute the suspension with 10–15 ml of medium. Subsequently, pipette the suspension to culture vessels to achieve a correct cell density.

(d) Carefully swirl and shake the vessel, or pipette the cell suspension gently, to distribute the cells evenly in the medium in the vessel.

(e) Incubate the cells for at least 4 h without disturbing to promote highest attachment.

(f) Replace the medium with fresh growth medium after 4–24 h to remove unattached cells and remaining DMSO.

Protocol 7.5. Determination of Colony Forming Efficiency of Oral Keratinocytes

Reagents and Materials

Sterile

- ❑ Growth medium (see Section 2.1 and Appendix A)
- ❑ Reagent or solution for testing
- ❑ Petri dishes, 6 cm

Nonsterile

- ❑ Formalin, 10%
- ❑ Aqueous crystal violet, 0.25%

Protocol

(a) Seed epithelial cells in growth medium at 50 cells per cm^2 in 6-cm dishes (surface area $\sim$20 cm^2).

(b) Incubate the dishes undisturbed for 24–48 h to allow for cell attachment and initiation of growth. Individual cells can then multiply into clones that can be counted as colonies under a microscope (see below). In principle, a seeding density that gives ≥50 but preferably <500 colonies per dish should be used. Within these colony numbers, enough colonies can be obtained to produce reliable data, whereas the risk of having too many colonies growing together is small.

(c) Exchange medium with fresh medium and incubate the cells with the reagent, mixture, or solution under study. Short-term exposure to agents, e.g., toxicants, is generally for 1–24 h, then followed by addition of fresh growth medium. Alternatively, cells might be exposed continuously during the colony forming efficiency (CFE) assay, e.g., to individual or mixtures of growth factor(s).

(d) Incubate the dishes until colonies are visible under the microscope, e.g., for 7–10 days. Usually, the medium is replaced with fresh medium at 4 days (in the middle of the experiment).

(e) Fix the cells with 10% formalin and then stain with 0.25% aqueous crystal violet.

(f) Determine the mean CFE from duplicate or triplicate dishes using a stereomicroscope. For a particular treatment or condition, CFE is calculated as the number of colonies as a percentage of the number of cells seeded. The surviving fraction is the mean CFE of the tests divided by the mean number of colonies in the control cultures.

Protocol 7.6. Preparation of Organotypic Cultures of Oral Epithelium

Reagents and Materials

Sterile

- ❑ Collagen type I (from rat tail tendon), 4 mg/ml in 0.1% sterile acetic acid (see Section 2.2.7)
- ❑ Hanks' balanced saline (with phenol red) 10×
- ❑ NaOH, 5 N (for neutralization)
- ❑ Fetal bovine serum (FBS)
- ❑ Growth medium (see Section 2.1 and Appendix A)
- ❑ Multiwell plates, 24-well, to act as molds
- ❑ Oral keratinocytes in monolayer culture

❑ Mesenchymal cells, e.g., oral fibroblasts, in monolayer culture (optional)

Protocol

(a) Precool a sterile beaker and stirring bar in an ice tray on a magnetic stirrer in the sterile hood.

(b) Mix 8 parts collagen and 1 part 10× Hanks' BSS, avoiding air bubbles. Keep the mixture on ice.

(c) Neutralize by adding 5 N NaOH (~50–100 μl per 10 ml mix) while stirring and keeping on ice. Color should turn to pale/light purple.

(d) Add 1 part FBS with stirring.
For incorporation of mesenchymal cells into the gels, detach the mesenchymal cells by trypsinization and suspend at 10-fold normal density in FBS (usually 10^5 cells are used per ml gel volume). Then add this suspension to the gel as for addition of FBS alone.

(e) Transfer 1-ml aliquots of the mix into the wells of 24-well plates and allow polymerization (a thermal solution-gel transition will take place) for 30–60 min at 37°C in a CO_2 incubator.

(f) Add 1 ml of cell culture medium and allow the gels to equilibrate overnight in the incubator.

(g) Seed oral keratinocytes at 3×10^5 on top of each gel.

(h) Allow the keratinocytes to adhere and to form a confluent monolayer (takes 24–48 h).

(i) Shift the gels to organotypic culture conditions by transferring them onto tablelike supports (made of stainless steel grid) in 6-cm culture dishes.

(j) Add growth medium (EMHA containing 1 mM Ca^{2+}) to the dish such that the epithelium is placed at the medium/air interface (the top of gel should be moist).

4. APPLICATIONS OF METHODS FOR CULTURE OF ORAL EPITHELIUM

The stepwise development of in vitro methods for oral mucosa in the author's laboratory and their application to various projects in environmental medicine and carcinogenesis research are briefly summarized in Table 7.3. The results span characterization of keratinocyte features, including basal and terminal features, and the responsiveness to factors that regulate growth and differentiation.

TABLE 7.3. Application of In Vitro Model Systems for Toxicity and Carcinogenesis Studies of Human Buccal Mucosa[a]

Cell Types/Method Development	Method/Culture Conditions/ Longevity[c]	Studies/Results	References[c]
Keratinocytes; conditions for keratinocyte culture from explants established	NOK: explant outgrowth; buccal epithelial growth (BEG) medium, fibronectin/collagen (FN/C) coating; cells used in passages 1–3	Areca nut extract, 4 areca nut-specific alkaloids and their respective N-nitrosamines variably influence cell cloning, membrane integrity, vital dye accumulation, glutathione content, and DNA integrity; areca nut extract and the nitroso compound 3-(N-nitrosomethylamino)-propionaldehyde are highly cytotoxic and genotoxic	Sundqvist et al., 1989
Keratinocytes; conditions for keratinocyte culture from digested tissue established	NOK: explant outgrowth; FN/C coating; BEG medium; longevity of explants for generation of primary cultures: 2 months; longevity of cell lines: 5 passages	Morphology, growth, cell surface area, and migration variably regulated by factors; Basal, activation, and simple keratins expressed; CFE: ≤6% (≥16 cells/colony); CGR: 0.8 PD/D; EGF, cholera toxin, retinoic acid, and pituitary extract increase clonal growth; GI by TGF-β; TD induction (assessed from involucrin and cross-linked envelopes) by Ca^{2+}, FBS, and the tumor promoting agent 12-O-tetradecanoylphorbol-13-acetate	Sundqvist et al., 1991b
Normal and malignant keratinocytes; serum-free strain of carcinoma line SqCC/Y1 established	NOK: trypsin digestion and mechanical scraping; FN/C coating; longevity of cell lines: ~7 months, 60 PD, (10 passages); EMHA; SqCC/Y1; no surface coating; DMEM:Ham's F12 (3:1) + 10% FBS or EMHA	Coating with FN/C promotes generation of primary cultures; CFE: ≤40% (≥16 cells/colony); CG: ≤1.2 PD/D; GI by TGF-β; TD by FBS; medium suitable also for growth of SqCC/Y1: carcinoma cells resistant to induction of GI and TD by TGF-β, Ca^{2+}, and FBS; diploid and aneuploid karyotypes of normal and SqCC/Y1 cells, respectively	Sundqvist et al., 1991a
Fibroblasts; conditions for culture of oral fibroblasts at different serum levels established	Explant outgrowth; low-serum medium (LSM; 1.25% FBS) and high-serum medium (HSM; 10% FBS); explant longevity for generation of primary cultures: 8–12 months; longevity of cell lines: ≥5 passages	Cells exhibit fibroblastic morphology and marker expression (vimentin); CFE assay/toxicity assessments preferable in LSM because of lower reaction with toxicants, higher growth, and lower cell migration than in HSM; content of low-molecular-weight thiols determined: glutathione is the major free thiol present primarily in its reduced state; cysteine is present in lower amounts and primarily in its oxidized form	Liu et al., 1991

TABLE 7.3. Application of In Vitro Model Systems for Toxicity and Carcinogenesis Studies of Human Buccal Mucosa[a] (continued)

Cell Types/Method Development	Method/Culture Conditions/ Longevity[c]	Studies/Results	References[c]
Keratinocytes and fibroblasts	NOK: explant outgrowth; BEG medium, FN/C coating; fibroblasts: explant outgrowth; LSM	Biocompatibility assessment of single crystal sapphire indicates that this material is well suited for dental implantation; cells proliferate in vitro on implant material; cell morphology, and growth in mass culture and at clonal density identical as on regular tissue culture plastic	Arvidson et al., 1991
Normal and malignant keratinocytes	NOK: trypsin digestion and mechanical scraping; FN/C coating; serum-free strain of SqCC/Y1; EMHA for both cell types	Areca nut extract induces morphologic alterations (plasma membrane ridges) associated with particle internalization and aberrant TD; DNA single strand breaks may accumulate because of inhibited DNA repair; similar toxicity in normal and SqCC/Y1 cells; 3-(N-nitrosomethylamino)-propionaldehyde causes DNA single strand breaks and protein cross-links	Sundqvist and Grafström, 1992
Fibroblasts	Explant outgrowth; sequential application of HSM and LSM	A corrosion product of amalgam, Hg^{2+}, decreases cell viability assessed by CFE, vital dye accumulation, cytosolic deoxyglucose retention, and mitochondrial reduction of tetrazolium; Hg^{2+} exhibits high affinity for protein thiols, and glutathione offers limited protection against toxicity	Liu et al., 1992
Explant culture, normal and malignant keratinocytes; conditions for explant culture established	Explant culture on tissue culture plastic or gelatin sponge (2–5 days longevity); BEX medium; NOK: trypsin digestion and mechanical scraping; EMHA; FN/C coating; serum-free strain of SqCC/Y1; EMHA	A tobacco-specific N-nitrosamine termed NNK undergoes metabolism through α-carbon hydroxylation, carbonyl reduction, and N-pyridine oxidation; reactive metabolites bind to macromolecules in explant and monolayer cultures; NNK and nicotine do not influence cell cloning below 1 mM in normal and carcinoma cells	Liu et al., 1993

Cell Types/Method Development	Method/Culture Conditions/ Longevity[c]	Studies/Results	References[c]
Exfoliated normal keratinocytes and malignant keratinocytes	Short-term incubation of exfoliated cells collected by scraping; BSA-enriched Hanks' BSS; serum-free strain of SqCC/Y1; EMHA	Sialylation of mucinlike glycoproteins shown to be critical for cell surface adhesion of the bacterial strain Streptococcus sanguis; a NeuNAcα2-3Gal$\beta\beta$1-3GalNAc O-linked carbohydrate chain located on a 23-kDa membrane glycoprotein identified as receptor in the adhesion mechanism	Neeser et al., 1995
Normal and malignant keratinocytes; serum-free strains of SV40T-transfected cell lines developed	Transfection of NOK with SV40T; FN/C coating; SqCC/Y1; establishment of immortalized line SVpgC2a; EMHA for all cell types	Several lines generated with extended life span; the immortalized line SVpgC2a exhibits stable integration of SV40 T gene and complex formation between SV40T and the p53 and Rb proteins, respectively; SVpgC2a resistant to induction of GI and TD by TGF-β and FBS; aneuploid karyotype; SVpgC2a and SqCC/Y1 nontumorigenic and tumorigenic, respectively, in athymic nude mice (Balb/c strain)	Kulkarni et al., 1995
Normal and malignant keratinocytes	NOK: trypsin digestion and mechanical scraping; FN/C coating; SqCC/Y1; EMHA for both cell types	Differential display optimized and applied to search for genes that show higher expression in carcinoma; cloning and sequence analysis identified 3 oral tumor-expressed (OTEX) genes; OTEX 2 identical to L26 ribosomal protein whereas OTEX 1 and -3 had unknown identity/functions	Sundqvist et al., 1995
Normal and SV40T-transfected keratinocyte lines	NOK: trypsin digestion and mechanical scraping; FN/C coating; SqCC/Y1; EMHA for all cell types	Karyotyping by G-banding and flow cytometry demonstrated gross chromosomal changes in early passage of SV40 T-transfected lines; SVpgC2a exhibit a stabilized DNA content in the near-diploid range and as well as a nonrandom component in the overall pattern of random change	Kulkarni et al., 1996

TABLE 7.3. Application of In Vitro Model Systems for Toxicity and Carcinogenesis Studies of Human Buccal Mucosa[a] **(continued)**

Cell Types/Method Development	Method/Culture Conditions/ Longevity[c]	Studies/Results	References[c]
Normal, immortalized and malignant keratinocytes; fibroblasts	NOK: trypsin digestion and mechanical scraping; FN/C coating; SVpgC2a; SqCC/Y1; EMHA for keratinocytes; LSM for fibroblasts	The DNA repair enzyme O^6-methylguanine DNA methyltransferase (MGMT) is expressed in oral tissue and the tested cell types; SVpgC2a and SqCC/Y1 show 50% and 10% activity of normal cells; extracts from products related to tobacco and areca nut usage inhibit MGMT in vitro	Liu et al., 1997
Normal and immortalized keratinocytes	NOK: trypsin digestion and mechanical scraping; FN/C coating; SVpgC2a; EMHA for both cell types	Acetaldehyde and methylglyoxal generally induce similar toxicity in normal and SVpgC2a cells; endogenous DNA adducts from both aldehydes demonstrated by ^{32}P-postlabeling in SVpgC2a; exposed cells show dose-dependent adduct formation at relatively nontoxic levels	Vaca et al., 1998
Keratinocytes and fibroblasts	NOK: trypsin digestion and mechanical scraping; FN/C coating; EMHA; fibroblasts: sequential application of HSM and LSM	Formaldehyde causes dose-dependent toxicity in both cell types; removal of serum and free medium thiols increase the sensitivity and reproducibility of the assessment protocol; thiols protect against formaldehyde toxicity; different sensitivity to formaldehyde toxicity correlates to differences in thiol state between both cell types	Nilsson et al., 1998
Normal, immortalized and malignant keratinocytes; fibroblasts	NOK: trypsin digestion and mechanical scraping; no surface coating; SVpgC2a; SqCC/Y1; EMHA for keratinocytes; fibroblasts: sequential application of HSM and LSM	Alcohol dehydrogenase 3 (ADH3) is expressed in oral epithelium and the tested cell types; mRNA is expressed in proliferative cells, whereas protein is expressed in both proliferative and terminally differentiated cells; activity measurements of various alcohol and aldehyde-oxidizing activities, as well as K_m determinations, indicate that ADH3 is the major enzyme involved in formaldehyde oxidation in oral mucosa	Hedberg et al., 2000

TABLE 7.3. Application of In Vitro Model Systems for Toxicity and Carcinogenesis Studies of Human Buccal Mucosa[a] (continued)

Cell Types/Method Development	Method/Culture Conditions/ Longevity[c]	Studies/Results	References[c]
Normal, immortalized, and malignant keratinocytes	NOK: trypsin digestion and mechanical scraping; no surface coating; SVpgC2a; SqCC/Y1; EMHA for all cell types	mRNA and activity detected for several xenobiotic metabolizing cytochrome *P450* enzymes (CYPs) in oral epithelium and the tested cell types; CYP-dependent activity can be preserved or even activated in immortalized keratinocytes; aflatoxin B$_1$ implicated as an oral carcinogen	Vondracek et al., 2001
Normal, immortalized, and malignant keratinocytes; fibroblasts; conditions for organotypic culture established	Monolayer culture as above in EMHA. Organotypic culture: collagen lattice + buccal fibroblasts; EMHA; submerged (2 days) followed by air-liquid interface (10 days)	Organotypic cultures of normal keratinocytes express many of the same keratins as tissue; loss of keratins in SVpgC2a and their retention in SqCC/Y1 have several features in common with the respective keratin profile of oral epithelial dysplasia and well-differentiated oral squamous cell carcinoma; the cell lines in organotypic culture may be used to model the multistep progression of oral cancer.	Hansson et al., 2001
Normal, immortalized, and malignant keratinocytes in organotypic culture	Organotypic culture: collagen lattice + buccal fibroblasts; EMHA; submerged (2 days) followed by air-liquid interface (10 days)	Epithelia regenerated with the different cell types show uniform expression of ADH3 similarly to tissue; The results indicate preservation of ADH3 during malignant transformation; NOK, SVpgC2a, and SqCC/Y1 likely represent functional models for studies of formaldehyde metabolism in oral epithelium	Hedberg et al., 2001

[a]The listing of these references is an effort to provide a chronological description of the developments of in vitro methods for oral mucosa for parallel studies of environmental medicine and carcinogenesis in the author's laboratory. Some studies overlap Tables 7.1 and 7.2, but the results are presented in more detail in the current table. Lesser detail for some reports may depend on an effort to avoid repetition from earlier part of table. [b]Under "Methods/Culture Conditions/Longevity" the information is presented in order of normal, immortalized, and malignant keratinocytes, or keratinocytes before fibroblasts, if studied. "Keratinocytes" without specification refers to cultures obtained from apparently normal tissue. Monolayer culture is implied unless specified. Abbreviations are variably used to save space in certain sections. Some abbreviations of terms are explained and then used in the sections, e.g., for enzymes. [c]Major findings are highlighted under "Studies/Results." The reader is referred to the original articles for in depth information. [c]The abbreviations used are: ADH3, alcohol dehydrogenase 3; BEG, buccal epithelial growth; BEX, buccal explant; BSA, bovine serum albumin; BSS, balanced salt solution; CFE, colony forming efficiency; CGR, clonal growth rate; CYP, cytochrome *P450* enzyme; EGF, epidermal growth factor; EMHA, epithelial medium with high levels of amino acids; FBS, fetal bovine serum; FN/C, fibronectin/collagen; GI, growth inhibition; HSM, high-serum medium; LSM, low-serum medium; MGMT, O^6-methylguanine DNA methyltransferase; NOK, normal oral keratinocytes; OTEX, oral tumor expressed; PD, population doublings; PD/D, population doublings per day; SV40T, Simian virus 40 T antigen; TD, terminal differentiation of the squamous type; TGF-β, human transforming growth factor β1.

Furthermore, a variety of chemicals believed to be potential causes of acute toxicity, or to initiate or promote cancer development, were studied. This work has been aimed at elucidating biochemical pathways and molecular mechanisms underlying pathological responses and establishing results in human cells that bridge information obtained from clinical and epidemiological studies or from experiments in laboratory animals. For example, chemicals/constituents/components or complex mixtures related to dental materials and usage of tobacco and areca nut were studied (see Table 7.3 for references). In this context, the protective function of cellular thiols such as glutathione was evaluated, and the roles of various enzymes were investigated by analysis of their expression and function. Notably, the results also involve the definition of suitable conditions for both short-term and longer-term exposure of oral cell types to various agents, including reactive chemicals.

Several points, of potential interest for those who consider initiating projects using in vitro methods for oral epithelium, can be made based on the results presented in Table 7.3. Many cellular functions are conserved among different cell types, and in this regard, oral fibroblast cell lines often show greater longevity and are easier to grow in culture than normal keratinocyte lines. Thus fibroblasts, or for that matter transformed keratinocyte lines (see Section 1.3.7), may be used concurrently with keratinocytes in the early phases of some projects. Various toxicity assessments involving the biochemical measurement of cell functions and DNA repair processes are examples where fibroblasts or immortalized lines may provide good preliminary indications for the actual outcome in normal keratinocytes. However, the type of project may require that all work demands the use of normal phenotypically competent cells, for example, studies of unique keratinocyte functions like terminal differentiation.

Interindividual variation may be a source of variation also in normal cell lines derived under standardized conditions in vitro. Therefore, the common standard of doing at least three experiments to allow for statistical analysis with permanent cell lines is often extended in the analysis of normal finite cell lines, typically involving lines from five donors. Some experiments also demand a large number of cells and may require pooling of normal cells from several donors. If pooling is employed it is important to adopt a consistent strategy, such that cells from different donors are pooled in equal proportions, usually at the first or second passage. For most laboratories, experiments that repeatedly utilize more than 50×10^6 cells require the use of cell lines that are more easily grown than normal keratinocytes.

Overall, the reports in Table 7.3 provide several examples that can aid in understanding the logistics involved in the application of the media, solutions, and protocols of this chapter in various experimental studies.

ACKNOWLEDGMENTS

After almost two decades of efforts with many appreciated co-workers, the author would like to especially thank Dr. Kristina Sundqvist and Ms. Å Elfwing for exceptional contributions to the establishment and realization of the methods described herein. The work was supported by the Swedish Cancer Society, Swedish Council for Forestry and Agricultural Research (EU Project AIR2-CT93-0860), the Swedish National Board of Laboratory Animals, the Swedish Fund for Research Without Animal Experiments, the Swedish Match, the Preem Environment Fund, and the Karolinska Institutet.

REFERENCES

Allen HB, Rheinwald JG (1984): Polycyclic aromatic hydrocarbon mutagenesis of human epidermal keratinocytes in culture. Proc Natl Acad Sci USA 81: 7802–7806.

D'Ambrosio SM, Gibson-D'Ambrosio R, Milo GE, Casto B, Kelloff GJ, Steele VE (2000): Differential response of normal, premalignant and malignant human oral epithelial cells to growth inhibition by chemopreventive agents. Anticancer Res 20: 2273–2280.

Arenholt BD, Jepsen A, MacCallum DK, Lillie JH (1987): The growth and structure of human oral keratinocytes in culture. J Invest Dermatol 88: 314–319.

Arvidson K, Fartash B, Moberg LE, Grafström RC, Ericsson I (1991): In vitro and in vivo experimental studies on single crystal sapphire dental implants. Clin Oral Impl Res 2: 47–55.

Autrup H, Grafström RC (1982): Comparison of carcinogen metabolism in different organs and species. In Hietanen E, Laitinen M and Hänninen O (eds): "Cytochrome P450: Biochemistry, Biophysics and Environmental Implications." Amsterdam: Elsevier Biomedical Press, pp 643–648.

Boyce ST, Ham RG (1983): Calcium-regulated differentiation of normal human epidermal keratinocytes in chemically defined clonal culture and serum-free serial culture. J Invest Dermatol 81(1 Suppl): 33s–40s.

Boyce ST, Ham RG (1986): Normal human epidermal keratinocytes. In Webber MM, Sekely L (eds): "In Vitro Models for Cancer Research." Boca Raton, FL: CRC Press, pp 245–274.

Boyd NM, Reade PC (1988): Mechanisms of carcinogenesis with particular reference to the oral mucosa. J Oral Pathol 17: 193–201.

Bradford MM (1976): A rapid and sensitive method for the quantitation of microgram quantities of protein utilizing the principle of protein-dye binding. Anal Biochem 7: 248–254.

Burkhart A, Maerker R (eds) (1981): "A Colour Atlas of Oral Cancers." London: Wolf Medical Publications

Burns JE, Clark LJ, Yeudall WA, Mitchell R, Mackenzie K, Chang SE, Parkinson EK (1994): The p53 status of cultured human premalignant oral keratinocytes. Br J Cancer 70: 591–595.

Chang SE (1991): Human oral keratinocyte cultures and in vitro model systems for studying oral carcinogenesis. In Johnson NW (ed): "Oral Cancer: Detection of Patients and Lesions at Risk." Cambridge: Cambridge University Press, Vol 2, pp 340–363.

Chang SE, Foster S, Betts D, Marnock WE (1992): DOK, a cell line established from human dysplastic oral mucosa, shows a partially transformed non-malignant phenotype. Int J Cancer 52: 896–902.

Cho KH, Ahn HT, Park KC, Chung JH, Kim SW, Sung MW, Kim KH, Chung PH, Eun HC, Youn JI (2000): Reconstruction of human hard-palate mucosal epithelium on de-epidermized dermis. J Dermatol Sci 22: 117–124.

Chopra DP, Xue-Hu IC (1993): Secretion of alpha-amylase in human parotid gland epithelial cell culture. J Cell Physiol 155: 223–233.

Chung JH, Cho KH, Lee DY, Kwon OS, Sung MW, Kim KH, Eun HC (1997): Human oral buccal mucosa reconstructed on dermal substrates: A model for oral epithelial differentiation. Arch Dermatol Res 289: 677–685.

Dale BA, Salonen J, Jones AH (1990): New approaches and concepts in the study of differentiation of oral epithelia. Crit Rev Oral Biol Med 1: 167–190.

Delcourt-Huard A, Corlu A, Joffre A, Magloire H, Bonnaure-Mallet M (1997): Reconstituted human gingival epithelium: Nonsubmerged in vitro model. In Vitro Cell Dev Biol Anim 33: 30–36.

De Luca M, Albanese E, Megna M, Cancedda R, Mangiante PE, Cadoni A, Franzi AT (1990): Evidence that human oral epithelium reconstituted in vitro and transplanted onto patients with defects in the oral mucosa retains properties of the original donor site. Transplantation 50: 454–459.

DiPaolo JA, Burkhardt A, Doniger J, Pirisi L, Popescu NC, Yasumoto S (1986): In vitro models for studying the molecular biology of carcinogenesis. Toxicol Pathol 14: 417–423.

Farin FM, Bigler LG, Oda D, McDougall JK and Omiecinski CJ (1995): Expression of cytochrome P450 and microsomal epoxide hydrolase in cervical and oral epithelial cells immortalized by human papillomavirus type 16 E6/E7 genes. Carcinogenesis 16: 1391–1401.

Formanek M, Millesi W, Willheim M, Scheiner O, Kornfehl J (1996): Optimized growth medium for primary culture of human oral keratinocytes. Int J Oral Maxillofac Surg 25: 157–160.

Freshney, RI (2000): "Culture of Animal Cells, a Manual of Basic Technique." New York: Wiley-Liss, pp 299–303.

Garlick JA, Parks WC, Welgus HG, Taichman LB (1996): Re-epithelialization of human oral keratinocytes in vitro. J Dent Res 75: 912–918.

Gilchrist EP, Moyer MP, Shillitoe EJ, Clare N, Murrah VA (2000): Establishment of a human polyclonal oral epithelial cell line. Oral Surg Oral Med Oral Pathol Oral Radiol Endod 90: 340–347.

Gosselin F, Gervaise M, Neveux Y, Portier MM (1989): Reconstitution in vitro of human gingiva. C R Acad Sci III 309: 323–329.

Gosselin F, Magloire H, Joffre A, Portier MM (1990): Cytokeratins as molecular markers in the evaluation of the precise differentiation stage of human gingival epithelium reconstituted in vitro. Arch Oral Biol 35: 17S–221S.

Grafström RC (1990): Carcinogenesis studies in human epithelial tissues and cells in vitro: Emphasis on serum-free culture conditions and transformation studies. Acta Physiol Scand Suppl 592: 93–133.

Grafström RC, Norén UG, Zheng X, Elfwing Å, Sundqvist K (1997): Growth and transformation of human oral epithelium in vitro. In: "Risk and Progression Factors in Carcinogenesis." Heidelberg: Springer-Verlag, Vol 143, pp 275–306.

Gron B, Andersson A, Dabelsteen E (1999): Blood-group-related carbohydrates are expressed in organotypic cultures of human skin and oral mucosa. APMIS 107: 779–790.

Hansson A, Bloor BK, Haig Y, Morgan PR, Ekstrand J, Grafström RC (2001): Expression of keratins in normal, immortalized and malignant oral epithelia in organotypic culture. Oral Oncol 37: 19–30.

Harris CC, Grafström RC, Shamsuddin AM, Sinopoli NT, Trump BF, Autrup H (1984): Carcinogen metabolism and carcinogen-DNA adducts in human tissues and cells. In Greim H, Jung R, Kramer M, Marquardt H, Oesch F (eds): "Biochemical Basis of Chemical Carcinogenesis." New York: Raven Press, pp 123–135.

Hedberg J, Höög JO, Nilsson JA, Zheng X, Elfwing Å, Grafström RC (2000): Expression of alcohol dehydrogenase 3 in tissue and cultured cells from human oral mucosa. Am J Pathol 157: 1745–1755.

Hedberg JJ, Hansson A, Nilsson JA, Höög JO, Grafström RC (2001): Uniform expression of alcohol dehydrogenase 3 (ADH3) in regenerated epithelia of normal, immortalized and malignant human oral keratinocytes. ATLA-Altern Lab Anim 29: 1–9.

Hibino Y, Hata K, Horie K, Torii S, Ueda M (1996): Structural changes and cell viability of cultured epithelium after freezing storage. J Craniomaxillofac Surg 24: 346–351.

Izumi K, Takacs G, Terashi H, Feinberg SE (1999): Ex vivo development of a composite human oral mucosal equivalent. J Oral Maxillofac Surg 57: 571–577.

Izumi K, Terashi H, Marcelo CL, Feinberg SE (2000): Development and characterization of a tissue-engineered human oral mucosa equivalent produced in a serum-free culture system. J Dent Res 79: 798–805.

Kang MK, Guo W, Park NH (1998): Replicative senescence of normal human oral keratinocytes is associated with the loss of telomerase activity without shortening of telomeres. Cell Growth Differ 9: 85–95.

Kang MK, Bibb C, Baluda MA, Rey O, Park NH (2000): In vitro replication and differentiation of normal human oral keratinocytes. Exp Cell Res 258: 288–297.

Kamata N, Yokoyama K, Fujimoto R, Ueda N, Hayashi E, Nakanishi H, Nagayama M (1999): Growth of normal oral keratinocytes and squamous cell carcinoma cells in a novel protein-free defined medium. In Vitro Cell Dev Biol Anim 35: 635–641.

Kasperbauer JL, Neel HB, Scott RE (1990): Proliferation and differentiation characteristics of normal human squamous mucosal cells of the upper aerodigestive tract. Ann Otol Rhinol Laryngol 99: 29–37.

Kasten FH, Pineda LF, Schneider PE, Rawls HR, Foster TA (1989): Biocompatibility testing of an experimental fluoride releasing resin using human gingival epithelial cells in vitro. In Vitro Cell Dev Biol 25: 57–62.

Kautsky MB, Fleckman P, Dale BA (1995): Retinoic acid regulates oral epithelial differentiation by two mechanisms. J Invest Dermatol 104: 546–553.

Kim MS, Shin KH, Baek JH, Cherrick HM, Park NH (1993): HPV-16, tobacco-specific N-nitrosamine, and N-methyl-N'-nitro-N-nitrosoguanidine in oral carcinogenesis. Cancer Res 53: 4811–4816.

Kulkarni PS, Sundqvist K, Betsholtz C, Höglund P, Wiman KG, Zhivotovsky B, Bertolero F, Liu Y, Grafström RC (1995): Characterization of human buccal epithelial cells transfected with the simian virus 40 T-antigen gene. Carcinogenesis 16: 2515–2521.

Kulkarni PS, Heiden T, Tribukait B, Grafström RC (1996): Non-tumorigenic SV40 T immortalized human buccal epithelial cells show aneuploidy and genetic instability. Anticancer Res 16: 2681–2686.

Lauer G, Otten JE, von Specht BU, Schilli W (1991): Cultured gingival epithelium. A possible suitable material for pre-prosthetic surgery. J Craniomaxillofac Surg 19: 21–26.

Lauer G (1994): Autografting of feeder-cell free cultured gingival epithelium. Method and clinical application. J Craniomaxillofac Surg 22: 18–22.

Lee H, Li D, Prior T, Casto BC, Weghorst CM, Shuler CF, Milo GE (1997): Ineffectiveness of the presence of H-ras/p53 combination of mutations in squamous cell carcinoma cells to induce a conversion of a nontumorigenic to a tumorigenic phenotype. Cell Biol Toxicol 13: 419–434.

Levine AJ, Momand J, Finlay CA (1991): The p53 tumour suppressor gene. Nature 351: 453–456.

Lindberg K, Rheinwald JG (1990): Three distinct keratinocyte subtypes identified in human oral epithelium by their patterns of keratin expression in culture and in xenografts. Differentiation 45: 230–241.

Liu Y, Arvidson K, Atzori L, Sundqvist K, Silva B, Cotgreave I, Grafström RC (1991): Development of low- and high-serum culture conditions for use of human oral fibroblasts in toxicity testing of dental materials. J Dent Res 70: 1068–1073.

Liu Y, Cotgreave I, Atzori L, Grafström R (1992): The mechanism of Hg^{2+} toxicity in cultured human oral fibroblasts: The involvement of cellular thiols. Chem Biol Interact 85: 69–78.

Liu Y, Sundqvist K, Belinsky SA, Castonguay A, Tjälve H, Grafström RC (1993): Metabolism and macromolecular interaction of the tobacco-specific carcinogen 4-(methylnitrosamino)-1-(3-pyridyl)-1-butanone in cultured explants and epithelial cells of human buccal mucosa. Carcinogenesis 14: 2383–2388.

Liu Y, Egyhazi S, Hansson J, Bhide SV, Kulkarni P, Grafström RC (1997): O^6-methylguanine-DNA methyltransferase activity in human buccal mucosal tissue and cell cultures. Complex mixtures related to habitual use of tobacco and betel quid inhibit the activity in vitro. Carcinogenesis 18: 1889–1895.

MacCallum DK, Lillie JH, Jepsen A, Arenholt BD (1987): The culture of oral epithelium. Int Rev Cytol 109: 313–330.

Neeser JR, Grafström RC, Woltz A, Brassart D, Fryder V, Guggenheim B (1995): A 23 kD membrane glycoprotein bearing NeuNAcα2-3Galβ1-3GalNac O-linked carbohydrate chains acts as a receptor for *Streptococcus sanguis* OMZ 9 on human buccal epithelial cells. Glycobiology 5: 97–104.

Neugebauer P, Bonnekoh B, Wevers A, Michel O, Mahrle G, Krieg T, Stennert E (1996): Human keratinocyte culture from the peritonsillar mucosa. Eur Arch Otorhinolaryngol 253: 245–51.

Nilsson J-A, Zheng X, Sundqvist K, Liu Y, Atzori L, Elfwing Å, Arvidson K, Grafström RC (1998): Toxicity of formaldehyde to human oral fibroblasts and epithelial cells: Influences of culture conditions and role of thiol status. J Dent Res 77: 1896–1903.

Oda D, Watson E (1990): Human oral epithelial cell culture. I. Improved conditions for reproducible culture in serum-free medium. In Vitro Cell Dev Biol 26: 589–595.

Oda D, Bigler L, Lee P, Blanton R (1996a): HPV immortalization of human oral epithelial cells: A model for carcinogenesis. Exp Cell Res 226: 164–169.

Oda D, Bigler L, Mao EJ, Disteche CM (1996b): Chromosomal abnormalities in HPV-16-immortalized oral epithelial cells. Carcinogenesis 17: 2003–2008.

Oda D, Savard CE, Eng L, Sekijima J, Haigh G, Lee SP (1998): Reconstituted human oral and esophageal mucosa in culture. In Vitro Cell Dev Biol Anim 34: 46–52.

Odioso LL, Doyle MJ, Quinn KW, Bartel RL, Zimber MP, Stevens-Burns D (1995): Development and characterization of an in vitro gingival epithelial model. J Periodont Res 30: 210–219.

Papaioannou W, Cassiman JJ, Van den Oord J, De Vos R, van Steenberghe D, Quirynen M (1999): Multi-layered periodontal pocket epithelium reconstituted in vitro: Histology and cytokeratin profiles. J Periodontol 70: 668–678.

Park NH, Min BM, Li SL, Huang MZ, Cherick HM, Doniger J (1991): Immortalization of normal human oral keratinocytes with type 16 human papillomavirus. Carcinogenesis 12: 1627–1631.

Park NH, Gujuluva CN, Baek JH, Cherrick HM, Shin KH, Min BM (1995): Combined oral carcinogenicity of HPV-16 and benzo(*a*)pyrene: An in vitro multistep carcinogenesis model. Oncogene 10: 2145–2153.

Pittelkow MR, Scott RE (1986): New techniques for the in vitro culture of human skin keratinocytes and perspectives on their use for grafting of patients with extensive burns. Mayo Clin Proc 61: 771–777.

Prime SS, Nixon SV, Crane IJ, Stone A, Matthews JB, Maitland NJ, Remnant L, Powell SK, Game SM, Scully C (1990): The behaviour of human oral squamous cell carcinoma in cell culture. J Pathol 160: 259–269.

Reid CB, Cloos J, Snow GB, Braakhuis BJ (1997): A simple and reliable technique for culturing of human oral keratinocytes and fibroblasts. Acta Otolaryngol (Stockh) 117: 628–633.

Rheinwald JG, Green H (1975): Serial cultivation of strains of human epidermal keratinocytes: The formation of keratinizing colonies from single cells. Cell 6: 331–343.

Rhim JS, Park JB, Kawakami T (1988): Techniques for establishing human epithelial cell cultures: Sensitivity of cell lines for propagation of herpesviruses. J Virol Methods 21: 209–222.

Rikimaru K, Toda H, Tachikawa N, Kamata N, Enomoto S (1990): Growth of the malignant and nonmalignant human squamous cells in a protein-free defined medium. In Vitro Cell Dev Biol 26: 849–856.

Sacks PG, Parnes SM, Price JC, Risemberg H, Goldstein JC, Marko M, Parsons DF (1985): In vitro modulation of differentiation by calcium in organ cultures of human and murine epithelial tissue. In Vitro Cell Dev Biol 21: 99–107.

Sacks PG (1996): Cell, tissue and organ culture as in vitro models to study the biology of squamous cell carcinomas of the head and neck. Cancer Metastasis Rev 15: 27–51.

Salonen JI, Kautsky MB, Dale BA (1989): Changes in cell phenotype during regeneration of junctional epithelium of human gingiva in vitro. J Periodont Res 24: 370–377.

Salonen J, Uitto VJ, Pan YM, Oda D (1991): Proliferating oral epithelial cells in culture are capable of both extracellular and intracellular degradation of interstitial collagen. Matrix 11: 43–55.

Schön M, Rheinwald JG (1996): A limited role for retinoic acid and retinoic acid receptors RARδ and RARβ in regulating keratin 19 expression and keratinization in oral and epidermal keratinocytes. J Invest Dermatol 107: 428–438.

Sexton CJ, Proby CM, Banks L, Stables JN, Powell K, Navsaria H, Leigh IM (1993): Characterization of factors involved in human papillomavirus type

16-mediated immortalization of oral keratinocytes. J Gen Virol 74: 755–761.

Shin KH, Min BM, Cherrick HM, Park NH (1994): Combined effects of human papillomavirus-18 and N-methyl-N'-nitro-N-nitrosoguanidine on the transformation of normal human oral keratinocytes. Mol Carcinog 9: 76–86.

Shuler C, Kurian P, French BT, Noyes I, Sital N, Hollering J, Trewyn RW, Schuller D, Milo GE (1990): Noncorrelative c-myc and ras oncogene expression in squamous cell carcinoma cells with tumorigenic potential. Teratog Carcinog Mutagen 10: 53–65.

Smulow JB, Glickman I (1966): An epithelial-like cell line in continuous culture from normal adult human gingiva. Proc Soc Exp Biol Med 121: 1294–1296.

Southgate J, Williams HK, Trejdosiewicz LK, Hodges GM (1987): Primary culture of human oral epithelial cells. Growth requirements and expression of differentiated characteristics. Lab Invest 56: 211–223.

Sundqvist K, Liu Y, Nair J, Bartsch H, Arvidson K, Grafström RC (1989): Cytotoxic and genotoxic effects of areca nut-related compounds in cultured human buccal epithelial cells. Cancer Res 49: 5294–5298.

Sundqvist K, Kulkarni P, Hybbinette SS, Bertolero F, Liu Y, Grafström RC (1991a): Serum-free growth and karyotype analyses of cultured normal and tumorous (SqCC/Y1) human buccal epithelial cells. Cancer Commun 3: 331–340.

Sundqvist K, Liu Y, Arvidson K, Ormstad K, Nilsson L, Toftgård R, Grafström RC (1991b): Growth regulation of serum-free cultures of epithelial cells from normal human buccal mucosa. In Vitro Cell Dev Biol 27A: 562–568.

Sundqvist K, Grafström RC (1992): Effects of areca nut on growth, differentiation and formation of DNA damage in cultured human buccal epithelial cells. Int J Cancer 52: 305–310.

Sundqvist K, Iotsova V, Shohreh SV, Wiman KG, Höög C, Grafström RC (1995): Identification of genes overexpressed in the SqCC/Y1 human buccal carcinoma cell line using the differential display method. Int J Oncol 7: 1123–1128.

Tomakidi P, Fusenig NE, Kohl A, Komposch G (1997): Histomorphological and biochemical differentiation capacity in organotypic co-cultures of primary gingival cells. J Periodont Res 32: 388–400.

Tomakidi P, Breitkreutz D, Fusenig NE, Zoller J, Kohl A, Komposch G (1998): Establishment of oral mucosa phenotype in vitro in correlation to epithelial anchorage. Cell Tissue Res 292: 355–366.

Tomakidi P, Breitkreutz D, Kohl A, Komposch G (1999): Normalization of keratinocyte-type integrins during the establishment of the oral mucosa phenotype in vitro. Anat Anz 181: 127–32.

Tomakidi P, Schuster G, Breitkreutz D, Kohl A, Ottl P, Komposch G (2000): Organotypic cultures of gingival cells: an epithelial model to assess putative local effects of orthodontic plate and occlusal splint materials under more tissue-like conditions. Biomaterials 21: 1549–1559.

Tomson AM, Scholma J, Blaauw EH, Rosingh HJ, Dikkers FG (1994): Improved in vitro generation of epithelial grafts with oral mucosa. Transplantation 58: 1282–1284.

Ueda M, Hata K, Horie K, Torii S (1995): The potential of oral mucosal cells for cultured epithelium: a preliminary report. Ann Plast Surg 35: 498–504.

Ueda M, Hata KI, Sumi Y, Mizuno H, Niimi A (1998): Peri-implant soft tissue management through use of cultured mucosal epithelium. Oral Surg Oral Med Oral Pathol Oral Radiol Endod 86: 393–400.

Vaca CE, Nilsson JA, Fang JL, Grafström RC (1998): Formation of DNA adducts in human buccal epithelial cells exposed to acetaldehyde and methylglyoxal in vitro. Chem Biol Interact 108: 197–208.

Vondracek M, Zheng X, Larsson P, Baker V, Mace C, Pfeifer A, Tjälve H, Grafström RC (2001): Cytochrome P450 expression and related metabolism in human buccal mucosa. Carcinogenesis 22: 481–488.

Weinberg RA (1991): Tumor suppressor genes. Science 254: 1138–1146.

Wille JJ, Mansson-Rahemtulla B, Rahemtulla F (1990): Characterization of human gingival keratinocytes cultured in a serum-free medium. Arch Oral Biol 35: 967–976.

Xu L, Schantz SP, Edelstein D, Sacks PG (1996): A simplified method for the routine culture of normal oral epithelial (NOE) cells from upper aerodigestive tract mucosa Methods Cell Sci 18: 31–39.

Yoo GH, Washington J, Piechocki M, Ensley J, Shibuya T, Oda D, Wei WZ (2000): Progression of head and neck cancer in an in vitro model. Arch Otolaryngol Head Neck Surg 126: 1313–8.

APPENDIX A: PREPARATION OF EMHA

EMHA is prepared from 500 ml of pre-MCDB 153 medium (made without Stock 4a, Stock 4b, Stock 7, Stock K2, and Stock L). To make EMHA, add the missing MCDB 153 stocks and the individual components as indicated:

Stocks and Supplements	Volume	Storage
Stock 4a	0.5 ml	Sterile, 4°C
Stock 4b	0.5 ml	Sterile, 4°C
Stock K2	0.5 ml	Sterile, 4°C
Hydrocortisone (HC), 1 mM	0.5 ml	Sterile, 4°C
Insulin, 5 mg/ml	0.5 ml	Sterile, 4°C
Epidermal growth factor (EGF), 10 μg/ml	0.5 ml	Sterile, 4°C
Ethanolamine, 0.1 M	0.5 ml	Sterile, 4°C
Phosphoethanolamine, 0.1 M	0.5 ml	Sterile, 4°C
Gentamicin, 50 mg/ml	0.5 ml	Sterile, 4°C
Stock L	5 ml	Sterile, 4°C
Stock 7	5 ml	Frozen, −20°C
High-amino acid (HAA) stock	15 ml	Frozen, −20°C
Pituitary extract (PEX)	20 μg/ml	Sterile, 4°C

Sterilize by membrane filtration (Nalgene 0.2 μm, 50 mm bottle-top) and store at 4°C. Do not freeze. The medium should be used for cell culture within 2 wk or discarded.

APPENDIX B: PREPARATION OF PRE-MCDB 153 MEDIUM

Pre-MCDB 153 is MCDB 153 without Stocks 4a, 4b, 7, K2, and L. To make 4 or 8 L of pre-MCDB 153, add 3 or 6 L, respectively, of water (purified for cell culture) to a 10-L flask. Use a magnetic stir plate and stir bar to dissolve the following solids in order at indicated amounts: glucose, NaCl, Na-acetate, L-glutamine, Na-pyruvate, and HEPES. Note that $NaHCO_3$ is added at a later step. (The solids are from Sigma and the product number is indicated).

Solids in Pre-MCDB 153

Component		For 4 L	For 8 L	Storage
Glucose	(G 7021)	4.32 g	8.65 g	Room temp.
NaCl	(S 5886)	30.40 g	60.80 g	Room temp.
Na-acetate	(S 5636)	1.20 g	2.40 g	Room temp.
L-Glutamine	(G 5763)	3.50 g	7.00 g	Room temp.
Na-pyruvate	(P 5280)	0.22 g	0.44 g	4°C
HEPES[a]	(H 9136)	26.40 g	52.80 g	Room temp.
$NaHCO_3$	(S 5761)	4.70 g	9.41 g	Room temp.

[a] N-2-Hydroxyethylpiperazine-N'-2-ethanesulfonic acid

When the solids are in solution add the stocks indicated below. Note that Stock 5 (phenol red) should be added as the last stock.

Stocks in Pre-MCDB 153

Component	For 4 L	For 8 L	Storage
The stocks are made as described in Appendix C			
Stock 1	40 ml	80 ml	−20°C
Stock 2	40 ml	80 ml	−20°C
Stock 3	80 ml	160 ml	−20°C
Stock 5 (add after other stocks)	4 ml	8 ml	−20°C
Stock 6c	4 ml	8 ml	−20°C
Stock 8	40 ml	80 ml	−20°C
Stock 9	40 ml	80 ml	−20°C
Stock 10	40 ml	80 ml	−20°C

Add water to almost final volume (~3.8 or 7.6 liter), and adjust pH to 7.3–7.4 with 10 M NaOH (~1 ml per liter medium). Add solid NaHCO3, do not adjust pH, and then add water to make up to final volume. Sterilize (VacuCap filter 0.2 μm) the medium and store at 4°C. Use batch for making EMHA within 2–3 wk.

APPENDIX C: EMHA AND PRE-MCDB 153 STOCK SOLUTIONS AND SUPPLEMENTS

Stock 1, 100×

Component	Product Number	Molecular Weight	g/L	Moles/L
L-Arginine · HCl	A 3909	210.7	21.07	1×10^{-1}
L-Histidine · HCl · H₂O	H 5659	209.06	1.677	8×10^{-3}
L-Isoleucine	I 7383	131.2	0.1968	1.5×10^{-3}
L-Leucine	L 1512	131.2	6.56	5×10^{-2}
L-Lysine · HCl	L 1262	182.6	1.826	1×10^{-2}
L-Methionine	M 2893	149.2	0.4476	3×10^{-3}
L-Phenylalanine	P 5030	165.2	0.4956	3×10^{-3}
L-Serine	S 4311	105.1	6.306	6×10^{-2}
L-Threonine	T 8441	119.1	1.191	1×10^{-2}
L-Tryptophan	T 0271	204.2	0.3063	1.5×10^{-3}
L-Tyrosine	T 1020	181.2	0.2718	1.5×10^{-3}
L-Valine	V 6504	117.1	3.513	3×10^{-2}
Choline chloride	C 7527	139.6	1.396	1×10^{-2}

For preparation of 1 liter, dissolve the chemicals one at a time under stirring and mild heating in about 600 ml of UPW. Then add UPW to make up to final volume. Stock 1 is stored frozen at −20°C in 40-ml aliquots for up to 3 months. Freshly thawed Stock 1 frequently contains a precipitate that will dissolve on gently warming.

Stock 2, 100×

Component	Product Number	Molecular Weight	g/L	Moles/L
d-Biotin	B 4639	244.3	0.00146	6×10^{-6}
Niacinamide	N 0636	122.1	0.003663	3×10^{-5}
D-Pantothenic acid	P 5155	238.3	0.02383	1×10^{-4}
Pyridoxine · HCl	P 6280	205.6	0.006168	3×10^{-5}
Thiamin · HCl	T 1270	337.3	0.03373	1×10^{-4}
KCl	P 5405	74.55	11.184	1.5×10^{-1}

For preparation of 1 liter, dissolve the chemicals one at a time under stirring and mild heating in about 700 ml UPW. Then add UPW to make up to final volume. Stock 2 is stored frozen at −20°C in 40-ml aliquots for up to 3 months.

Stock 3, 50×

Component	Product Number	Molecular Weight	g/2 L	Moles/L
Folic acid	F 8758	441.4	0.790	9×10^{-5}
Na₂HPO₄	S 5136	142.0	28.392	1×10^{-1}

For preparation of 2 liters, initially dissolve Na$_2$HPO$_4$ with stirring in 1500 ml of UPW. Then dissolve folic acid and add UPW to make up to final volume. Stock 3 is stored frozen at -20°C in 40-ml aliquots for up to 3 months.

Note that disodium phosphate provides the alkaline conditions necessary to dissolve the folic acid. In experimental media where the folic acid is prepared separately, great care must be taken to be certain that the folic acid has dissolved. Under neutral or slightly acid conditions, folic acid tends to form a fine particulate suspension that is not easily seen in the medium but is retained on the sterilizing filter. Once the folic acid has been dissolved completely, however, it will normally remain in solution in the final medium even under slightly acidic conditions.

Stock 4a, 1000×

Component	Product Number	Molecular Weight	g/100 ml	Moles/L
CaCl$_2 \cdot$2H$_2$O	C 7902	147.0	1.470	1×10^{-1}

For preparation of 100 ml, dissolve the chemical with stirring in 90 ml of UPW. Then add UPW to make up to final volume and sterilize. Stock 4a is stored at 4°C in 10-ml aliquots for up to 3 months.

Stock 4b, 1000×

Component	Product Number	Molecular Weight	g/100 ml	Moles/L
MgCl$_2 \cdot$6H$_2$O	M 2393	203.3	12.20	6×10^{-1}

For preparation of 100 ml, dissolve the chemical with stirring in 90 ml of UPW. Then add UPW to make up to final volume and sterilize. Stock 4a is stored at 4°C in 10-ml aliquots for up to 3 months.

Stock 5, 1000×

Component	Product Number	Molecular Weight	g/100 ml	Moles/L
Phenol red	P 5530	376.4	0.1242	3.3×10^{-3}

For preparation of 100 ml, dissolve the chemical with stirring in 90 ml of UPW. Then add UPW to make up to final volume and sterilize. Stock 5 is stored at $-20°C$ in 4-ml aliquots for up to 3 months.

Stock 6c, 1000×

Component	Product Number	Molecular Weight	g/L	Moles/L
Riboflavin	R 9504	376.4	0.03764	1×10^{-4}

For preparation of 1 liter, dissolve the chemical with stirring in 700 ml of UPW. Then add UPW to make up to final volume and sterilize. Stock 5 is stored at $-20°C$ in 4-ml aliquots (make 20 such aliquots only) for up to 3 months (note that Stock 6c is made up to 1 liter to ensure accuracy when weighing).

Stock 7, 100×

Component	Product Number	Molecular Weight	g/L	Moles/L
L-Cysteine HCl · H$_2$O	C 6852	175.6	4.214	2.4×10^{-2}

For preparation of 1 liter, dissolve the chemical with stirring in 900 ml of UPW. Then add UPW to make up to final volume. Stock 7 is stored frozen at $-20°C$ in 20-ml aliquots for up to 3 months. Thawed stock solution is kept at 4°C and used within 2 wk.

Stock 7 is added when making EMHA from pre-MCDB 153, to facilitate making a cysteine-free medium when needed. Cysteine autooxidizes to cystine when stored in solution. Short-term toxicity assessments are made in cysteine-free media to increase reproducibility (reactive chemicals commonly bind to the sulfhydryl group of free cysteine, and uncontrolled cysteine oxidation will prejudice experimental reproducibility).

Stock 8, 100×

Component	Product Number	Molecular Weight	g/L	Moles/L
L-Asparagine · H$_2$O	A 4284	150.1	1.501	1×10^{-2}
L-Proline	P 5607	115.1	3.453	3×10^{-2}
Putrescine	P 5780	161.1	0.01611	1×10^{-4}
Vitamin B$_{12}$	V 6629	1355.4	0.04066	3×10^{-5}

For preparation of 1 liter, dissolve the chemicals one at a time with stirring in about 700 ml of UPW. Then add UPW to make up to final volume. Stock 8 is stored frozen at −20°C in 40-ml aliquots for up to 3 months.

Stock 9, 100×

Component	Product Number	Molecular Weight	g/L	Moles/L
L-Alanine	A 3534	89.09	0.891	1×10^{-2}
L-Aspartic acid	A 4534	133.1	0.399	3×10^{-3}
L-Glutamic acid	G 5638	147.1	1.471	1×10^{-2}
Glycine	G 6388	75.07	0.751	1×10^{-2}

For preparation of 1 liter, initially add L-aspartic acid and L-glutamic acid with stirring to about 700 ml of UPW. Then add 1 ml of phenol red (Stock 5). Neutralize the solution with drop-wise addition of 1 M NaOH (until orange color); L-aspartic acid and L-glutamic acid will dissolve under neutral conditions. Then add and dissolve alanine and glycine. Add UPW to make up to final volume. Stock 9 is stored frozen at −20°C in 40-ml aliquots for up to 3 months.

Stock 10, 100×

Component	Product Number	Molecular Weight	g/L	Moles/L
Adenine	A 2786	135.1	2.432	1.8×10^{-2}
myo-Inositol	I 7508	180.2	1.802	1×10^{-2}
DL-6,8-Thioctic acid	T 1395	206.3	0.02063	1×10^{-4}
Thymidine	T 1895	242.2	0.07266	3×10^{-4}
$CuSO_4 \cdot 5H_2O$	C 8027	249.7	0.000249	1×10^{-6}

For preparation of 1 liter, add about 400 ml of UPW to a flask. The chemicals are then prepared, added, and/or dissolved as described below with stirring and mild heating (~40°C). Adenine is dissolved in 25 ml of 4 M HCl and the solution added to the stock solution in the main flask. Thioctic acid is dissolved in a few drops of 1 M NaOH and then added to the solution in the main flask (the solution becomes rather opaque). Make a 0.5 mM $CuSO_4$ stock by dissolving 0.01245 g of $CuSO_4$ in 100 ml of UPW, and add only 2 ml of this stock to the solution in the main flask. Dissolve the remaining components one by one, and then add UPW to make up to final volume. Leave solution to stir over-night at room temperature (to ensure that all components completely dissolve). Stock 10 is stored frozen at $-20°C$ in 40-ml aliquots for up to 3 months.

Stock K2 1000×

Component	Product Number	Molecular Weight	g/100 ml	Moles/L
$FeSO_4 \cdot 7H_2O$	F 8633	278.0	0.139	5×10^{-3}

For preparation of 100 ml, dissolve the $FeSO_4 \cdot 7H_2O$ in 2.0 ml of 0.5 M HCl. Then add UPW to make up to final volume (final conc. 10 mM HCl) and sterilize by filtration through 0.22 μm. Stock K2 is stored at 4°C in 10-ml aliquots for up to 3 months. Discard the solution if a precipitate or yellow/orange color occurs.

Stock L 100×

Component	Product Number	Volume (ml)	Moles/L
$CuSO_4 \cdot 5H_2O$	C 8027	0.10	1.0×10^{-7}
Selenious acid	KEBO-652	3.0	3.0×10^{-6}
Manganese sulfate $\cdot H_2O$	M 1144	0.10	1.0×10^{-7}
Sodium metasilicate $\cdot 9H_2O$	S 4392	50.0	5.0×10^{-5}
Molybdic acid $\cdot 4H_2O$	M 1019	0.10	1.0×10^{-7}
Ammonium metavanadate	A 8175	0.50	5.0×10^{-7}
Nickel chloride $\cdot 6H_2O$	N 6136	0.05	5.0×10^{-8}
Stannous chloride $\cdot 2H_2O$	S 9262	0.50	5.0×10^{-8}
Zinc sulfate $\cdot 7H_2O$	Z 0251	50.0	5.0×10^{-5}

The instructions for the individual components to Stock L, including molecular weights, are shown in Appendix D. Make up individual stocks in 10 mM HCl. For preparation of 1 liter, add 895.65 ml of 10 mM HCl to a flask. Then add the indicated volume of each individual stock. Sterile filter and store Stock L at 4°C in 30- to 40-ml aliquots for up to 12 months. Note that Stock 10 is the major contributor of cupric sulfate to EMHA.

High-Amino Acid Stock

Increase in Concentration[a]	Component	Product Number	Molecular Weight	g/L	Moles/L
3×	L-Histidine $\cdot$ HCl $\cdot H_2O$	H 5659	209.6	1.6778	8×10^{-3}
50×	L-Isoleucine	I 7383	131.2	3.2800	2.5×10^{-2}
3×	L-Methionine	M 2893	149.2	0.4477	3×10^{-3}
3×	L-Phenylalanine	P 2126	165.2	0.4957	3×10^{-3}
3×	L-Tryptophan	T 0271	204.2	0.3063	1.5×10^{-3}
5×	L-Tyrosine	T 1020	181.2	0.4530	2.5×10^{-3}

[a] Increase in concentration compared with the concentration provided through Stock 1.

For preparation of 1 liter, dissolve the chemicals one at a time with stirring and mild heating (~55°C) in about 400 ml of UPW. Then add UPW to make up to final volume and leave the solution stirring for 2 h (to ensure that all components completely dissolve). The High-Amino Acid Stock is stored frozen at −20°C in 35-ml aliquots for up to 3 months. Freshly thawed stock is kept at 4°C and used within 2 wk to make EMHA.

Epidermal Growth Factor (EGF)

Stock	Molecular Weight	Amount
EGF, human, recombinant	~6000	100 μg
Bovine serum albumin (BSA, 1 mg/ml)	—	1 ml
Phosphate-buffered saline (PBSA)	—	9 ml

Dissolve the EGF in a mixture of BSA and PBSA. Sterilize with a low-protein-binding filter. Store at 4°C in 5-ml aliquots. Concentration 10 μg/ml (1.64 μM). The stock is generally used within 4 months.

Insulin

Stock	Molecular Weight	Amount
Insulin, porcine, Zn-free	5778	100 mg
PBSA	—	20 ml

Dissolve at 5 mg/ml in PBSA in beaker placed on a magnetic stir plate. Sterilize with a low-protein-binding filter. Store at 4°C in 5-ml aliquots. A new stock should be made after 6 months.

Hydrocortisone Superstock

Component	Product Number	Molecular Weight	Amount	Concentration
Hydrocortisone	H 0888	362.5	36 mg	10 mM
Ethanol 95%			10 ml	

Sterilize and store at 4°C in 2 × 5-ml aliquots. A new superstock should be made after 6 months.

Hydrocortisone Stock

Component	Amount	Concentration
Hydrocortisone superstock	1 ml	1 mM
Ethanol (95%)	9 ml	

Store at 4°C in 2 × 5-ml aliquots. The stock is generally used within 2 months.

Ethanolamine Superstock

Component	Product Number	Molecular Weight	Amount	Concentration
Ethanolamine	E 0135	61.08	1 ml	1 M
PBSA			15.25 ml	

Sterilize and store at 4°C in ~5-ml aliquots. A new superstock should be made after 6 months.

Ethanolamine Stock

Component	Amount	Concentration
Ethanolamine, 1 M	1 ml	0.1 M
PBSA (sterile)	9 ml	

Store at 4°C in 2 × 5-ml aliquots. The stock is generally used within 2 months.

***o*-Phosphoethanolamine Stock**

Component	Product Number	Molecular Weight	Amount	Concentration
o-Phosphoethanolamine	P 0503	141.1	0.1411 g	0.1 M
PBSA			10 ml	

Sterilize and store at 4°C in 2 × 5-ml aliquots. The stock is generally used within 2 months.

Pituitary Extract (PEX)

Prepare from bovine pituitaries according to separate protocol (see Appendix E). The dialysis usually results in a stock solution at 3–5 mg/ml. Store at −20°C. After thawing a PEX aliquot, it is stored at 4°C and not refrozen. One preparation from 100 pituitaries usually provides extract for 1 year of cell culture.

Gentamicin Stock

Component	Product Number	Amount	Concentration
Gentamicin sulfate	G 3632	0.5 g	50 mg/ml
PBSA		10 ml	

Store at 4°C in 2 × 5-ml aliquots. The stock is generally used within 2 months.

APPENDIX D: SOLUTIONS FOR PREPARATION OF STOCK L

Copper

Component	Product Number	Molecular Weight	g/100 ml	Moles/L
Cupric sulfate·5H$_2$O	C 8027	249.7	0.02497	1.0×10^{-3}

For preparation of 100 ml, dissolve the chemical with stirring in about 90 ml of 10 mM HCl. Then add 10 mM HCl to make up to final volume.

Selenium

Component	Product Number	Molecular Weight	g/100 ml	Moles/L
Selenious acid	KEBO 652	128.97	0.0129	1.0×10^{-3}

Δ*Safety note.* This stock is prepared in a fume cabinet because selenious acid is considered to be poisonous.

For preparation of 100 ml, dissolve the chemical with stirring in about 90 ml of 10 mM HCl. Then add 10 mM HCl to make up to final volume.

Manganese

Component	Product Number	Molecular Weight	g/100 ml	Moles/L
Manganese sulfate·H$_2$O	M 1144	151.0	0.0151	1.0×10^{-3}

For preparation of 100 ml, dissolve the chemical with stirring in about 90 ml of 10 mM HCl. Then add 10 mM HCl to make up to final volume. The chemical is hydroscopic (H$_2$O content 1 mol/mol), i.e., the molecular weight becomes 169.0 in opened containers.

Silica

Component	Product Number	Molecular Weight	g/500 ml	Moles/L
Sodium metasilicate $\cdot$ 9H$_2$O	S 4392	284.2	0.1421	1.0×10^{-3}

For preparation of 500 ml, dissolve the chemical with stirring in about 400 ml of 10 mM HCl. Then add 10 mM HCl to make up to final volume.

Molybdenum

Component	Product Number	Molecular Weight	g/100 ml	Moles/L
Molybdic acid $\cdot$ 4H$_2$O	M 1019	1235.9	0.12359	1.0×10^{-3}

For preparation of 100 ml, dissolve the chemical with stirring in about 90 ml of 10 mM HCl. Then add 10 mM HCl to make up to final volume.

Vanadium

Component	Product Number	Molecular Weight	g/100 ml	Moles/L
Ammonium metavanadate	A 8175	117.0	0.0117	1.0×10^{-3}

For preparation of 100 ml, dissolve the chemical with stirring in about 90 ml of 10 mM HCl. Then add 10 mM HCl to make up to final volume.

Nickel

Component	Product Number	Molecular Weight	g/100 ml	Moles/L
Nickel chloride $\cdot$ 6H$_2$O	N 6136	237.7	0.02377	1.0×10^{-3}

For preparation of 100 ml, dissolve the chemical with stirring in about 90 ml of 10 mM HCl. Then add 10 mM HCl to make up to final volume.

Tin

Component	Product Number	Molecular Weight	g/100 ml	Moles/L
Stannous chloride·2H$_2$O	S 9262	225.6	0.00226	1.0×10^{-4}

For preparation of 100 ml, dissolve the chemical with stirring in about 90 ml of 10 mM HCl. Then add 10 mM HCl to make up to final volume.

Zinc

Component	Product Number	Molecular Weight	g/500 ml	Moles/L
Zinc sulfate·7H$_2$O	Z 0251	287.5	0.14377	1.0×10^{-5}

For preparation of 500 ml, dissolve the chemical with stirring in about 400 ml of 10 mM HCl. Then add 10 mM HCl to make up to final volume.

APPENDIX E: PREPARATION OF PITUITARY EXTRACT (PEX) STOCK

Use protective gloves throughout the work for your own protection and to avoid contaminating the PEX. Use the Assessment Protocol to record details about the pituitaries and the PEX preparation.

  (i)   Thaw one package of bovine pituitaries (~100 pieces) in a 200-ml beaker overnight in refrigerator.
 (ii)   Fill a 10-L flask with UPW and place it in the cold room over night (will be used for dialysis of PEX).
(iii)   Rinse the pituitaries with cold PBSA to remove excess blood and maintain them in PBSA on ice.
 (iv)   Remove any hard tissue around each pituitary, including the capsule of connective tissue and vessels. Work in a Petri dish on ice. Collect the cleaned pituitary tissue in a beaker on ice.
  (v)   Weigh the pituitary tissue, and add 227 ml of PBSA per 100 g of tissue.
 (vi)   Fragmentize the tissue using an ordinary kitchen mixer or a Waring blender. Run until it forms a slurry. Avoid heating of the suspension!
(vii)   Leave in refrigerator for 1 h.

(viii)   Filter the suspension through gauze, and squeeze thoroughly to optimize the yield.

(ix)   Centrifuge the filtrate at 10,000 g for 20 min at 4°C. Start at a lower rpm and gradually increase the velocity to final speed during the first few minutes. (Centrifuge Beckman J-21B and rotor JA-20; hard plastic 50-ml tubes, 9000 rpm).

(x)   Prepare dialysis tubing (dry cylinder 16 mm, molecular weight cutoff 12,000–14,000) by placing it in cold UPW. Cut the tubing, i.e., prepare 7 pieces that are 30 cm in length.

(xi)   Collect the supernatants and the pellets separately after centrifugation. (The pellets are frozen in case of failure with the preparation; if so, consider redoing the protocol from step (vi).)

(xii)   Close one end of the dialysis tubes, e.g., by making two knots. Transfer the supernatant into dialysis tubes with the aid of a 20- or 50-ml syringe (without needle). Work in a beaker in case the tubing bursts. As the PEX will approximately double its volume during dialysis, fill only half of the tube.

(xiii)   Remove air from the dialysis tube before closing it with two separate knots.

(xiv)   Tie a string to each tube; adjust the length of the string so the tubes are suspended 2–3 cm above the bottom in the 10-L flask containing 10 L of the cold UPW. Secure strings with tape on the outside of the flask and seal/cover the opening of the flask with aluminum foil.

(xv)   Exchange the dialysis water on a daily basis for 7 consecutive days with fresh cold UPW (flasks that take ~12 L of UPW must be filled up and placed in the cold room in advance). Precipitation of PEX components is a normal phenomenon during dialysis.

(xvi)   Collect the dialysate by cutting the tubes in a large beaker. Centrifuge at 10,000 g for 20 min, as in step (ix).

(xvii)   Filter the PEX, using a water suction device, initially through a 1.2-μm glass fiber filter (Whatman GF/C), followed by a 0.7-μm filter (Whatman GF/F). The reddish color of the PEX changes to brown.

(xviii)   Sterilize the PEX (0.2-μm filter with low protein binding).

(xix)   Store the PEX in aliquots of 10 ml in 50-ml tubes at −20° C. Consider storing the PEX preparations in different freezers in case of freezer failure.

(xx)   Determine the protein concentration of the preparation (usually ~3–5 mg/ml). The Bradford method [Bradford, 1976] is an option.

(xxi) Perform a colony forming efficiency assay using oral keratinocytes (according to separate protocol) for assessment of optimal concentration of the PEX. Routinely use a concentration that gives optimal growth without a very rapid consumption of the batch. Usually 20 μg/ml is sufficient for mass cultures of oral keratinocytes [Sundqvist et al., 1991b].

Bovine Pituitary Extract (PEX) Quality Control

Record of Preparation

Batch no:
Source:
Date of excision:
Number of pituitaries used:
Preparation dates, start: end:
Weight of pituitary tissue without superfluous tissue:
No. of days of dialysis:
Final volume of PEX:
Protein concentration in sterilized PEX:

Record of Effect of PEX on Growth

The activity of each batch should be assessed from colony forming efficiency (see Protocol 7.5) and recorded as suggested below:

Cells used, etc: _____ Date _____		
Concentration of PEX Protein in Growth Medium (μg/ml)	No. of Colonies in Each Duplicate Dish	Mean
0.0		
3.0		
10		
20		
30		
60		
100		
Concentration that will be used routinely: _____ μg/ml		

APPENDIX F: SOURCES OF MATERIALS

Material	Catalog #	Supplier
Bovine serum albumin (BSA)	A 4378	Sigma
Centrifuge rotor	J-21B JA-20	Beckman Coulter Beckman Coulter
Centrifuge tubes, high g, polycarbonate, 50 ml	03146	Sorvall
Centrifuge tubes, 15 ml, polystyrene, sterile	28-009.115	Techno Plastic Products
Chemicals listed in Appendixes	See relevant appendix	Sigma
Collagen: Vitrogen 100	—	Celtrix; KeLab
Dialysis tubing	132 706	Spectrum
EDTA	E 6511	Sigma
EGTA	E 4378	Sigma
Epidermal growth factor	GF-010-8	Austral Biologicals, USA.
Ethanolamine	E 0135	Sigma
Fibronectin (from bovine plasma)	33010-018	GIBCO
Fungizone	15290-026	GIBCO
Glass fiber filters	GF/C; GF/F	Whatman
Hydrocortisone	H 0888	Sigma
Gentamicin	G 3632	Sigma
Insulin	—	Gift from Eli Lilly Co., Stockholm. Request using a form from Lilly Corporate Center, Drop Code 2223, Indianapolis, IN 46285, USA (the batch of insulin is often provided in sealed glass containers containing 100 mg).
Leibovitz L-15 medium without glutamine	11415-049	GIBCO
Penicillin-streptomycin	15145-014	GIBCO
o-Phosphoethanolamine	P 0503	Sigma
Polyvinylpyrrolidone	P 0930	Sigma
Selenious acid	KEBO-652	Merck KGaA

Appendix F continues

APPENDIX F: SOURCES OF MATERIALS (continued)

Material	Catalog #	Supplier

Sterilization filters
    Nalgene 50-mm bottle-top
    VacuCap
	101.103-45/33
	35-004622
		Nalge-Nunc
		Gelman Sciences

Trypsin, 1:250, 2.5% in normal saline, 10×	25090-028	GIBCO
Vials for freezing cells, 2 ml	CC 430659	Corning

8

Normal Human Bronchial Epithelial Cell Culture

John Wise[1] and John F. Lechner[2]

[1]Yale University, School of Medicine, New Haven, CT 06520, and
[2]Bayer Diagnostics, NAD, Emeryville, CA 94608, USA.
John.Lechner.B@bayer.com

I. OVERVIEW

Hyperplasia, squamous metaplasia, and dysplasia are common reactions of human airway epithelia to chemical and physical cytotoxic agents. These processes demand strict interregulation of cell replication and squamous and mucoepidermoid differentiation control mechanisms. Aberrations in these processes positively correlate with a high risk for neoplastic transformation [Terzaghi and Nettesheim, 1979; Farber, 1984; Harris, 1987; Pierce and Speers, 1988; Yuspa and Poirier, 1988]. Replicative cultures of normal human bronchial epithelial (NHBE) cells offer opportunities to study these phenomena. This chapter reviews methodologies commonly used to establish these cultures and briefly describes potential modifications.

2. REAGENTS

2.1. Nutrient Media

The three nutrient media used are L-15, CMRL 1066, and LHC (Laboratory of Human Carcinogenesis) basal [Lechner et al., 1982]. The latter two media are supplemented with additives according to the formula for HB medium (see Section 2.1.1) and LHC-9 medium (see Section 2.1.2 and Chapter 7). LHC basal medium is a version of nutrient medium MCDB 151 [Peehl and Ham, 1980]. Specifically, MCDB 151 has been modified as follows: The concentrations of MCDB 151 stock 1 (amino acids) are doubled; the concentration of $CaCl_2 \cdot 2H_2O$ is increased to 0.11 mM; and the osmolality is lowered from 345 to 285 mOsm/kg by reducing the concentrations of NaCl, HEPES, and sodium bicarbonate by 20%, 18%, and 15%, respectively [Lechner and LaVeck, 1985].

2.1.1. HB Medium

To medium CMRL 1066 add the following:

Component		Final Concentration in HB Medium	
		μM	μg/ml
Insulin		0.87	5
Hydrocortisone		0.10	0.036
β-Retinyl acetate		0.318	0.104
Glutamine	0.117		

Penicillin[a]	50 U/ml
Streptomycin[a]	50
Gentamicin[a]	50
Fungizone[a]	1

[a]The medium contains 2× these concentrations and chloramphenicol (150 μg/ml) when tissue is first placed into culture, for the first 2–3 days of incubation.

2.1.2. LHC-9 Medium

Component	Final Concentration in Basal Medium	
	μM	/ml

LHC basal nutrients (see Chapter 7 and Table 3 of Lechner and LaVeck [1985])

Stock 4 (see Chapter 7 and Table 3 of Lechner and LaVeck [1985])

Stock 11 (see Chapter 7 and Table 3 of Lechner and LaVeck, 1985)

Trace elements solution (see Chapter 7 and Table 4 of Lechner et al., 1986b)

Insulin	0.87	5 μg/ml
EGF	0.000825	5 ng/ml
Transferrin	0.125	10 μg/ml
Phosphoethanolamine	0.50	0.07 μg/ml
Ethanolamine	0.50	0.03 μg/ml
Hydrocortisone	0.20	0.07 μg/ml
Gentamicin	50 ng/ml	
Pituitary extract[a]	35 μg protein/ml	
Triiodothyronine (T_3)	0.01	6.73 ng/ml
Retinoic acid	0.00033	0.1 μg/ml
Epinephrine	2.7	0.5 μg/ml

[a]Pituitary extract is undefined, but it markedly enhances the growth rate, especially when T_3 is also present.

2.1.3. Transport Medium, 2 × AL-15

Leibowitz L-15 medium supplemented as follows:

| Penicillin | 100 U/ml |
| Streptomycin | 100 μg/ml |

Gentamicin	100 μg/ml
Fungizone	2 μg/ml
Chloramphenicol	150 μg/ml

2.1.4. Freezing Medium

DMSO	7.5%
Polyvinylpyrrolidine	1%
HEPES	20 mM
FBS	10%
Penicillin	100 U/ml
Streptomycin	100 μg/ml

Made up in L-15 medium.

2.2. Preparation of Bovine Pituitary Extract

Bovine pituitary extract is prepared by blending 110 g of quick-frozen bovine pituitaries in 250 ml of HEPES-buffered saline. The blended material is then centrifuged (10,000 g, 20 min), dialyzed against UPW (2 days; 1:24, 4–5 times), recentrifuged (10,000 g, 20 min), and sterilized through a 0.22-μm hydrophobic filter. All procedures are carried out at 4°C. The extract, which normally contains 70 mg protein per 1 ml, is stored at -70°C in 10-ml aliquots until used.

2.3. Enzymes, Salt Solution, and Matrix

2.3.1. Trypsin Solution (PET)

Trypsin, crystalline	0.05%	0.5 mg/ml
EGTA	0.5 mM	0.2 mg/ml
Polyvinylpyrrolidone	1%	10 mg/ml

Made up in HBS [Lechner and LaVeck, 1985].

2.3.2. Soybean Trypsin Inhibitor (SBTI)

SBTI 30 mg/ml in HBS.

2.3.3. DNase

DNase I, 4 mg/ml in HBS

2.3.4. FN/V/BSA solution

| Human fibronectin | 10 μg/ml |
| Collagen (Vitrogen 100) | 30 μg/ml |

Crystalline BSA	10 μg/ml

Made up in LHC basal medium. (Available complete from BRFF.)

2.3.5. HEPES-Buffered Saline (HBS)

HEPES	20.00 mM
NaCl	120.00 mM
KCl	2.70 mM
D-glucose	9.44 mM
Sodium phosphate (monobasic)	14.00 mM
Phenol red	3.00 μM

3. CULTURE PROCEDURES

These protocols are condensed from Lechner and LaVeck [1985], which provides a more detailed description.

3.1. Tissue Sources

Replicative cultures of NHBE cells can be established from several sources of donated airway specimens, including surgeries and autopsies [Lechner et al., 1986a,b]. Of these, tissue recovered by surgery from noncancerous patients or donors undergoing "immediate" autopsies yield the greatest quantity of culturable cells and are least likely to harbor malignant cells. However, obtaining tissues from these sources can be sporadic and difficult. A more readily obtainable source of lung tissue is from local medical examiners. Specimens can be collected from autopsies of noncancerous individuals within 12 h of death, but investigators should be aware that it becomes progressively more difficult to establish these cultures if the postmortem interval exceeds 6 h.

Culturable NHBE cells can also be obtained by biopsy [Al-Batran et al., 1999] or brushing [Crowell et al., 1996] of airways during bronchoscopy. However, the quantity of cells recovered with this approach significantly limits the numbers of cultures that can be established. Another source that is frequently exploited is uninvolved tissue obtained at surgery of a cancer-bearing lung. However, for these cultures, the investigator must remember that there is a significant possibility of abnormal or malignant cell contamination.

3.2. Avoiding Contamination and Ischemia

3.2.1. Contamination

When culturing NHBE, an immediate concern is the potential for microbial contamination, particularly for those tissues obtained from medical examiners. For surgery or autopsy samples, this potential can be significantly reduced by repeatedly washing the tissue in ice-cold 2 × AL-15 medium, which is L15 medium supplemented with "2×" concentrations of the antibiotics listed in Section 2.1.1 (see Section 2.1.3), followed by careful prosection. This prosection should be performed with sterile technique, and the tissue should be kept in ice-cold 2 × AL-15 medium. Prosection will also reduce the likelihood of contamination with adventitious cell types. For samples from bronchial brushings, the cells should be washed in 2 × AL-15 medium through repeated centrifugations at 4°C.

When these steps are followed, surgery- and brushing-derived specimens rarely produce contaminated cultures. Good success can be had for those specimens obtained from medical examiners; however, even with these precautions, some cell cultures will still become contaminated, particularly if the donor was septic at the time of death.

3.2.2. Ischemia

Ischemia-induced cell injury develops as soon as the blood supply to the tissue/epithelium ceases and reduces the ability to culture human airway epithelial cells [Trump and Harris, 1979]. The first step to minimize ischemic injury is to transport the tissue from the donor to the laboratory in ice-cold L-15. This is because L-15 is formulated to maintain a nearly neutral pH in equilibrium with an air atmosphere.

To further reduce ischemic injury, small fragments (2 cm^2) of opened airways, epithelium side up, should be placed at the edge of a 60-mm culture dish and incubated for 5–7 days in a 50% oxygen partial pressure atmosphere on a rocking platform [Trump and Harris, 1979] (see Protocol 8.1). The optimized medium for this procedure is HB medium [Stoner et al., 1980] (see Section 2.1.1). Each dish receives 3 ml of medium, and because these tissues initially elaborate copious amounts of mucin, it is recommended that the medium, containing 2× antibiotics, be replaced daily for the first few days and then every other day with 1× antibiotics. Ischemia does not appear to be a major consideration for the cells recovered by bronchial brushing, although experiments have not been done to ascertain whether a short incubation in 50% O_2 would improve plating efficiency.

Protocol 8.1. Reversal of Ischemic Injury in Airway Epithelium

Reagents and Materials

Sterile

- ❑ L-15 medium (see Section 2.1.3)
- ❑ HB medium (see Section 2.1.1)
- ❑ Petri dishes, 6 cm
- ❑ Scalpel
- ❑ Scissors, dissecting
- ❑ Forceps, slightly curved, microdissecting
- ❑ High-O_2 gas mixture: 50% O_2, 45% N_2, 5% CO_2

Nonsterile

- ❑ Controlled atmosphere chamber
- ❑ Rocker platform

Protocol

(a) Before culturing, scratch, with a scalpel blade, a 1-cm^2 area at the edge of the surface of 6-cm culture dishes.

(b) Open the airways, submerged in L-15 medium, with scissors and cut (by a knifing as opposed to a sawing action) with a scalpel into 2 × 3-cm pieces.

(c) Pick up the moist fragments by a scooping motion with the curved microdissecting forceps and place epithelium side up onto the scratched area in the 6-cm culture dish.

(d) Incubate the fragments at room temperature without medium for 3–5 min to allow time for them to adhere to the scratched areas of the culture dishes.

(e) Add 3 ml of HB medium [Lechner et al., 1981, 1986a; Brent, 1986] (see Section 2.1.1) and place the dishes in the controlled atmosphere chamber.

(f) Flush the chamber with the high-O_2 gas mixture, and place on the rocker platform.

(g) Rock the chamber at 10 cycles/min, causing the medium to flow intermittently over the epithelial surface, while incubating at 36.5°C.

(h) Replace the medium and atmosphere after 1 day and then at 2-day intervals for 6–8 days.

3.3. Isolating Cells from Explants

After completion of the ischemia-reversal procedure, the tissue is further cut into 0.5-cm^2 fragments, and then several pieces are explanted onto the surface of each culture dish (see Protocol 3.2 and Section 2.1.2). Within 4–8 days, replicating epithelial cells will emigrate from these fragments. Once this outgrowth expands to 1–3 cm in diameter, the remaining tissue can be gently removed with forceps and transferred to a new dish to obtain additional outgrowth cultures. This explant transfer step can be repeated at least 7 times with a robust outgrowth of epithelial cells developing each time. Occasionally, productive fragments can be transferred biweekly for over a year [Lechner et al., 1981].

Early observations suggested an important need for the inoculation of Swiss mouse 3T3 feeder cells into the culture [Lechner et al., 1981, 1986a]. Specifically, the airway epithelial cells that grew from explants rapidly differentiated into terminal squamous epithelia when the explant was removed unless these feeder cells were present. In addition, secondary and subsequent passages of the outgrowth cells could be propagated if the dissociated cells were maintained on feeder layers. Furthermore, it was found that if these subcultured cells were seeded at cell densities of 150 cells per cm^2, then colonies of pure epithelial morphology cells would develop at a plating efficiency of 15%. Indeed, this feeder cell technique supported robust and rapid (1 population doubling per day) growth of NHBE cells.

However, the feeder layer method is costly and labor-intensive. Fortunately, medium optimization investigations formulated a medium that maintained robust cell growth in the absence of feeder cells. This medium, LHC-9, was derived with relatively minor changes from MCDB 151 medium [Peehl and Ham, 1980], which had been designed to propagate human epidermal keratinocytes. A complete "cookbook" description of LHC-9 can be found in Lechner and LaVeck [1985].

Protocol 8.2. Explant Outgrowth Cultures

Reagents and Materials

Sterile

❑ FN/V/BSA coating solution (see Section 2.3.4)
❑ Petri dishes, 6 cm

❑ Scalpel

Protocol

(a) Before explanting, scratch 4 areas (0.3 cm^2) of the surface of 6-cm culture dishes with a scalpel blade.

(b) Coat the culture dish surfaces with the FN/V/BSA coating solution.

(c) Cut the moist ischemia-reversed fragments into 0.5 × 0.5-cm pieces and explant epithelium side up onto the scratched areas.

(d) Incubate the fragments at room temperature without medium for 3–5 min to allow time for them to adhere to the scratched areas of the culture dishes.

(e) Add 4 ml of LHC-9 medium to the dishes and incubate the explants at 36.5°C in a humidified CO_2 incubator.

(f) Replace the medium with fresh medium every 3–4 days. After 8–11 days of incubation the epithelial cell outgrowths radiate from the tissue fragments more than 0.5 cm; fibroblastic cell contamination, as determined by phase contrast microscopy, is rare.

(g) Transfer the tissue fragments to new scratched and FN/V/BSA-coated culture dishes for new outgrowths of epithelial cells. Routinely, the tissue can be reexplanted up to 7 times with a high yield of NHBE cells.

(h) The postexplant outgrowth cultures are incubated in LHC-9 medium for an additional 2–4 days before they are enzyme dissociated and subcultured, used in experimental protocols, or cryopreserved.

3.4. Subculture

Having established outgrowths of primary cells, the next goal is to subculture them (see Protocols 3.3 and 3.4). Several considerations underpin the subculturing procedure. These include removing cells from the culture dish, improving colony forming efficiency, and avoiding terminal differentiation.

3.4.1. Removing Cells from Culture Dish

There are a couple of ways to remove the cells from the culture dish. Urea can be used to denature glycocalyx elaborated by the cells to augment their attachment to the culture dish. However, relatively good subculturing can still be attained if the urea bath is omitted. The best agent is PET [polyvinylpyrrolidone (PVP),

EGTA, and trypsin dissolved in HBS] [Lechner and LaVeck, 1985]. PET was specifically formulated for bronchial epithelial cells. It has: 1) a minimal concentration of trypsin, 2) EGTA to augment depolymerization of microtubules, and 3) PVP to protect the cell membrane. The cells are usually incubated in PET at room temperature until they float free (usually 5–10 min). It is not altogether uncommon that the cells will fail to dissociate within 10 min of incubation. In this instance, the PET should be replaced with fresh PET and the cells should then rapidly release from the culture dish surface.

When the cells lift off the dish, it is important to quickly neutralize any remaining trypsin. Experience has shown that pelleting the cells, then resuspending them in a few milliliters of soybean trypsin inhibitor (SBTI), and incubating at room temperature for 2–4 min markedly enhances the colony forming efficiency (CFE). Adding DNase will augment single cell formation.

Protocol 8.3. Dissociation and Subculture of Bronchial Epithelium

Reagents and Materials

- ❑ HEPES-buffered saline (HBS) (see Section 2.3.5)
- ❑ Urea, 0.5 M in HBS
- ❑ PET (see Section 2.3.1)
- ❑ SBTI (see Section 2.3.2)
- ❑ DNase (see Section 2.3.3)

Protocol

(a) Aspirate the medium and bathe the culture two times with HBS [Lechner et al., 1980].

(b) Remove the HBS and incubate the culture at room temperature in 0.5 M urea [Lechner et al., 1980] for 5 min.

(c) Remove the urea solution by aspiration and bathe the cells in a minimal volume of PET and incubate at room temperature until the cells float free (usually 5–10 min).

(d) Remove the cells from the culture with 10 volumes of HBS and pellet by centrifugation (125 g for 5 min).

(e) Resuspend the pellet of cells in 0.3 ml of SBTI and 0.1 ml of DNase I.

(f) Enumerate the cells and reinoculate at the desired cell density into culture dishes that have been coated with FN/V/BSA.

3.4.2. Improving CFE

CFE can be augmented by coating the culture dishes with a FN/V/BSA solution (see Section 2.3.4). In addition, speed increases CFE, as prolonged suspension times promote terminal squamous differentiation of the cells [Lechner et al., 1982]. Optimally, the CFE should be 15%, and normally the cells can be subcultured five times (30–35 population doublings) before senescence.

Protocol 8.4. Matrix-Coating Culture Dish Surfaces

Reagents and Materials

Sterile

- ❑ FN/V/BSA (see Section 2.3.4)
- ❑ Petri dishes
- ❑ Culture medium: LHC-9 (see Section 2.1.2)

Protocol

(a) Coat culture dish surfaces with FN/V/BSA by adding FN/V/BSA to culture dish surfaces at a ratio of 2 ml/10 cm^2 of surface area.

(b) Incubate the plates in a humidified CO_2 incubator at 36.5°C for at least 2 h (2- to 72-h incubations are statistically identical).

(c) Vacuum aspirate the mixture.

(d) Add the normal volume of medium to the dish.

3.4.3. Additional Methods to Avoid Terminal Differentiation

Replicative cultures of NHBE cells require a medium formula and culture conditions that not only will promote cell replication but will impede the cells from undergoing terminal differentiation. NHBE cells spontaneously undergo squamous differentiation if maintained at confluence in serum-free culture medium for extended periods of time (2–4 days), even if the medium is replaced with fresh medium daily. In addition, a significant proportion of the cells will differentiate if they are maintained in suspension for a prolonged period. Furthermore, cells growing at clonal density will fail to enter the S phase of the cell cycle and differentiate, if the medium is supplemented with >1–2% FBS [Ke et al., 1989; Lechner et al., 1983a, 1984].

The mechanistic steps for squamous differentiation involve TGF-β_1, particularly for sparse cell density cultures of NHBE cells. This is evidenced by experiments showing inhibition of terminal differentiation of NHBE cells after incorporating anti-transforming growth factor type β_1 (TGF-β_1) antibodies into medium containing FBS and stimulation of terminal differentiation by direct TGF-β_1 dose-response titration experiments [Masui et al., 1986]. Other putative endogenous serum-borne squamous differentiation-inducing factors may be involved, but they remain to be identified. Similarly, certain xenobiotics, most notably phorbol esters such as 12-O-tetradecanoylphorbol-13-acetate (TPA), induce NHBE to undergo squamous differentiation [Willey et al., 1984]. Medium supplements, such as epinephrine and cholera toxin, can antagonize the differentiation-inducing effects of TGF-β_1 and TPA [Willey et al., 1985; Masui et al., 1986]. Of course, epinephrine also interacts with other medium supplements in complex ways; for example, it is not growth stimulating unless the medium contains both EGF and BPE, and BPE is inactive unless EGF is also present [Willey et al., 1985].

It has been found that the cell density of the culture affects the probability that a cell will respond to TGF-β_1 [Ke et al., 1989]. Irreversible inhibition of DNA synthesis occurs in sparse cell density cultures within 24 h after exposure. In high-density cultures (>10,000 cells per cm^2) this effect is only transient ($\sim$36 h). Moreover, phase-contrast microscope image analysis of high-density cultures reveals that virtually all of the cells display a squamous morphology within 1 h after exposure to FBS or TGF-β_1, but after 48–72 h clusters of small prolate spherical cells surrounded by numerous involucrin-positive squamous-appearing cells are present. Only these small cells are capable of DNA synthesis and cell division, as determined by autoradiography and time-lapse photomicrographic images. These small replicating cells will immediately undergo squamous differentiation if they are subcultured and reinoculated at low cell density and incubated in medium supplemented with FBS or TGF-β_1. No medium or matrix conditioning effects can be detected. Therefore, whether or not a human bronchial epithelial cell will be refractive to squamous terminal differentiation by FBS or TGF-β_1 seems to be solely a function of the cell density of the culture.

A similar but opposite cell density effect has been found for Ca^{2+}. Specifically, variations in the concentration of Ca^{2+} in the medium between 0.1 mM and 1.0 mM have no significant effect on the clonal growth rate of the cells [Lechner et al., 1982]. However, if the cell density exceeds 10,000 cells per 1 cm^2, Ca^{2+} concentrations greater than 0.4 mM cause the cells to undergo squamous differentiation [Pfeifer et al., 1989].

Interestingly, lung carcinoma cells of various histopathologies are significantly different from their normal counterparts with respect to growth and differentiation control. Specifically, when incubated in the growth-optimized serum-free medium, they either fail to proliferate or grow at rates that are markedly slower than that of their normal counterparts. Carcinoma cells do not undergo squamous differentiation when FBS is added to the medium but exhibit clonal growth rates that are nearly equal to that of the NHBE cells [Lechner et al., 1983a]. On the basis of these observations, it was concluded that most human lung carcinoma cells differ from their normal counterparts in two critical areas of growth control. First, they have gained a requirement for serum-borne mitogens for growth, and second, they have lost the ability to respond to FBS-contained agents as endogenous inducers of terminal squamous differentiation.

3.5. Distinguishing and Identifying Epithelial Cells

NHBE are identified by several criteria based on the characteristic structure and function of normal epithelium. In explant outgrowth cultures, polygon-shaped epithelial cells grow out from the periphery of the explant onto the culture dish before the fusiform fibroblast cells [Stoner et al., 1980]. Cytochemical stains can further distinguish epithelial cells and fibroblasts in primary cultures. Squamous epithelial cells stain positively with the immunoperoxidase method for prekeratin and keratin, whereas fibroblasts stain negatively. In some cultures, epithelial cells will stain positively with alcian blue-PAS before and after treatment with diastase, indicating the production of acidic and neutral mucopolysaccharides, two components of mucus. Most cultures, however, will not exhibit positive staining for mucous substances. Epithelial cells in first-passage cultures are similar in appearance to those in explant outgrowth cultures, and they continue to react positively with the keratin antibodies.

Scanning electron microscopy of subcultures shows colonies composed of prolate spherical cells covered with varying numbers of microvilli [Lechner et al., 1983a, 1984] and apposed cell borders. Ultrastructural studies show that the epithelial cells have tight junctions, desmosomes, and tonofilaments [Lechner et al., 1982, 1984; Stoner et al., 1981]. Epithelial cells initiated from explants taken from blood type A or type B patients possess A or

B blood group antigen-specific reactivity for periods of at least 90 days in primary culture [Stoner et al., 1981; Katoh et al., 1979]; fibroblast cells are negative. In addition, epithelial cells can be distinguished from fibroblasts in secondary and tertiary cultures of mixed cell types, because only the epithelial cells react with antibodies to blood group A or group B antigens. However, neither the epithelial cells nor the fibroblasts from patients with blood type O [H] reacted with the human anti-H antisera; this antiserum has a low affinity, and negative results should be viewed with caution.

Epithelial cells react with antibodies to prekeratin proteins from both human stratum corneum and mouse epidermis [Lechner et al., 1982; Stoner et al., 1981]; fibroblasts do not react. Epithelial cells and fibroblasts can also be identified by their reactivity to anti-collagen antibodies [Stoner et al., 1981]. Fibroblasts react with antibodies to types I and III collagen, but epithelial cells are negative. Epithelial cells react weakly with antibodies to type IV collagen, and fibroblasts do not react. Human bronchial epithelial cells do not form colonies in soft agar when plated at a density of 100,000 per 1 ml, and chromosome analysis shows that the cells retain the normal human karyotype (2N = 46) throughout the replicative phase [Lechner et al., 1982, 1983b]. Additionally, these cells are metabolically active and capable of converting xenobiotics to DNA adducts [Lechner et al., 1981].

3.6. Cryopreservation

Both dissociated NHBE cells and bronchial tissue fragments can be cryopreserved with good viability using relatively routine procedures, as follows.

Protocol 8.5. Cryopreservation of Bronchial Epithelium

Reagents and Materials

Sterile

❑ 2 × AL-15 medium (see Section 2.1.3) [Lechner and LaVeck, 1985]
❑ DMSO freezing medium (see Section 2.1.4)
❑ Freezer vials
❑ Controlled-rate freezer

Protocol

(a) Suspend the tissue (0.5-cm^3 fragments) or pelleted NHBE cells ($2-5 \times 10^6$) in 0.5 ml of cold $2 \times$ AL-15 in a freezing vial.

(b) Add 0.5 ml of DMSO freezing medium to the vial, swirl the mixture, and close the vial.

(c) Transfer vial(s) to a controlled-rate freezer and freeze the cells/tissues at 1°C/min according to the manufacturer's directions.

(d) Transfer the frozen vials to liquid N_2 for storage.

Δ *Safety note.* A transparent face mask, cryoprotective gloves and a fastened lab coat must be worn when placing any material into liquid nitrogen.

(e) Resurrect the cells/tissues by rapidly warming the vial to 37°C.

Δ *Safety note.* An ampoule that has been stored in liquid nitrogen can inspire liquid nitrogen if not properly sealed. The ampoule will then explode violently when warmed. To protect from potential explosion of ampoules, thaw in a covered container, such as a large plastic bucket with a lid, or store in the vapor phase. Wear gloves, a face mask, and a closed lab coat.

(f) Swab the vial with 70% alcohol, open it, and transfer the cells to 10 ml of LHC-9 medium.

(g) Pellet the cells, resuspend in LHC-9 medium, and inoculate into FN/V/BSA surface-coated culture dishes containing LHC-9 medium.

3.7. Alternative Protocols

Collagen matrices and the presence of mesenchymal cells alter the response of NHBE cells to squamous differentiation-inducing agents and conditions. For example, cultured cells will reconstitute a regular mucociliary epithelium if inoculated onto the luminal surface of a deepithelialized rat trachea that is xenotransplanted subcutaneously into a nude mouse [Baba et al., 1987]. To mimic the conditions of the deepithelialized trachea in vitro, we have found that NHBE cells that have been transferred from plastic dishes to these structures and incubated in the same serum-free medium synthesize neutral and acid mucin after 2 wk of incubation. Surprisingly, the mucin-synthesizing cells also do not undergo squamous differentiation when TGF-β_1, FBS, or TPA is added to the medium [Murakami and Lechner, unpublished observations]. The mechanisms responsible for the induction of mucin differentiation and the loss of the ability of the cells to undergo squamous differentiation are being sought.

The method of obtaining bronchial epithelial cells from explant tissue has been modified and used by other investigators [Siegfried and Nesnow, 1984; Bernal et al., 1988]. Siegfried and others have obtained human bronchial and rodent epithelial cells from outgrowths of explanted tissue and have used them to study cytotoxicity and carcinogenicity in clonal assays [Mass et al., 1985; Siegfried et al., 1986; Beeman et al., 1987]. Other culture systems that support the growth and differentiation of normal respiratory epithelial cells have been defined [Vollberg et al., 1990]. For example, rodent and nonhuman primate tracheal epithelial cells can be isolated by enzymatic digestion of the tracheal lumen and can be seeded onto collagen-coated culture dishes or collagen gels [Lee et al. 1984; Chang et al., 1985; Wu et al., 1986; Xu et al., 1986; Huang et al., 1989; Edmondson et al., 1990]. Everitt and co-workers [Everitt et al., 1989] have evolved a tracheal implant xenograft model in which normal human bronchial epithelial cells are grown from explanted tissue pieces previously frozen and stored in liquid nitrogen. Briefly, 0.5-cm^3 pieces of bronchus are thawed and placed on culture dishes coated with collagen, fibronectin, and bovine serum; epithelial cells are harvested 4–5 days later as an outgrowth from the explant. The cells are then used to repopulate deepithelialized rabbit tracheas and subsequently implanted into the subcutis of athymic nude mice. More recently, Al-Batran et al. [1999] published an extensive report of their methodologies for an organ culture model of airways.

REFERENCES

Al-Batran SE, Astner ST, Supthut M, Gamarra F, Brueckner K, Welsch U, Knuechel R, Huber RM (1999): Three-dimensional in vitro cocultivation of lung carcinoma cells with human bronchial organ culture as a model for bronchial carcinoma. Am J Respir Cell Mol Biol 21: 200–208.

Baba M, Klein-Szanto AJ, Trono D, Obara T, Yoakum GH, Masui T, Harris CC (1987): Preneoplastic and neoplastic growth of xenotransplanted lung-derived human cell lines using deepithelialized rat tracheas. Cancer Res 47: 573–578.

Beeman DK, Siegfried JM, Mass MJ (1987): Effect of phorbol esters on clonal cultures of human, hamster, and rat respiratory epithelial cells. Cancer Res 47: 541–546.

Bernal S, Weinberg K, Kakefuda M, Stahel R, O'Hara C, Wong YC (1988): Membrane antigens of human bronchial epithelial cells identified by monoclonal antibodies. In Vitro Cell Dev Biol 24: 117–125.

Brent TP (1986): Inactivation of purified human O^6-alkylguanine-DNA alkyltransferase by alkylating agents or alkylated DNA. Cancer Res 46: 2320–2323.

Chang LY, Wu R, Nettesheim P (1985): Morphological changes in rat tracheal cells during the adaptive and early growth phase in primary cell culture. J Cell Sci 74: 283–301.

Crowell RE, Gilliland FD, Temes RT, Harms HJ, Neft RE, Heaphy E, Auckley DH, Crooks LA, Jordan SW, Samet JM, Lechner JF, Belinsky SA (1996): Detection of trisomy 7 in nonmalignant bronchial epithelium from lung cancer patients and individuals at risk for lung cancer. Cancer Epidemiol Biomarkers Prev 5: 631–637.

Edmondson SW, Wu R, Mossman BT (1990): Regulation of differentiation and keratin protein expression by vitamin A in primary cultures of hamster tracheal epithelial cells. J Cell Physiol 142: 21–30.

Everitt JJ, Boreiko CJ, Mangum JB, Martin JT, Iglehart JD, Hesterberg TW (1989): Development of a tracheal implant xenograft model to expose human bronchial epithelial cells to toxic gases. Toxicol Pathol 17: 465–473.

Farber E (1984): Chemical carcinogenesis: A current biological perspective. Carcinogenesis 5: 1–5.

Ham RG, McKeehan WL (1979): Media and growth requirements. Methods Enzymol 58: 44–93.

Harris CC (1987): Human tissues and cells in carcinogenesis research. Cancer Res 47: 1–10.

Huang TH, St. George IA, Plopper CG, Wu R (1989): Keratin protein expression during the development of conducting airway epithelium in nonhuman primates. Differentiation 41: 78–86.

Katoh Y, Stoner GD, McIntire KR, Hill TA, Anthony R, McDowell EM, Trump BF, Harris CC (1979): Immunologic markers of human bronchial epithelial cells in tissue sections and in culture. J Natl Cancer Inst 62: 1177–1185.

Ke Y, Gerwin BI, Ruskie SE, Pfeifer AMA, Harris CC, Lechner JF (1989): Cell density governs the ability of human bronchial epithelial cells to recognize serum and transforming growth factor β as squamous differentiation inducing agents. Am J Pathol 137: 833–843.

Lechner JF, LaVeck MA (1985): A serum-free method for culturing normal human bronchial epithelial cells at clonal density. J Tissue Culture Methods 9: 43–48.

Lechner JF, Babcock MS, Marnell MM, Narayan KS, Kaighn ME (1980): Normal human prostate epithelial cell cultures. In Harris CC, Trump BF, Stoner GD (eds): "Methods in Cell Biology." New York: Academic Press, pp 195–225.

Lechner JF, Haugen A, Autrup H, McClendon IA, Trump BF, Harris CC (1981): Clonal growth of epithelial cells from normal adult human bronchus. Cancer Res 41: 2294–2304.

Lechner JF, Haugen A, McClendon IA, Pettis EW (1982): Clonal growth of normal adult human bronchial epithelial cells in a serum-free medium. In Vitro 18: 633–642.

Lechner JF, McClendon IA, LaVeck MA, Shamsuddin AKM, Harris CC (1983a): Differential control by platelet factors of squamous differentiation in normal and malignant human bronchial epithelial cells. Cancer Res 43: 5915–5921.

Lechner JF, Haugen A, Tokiwa T, Trump BF, Harris CC (1983b): Effects of asbestos and carcinogenic metals on cultured human bronchial epithelium. In Harris CC, Autrup H (eds): "Human Carcinogenesis." New York: Academic Press, pp 561–585.

Lechner JF, Haugen A, McClendon IA, Shamsuddin AKM (1984): Induction of squamous differentiation of normal human bronchial epithelial cells by small amounts of serum. Differentiation 25: 229–237.

Lechner JF, Stoner GD, Haugen A, Autrup H, Willey JC, Trump BF, Harris CC (1986a): In vitro human bronchial model systems for carcinogenic studies. In Webber MM, Sekely L (eds): "In Vitro Models for Cancer Research." New York: CRC Press, pp 143–159.

Lechner JF, Stoner GD, Yoakum GH, Willey JC, Grafström RC, Masui T, LaVeck MA, Harris CC (1986b): In vitro carcinogenesis with human tracheobronchial tissues and cells. In Schiff LJ (ed): "In Vitro Models of Respiratory Epithelium." New York: CRC Press, pp 143–160.

Lee TC, Wu R, Brody AR, Barrett JC, Nettesheim P (1984): Growth and differentiation of hamster tracheal epithelial cells in culture. Exp Lung Res 6: 27–45.

Mass MI, Siegfried JM, Beeman DK, Leavitt SA (1985): Heterogeneity in responses of human and rodent respiratory epithelial cells to tumor promoters in culture. Carcinog Compr Surv 8: 173–189.

Masui T, Wakefield LM, Lechner JF, LaVeck MA, Sporn MB, Harris CC (1986): Type beta transforming growth factor is the primary differentiation-inducing serum factor for normal human bronchial epithelial cells. Proc Nail Acad Sci USA 83: 2438–2442.

Peehl DM, Ham RG (1980): Clonal growth of human keratinocytes with small amounts of dialyzed serum. In Vitro 16: 526–540.

Pfeifer A, Lechner JF, Masui T, Reddel RR, Mark GE, Harris CC (1989): Control of growth and squamous differentiation in normal human bronchial epithelial cells by chemical and biological modifiers and transferred genes. Environ Health Perspect 80: 209–220.

Pierce GB, Speers WC (1988): Tumors as caricatures of the process of tissue renewal: Prospects for therapy by directing differentiation. Cancer Res 48: 1996–2004.

Siegfried JM, Nesnow S (1984): Cytotoxicity of chemical carcinogens towards human bronchial epithelial cells evaluated in a clonal assay. Carcinogenesis 5: 1317–1322.

Siegfried JM, Rudo K, Bryant BJ, Ellis S, Mass MJ, Nesnow S (1986): Metabolism of benzo(a)pyrene in monolayer cultures of human bronchial epithelial cells from a series of donors. Cancer Res 46: 4368–4371.

Stoner GD, Katoh Y, Foidart JM, Myers GA, Harris CC (1980): Identification and culture of human bronchial epithelial cells. In Harris CC, Trump BE, Stoner GD (eds): "Methods in Cell Biology. Vol 21A: Normal Human Tissue and Cell Culture." New York: Academic Press, pp 15–35.

Stoner GD, Katoh Y, Foidart JM, Trump BF, Steinert PM, Harris CC (1981): Cultured human bronchial epithelial cells: Blood group antigens, keratin, collagens, and fibronectin. In Vitro 17: 577–587.

Terzaghi M, Nettesheim P (1979): Dynamics of neoplastic development in carcinogen-exposed tracheal mucosa. Cancer Res 39: 4003–4010.

Trump BF, Harris CC (1979): Human tissues in biomedical research. Hum Pathol 10: 245–248.

Vollberg TM, Nervi C., George MA, Jetten AM (1990): Identification of multiple stages in the program of squamous differentiation in tracheobronchial epithelial cells. In Thomassen D, Nettesheim P (eds): "Biology, Toxicology, and Carcinogenesis of Respiratory Epithelium." New York: Hemisphere Publishing, pp 74–87.

Willey JC, Saladino AJ, Ozanne C, Lechner JF, Harris CC (1984): Acute effects of 12-O-tetradecanoylphorbol-13-acetate, teleocidin B, or 2,3,7,8-tetrachlorodibenzo-p-dioxin on cultured normal human bronchial epithelial cells. Carcinogenesis 5: 209–215.

Willey JC, LaVeck MA, McClendon LA, Lechner JF (1985): Relationship of ornithine decarboxylase activity and cAMP metabolism to proliferation of normal human bronchial epithelial cells. J Cell Physiol 124: 207–212.

Wu R, Wu MM (1986): Effects of retinoids on human bronchial epithelial cells: Differential regulation of hyaluronate synthesis and keratin protein synthesis. J Cell Physiol 127: 73–82.

Wu R, Groelke JW, Chang LY, Proter ME, Smith D, Nettesheim P (1982): Effects of hormones on the multiplication and differentiation of tracheal epithelial cells in culture. In Sirbasku D, Sato GH, Pardee A (eds): "Growth of Cells in Hormonally Defined Media." Cold Spring Harbor, NY: Cold Spring Harbor Laboratory, pp 641–656.

Wu R, Yankaskas J, Cheng E, Knowles MR, Boucher R (1985): Growth and differentiation of human nasal epithelial cells in culture. Serum-free, hormone-supplemented medium and proteoglycan synthesis. Am Rev Respir Dis 132: 311–320.

Wu R, Sato GH, Whitcutt MJ (1986): Developing differentiated epithelial cell cultures: Airway epithelial cells. Fundam Appl Toxicol 6: 580–590.

Xu GL, Sivarajah K, Wu R, Nettesheim P, Eling T (1986): Biosynthesis of prostaglandins by isolated and cultured airway epithelial cells. Exp Lung Res 10: 101–114

Yuspa SH, Poirier MC (1988): Chemical carcinogenesis: From animal models to molecular models in one decade. Adv Cancer Res 50: 25–70.

APPENDIX: SOURCES OF MATERIALS

Material	Catalog No.	Supplier
Bovine pituitaries	57133-2	Pel-Freez Biologicals
Bovine serum albumin, crystalline	—	Miles Biochemical (Bayer)
Chloramphenicol	C3175	Sigma
CMRL-1066	21530	GIBCO BRL
Controlled-atmosphere chamber	7441	Bellco, Vineland, NJ
Controlled-rate freezer	8001	Biofluids, Rockville, MD
DMSO	D2650	Sigma
DNase I	D4263	Sigma
EGTA	E4378	Sigma
Epidermal growth factor (EGF), human recombinant	40052	Becton Dickinson
Epinephrine	E4250	Sigma
Ethanolamine	E9508	Sigma
Fetal bovine (calf) serum (FBS)	—	HyClone

Appendix continues

APPENDIX: SOURCES OF MATERIALS (continued)

Material	Catalog No.	Supplier
Forceps, microdissecting, curved	RS-5135	Roboz
Freezing vial	25702	Corning
Fungizone (amphotericin B)	15290	GIBCO
Gas mixture, high-O_2 (50% O_2; 45% N_2 5% CO_2 special order)	—	Matheson Gas
Gentamicin	15710	GIBCO
Glutamine	25030	GIBCO
HEPES	16530	GIBCO
Human fibronectin	40008	Becton Dickinson (Collaborative Research)
Hydrocortisone	H4001	Sigma
Insulin	I1882	Sigma
Leibowitz L-15 medium	11415	GIBCO
LHC basal medium	—	Biofluids
LHC-9 medium	181-500	Biofluids
Penicillin	15070	GIBCO
Petri dishes	Lux 52 10	Bayer
Phosphoethanolamine	P0503	Sigma
Pituitary extract, bovine	CC4009	BioWhittaker (Clonetics)
Polyvinylpyrrolidone	—	USB
Retinoic acid, all *trans*	R2625	Sigma
β-Retinol acetate, all *trans*	R4632	Sigma
Rocker platform	7740	Bellco
SBTI	S9003	Sigma
Scalpel	1621	Becton Dickinson
Sterilizing filter, low protein binding	PES	Millipore
Streptomycin	15070	GIBCO
Transferrin, human	40204	Becton Dickinson
Triiodothyronine	T2877	Sigma
Trypsin	—	Cooper Biomedical
Urea	U4128	Sigma
Vitrogen 100	—	Collagen Corporation

9

Isolation and Culture of Pulmonary Alveolar Epithelial Type II Cells

---

Leland G. Dobbs[1]* and Robert F. Gonzalez[2]

[1]Professor of Medicine and Pediatrics, Adj. Cardiovascular Research Institute and Departments of Medicine and Pediatrics, University of California San Francisco,[2] Cardiovascular Research Institute, University of California San Francisco
*Corresponding author: Leland G. Dobbs, Suite 150, University of California Laurel Heights Campus, 3333 California Street, San Francisco, CA 94118. dobbs@itsa.ucsf.edu

I. INTRODUCTION

In this chapter, we describe current methods of isolating and culturing pulmonary alveolar epithelial type II cells. The pulmonary alveolar epithelium, which covers more than 99% of the internal surface area of the lungs, is comprised of two morphologically distinct types of cells, called type I and type II cells. Both cell types are believed to be essential for mammalian life. Each cell type has been characterized by distinctive ultrastructural morphologic features. Type I cells are very large squamous cells with calculated diameters of 50–100 μm and volumes of 3000 μm^3 [Stone et al., 1992]. Although type I cells comprise only ~8% of all lung cells, this very large cell type has thin cytoplasmic extensions that cover 95–98% of the alveolar surface. Type II cells are smaller, cuboid cells (diam. ~10 μm). There are approximately twice as many type II cells as type I cells; however, because of their smaller size and cuboid shape, type II cells cover only 2–5% of the alveolar surface [Stone et al., 1992]. Morphologically, type II cells are identified by an unusual intracellular organelle, the lamellar body, which is the storage granule for pulmonary surfactant (see Fig. 9.1). Type II cells have several important functions, which include synthesis, secretion, and recycling of surfactant; transport of ions [Goodman and Crandall, 1982; Mason et al., 1982] and water [Folkesson et al., 1994]; synthesis of immune effector molecules [Mager et al., 1999; Paine et al., 1993]; and repair of injury to the alveolar epithelium. During the course of alveolar repair in vivo, type II cells transdifferentiate into type I cells [Evans et al., 1975].

Despite efforts by a number of different laboratories to develop stable cell lines that would be good models for type II cells, the results to date have been discouraging. Initial reports of some passaged cells, such as the A549 [Giard et al., 1973; Lieber et al., 1976] and L2 [Douglas and Kaighn, 1974] lines, appeared promising; however; subsequent careful evaluation has shown that these cells do not display important morphologic [Mason and Williams, 1980], lipid [Mason and Williams, 1980] and molecular

[Korst et al., 1995; Li et al., 1998; Mason, personal communication] markers of the type II cell phenotype. Other cell lines (MLE 12 and 15 [Wikenheiser et al., 1993] and NIH H-441 [Gazdar et al., 1990]) express a few characteristics of type II cells but do not express the full spectrum of type II cell differentiated characteristics (i.e., they contain typical lamellar bodies, express high levels of surfactant proteins A, B, C, and D, and synthesize and secrete appropriate surfactant phospholipids). Therefore, none of these cell lines has been accepted to be a good model for studying general properties of type II cells; it continues to be necessary to use isolated and cultured type II cells to investigate type II cell-specific functions.

Because the intercellular junctions of the alveolar epithelium are among the "tightest" [Schneeberger, 1978] and because type II cells comprise only a small percentage of all lung cells, it is necessary to use both enzymatic digestion and cell selection to obtain homogeneous populations of type II cells. Kikkawa and Yoneda [1974] developed the first method of isolating type II cells from rodent lungs. In subsequent years, various modifications of this method have resulted in improved cell yields and purities

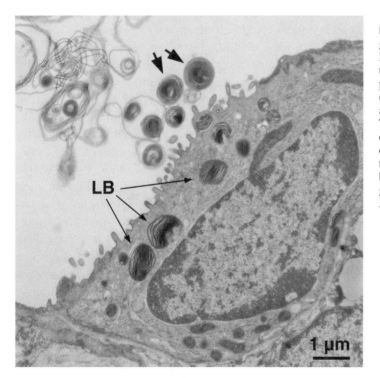

Fig 9.1. Electron micrograph of a rat type II cell. Hallmarks of the typical type II cell morphologic appearance are lamellar bodies (LBs), which contain lipid and protein components. The dense proteinaceous cores of the lamellar bodies can be readily visualized in the secreted LBs (indicated by arrowheads). The micrograph was taken by Lennell Allen, CVRI, UCSF.

[reviewed in Dobbs, 1990]. The majority of published studies of type II cell functions have been performed with type II cells obtained from adult rats. Type II cells have also been successfully isolated from other species, including rabbits [Kikkawa et al., 1975], mice [Corti et al., 1996], guinea pigs [Sikpi et al., 1986], hamsters [Pfleger, 1977], cows [Augustin-Voss et al., 1989], and humans [Robinson et al., 1984].

Type II cells maintained for several days on tissue culture plastic (TCP), in the presence of fetal bovine serum, undergo progressive morphologic and biochemical changes. The mitotic index of cells grown under these conditions is <1% [Leslie et al., 1993], the practical result of which is that proliferation is essentially nil. (It should be noted, however, that very low-density culture conditions [Leslie et al., 1993] and hepatocyte growth factor [Mason et al., 1994] permit low-level proliferation of type II cells.) In culture, type II cells flatten, lose specific type II cell morphologic characteristics, and stop synthesizing and secreting surfactant [Diglio and Kikkawa, 1977; Mason and Dobbs, 1980]. It was initially hypothesized that type II cells behaved similarly to mammary, hepatic, and pancreatic epithelia in that these cells all simply ceased to express differentiated characteristics in culture. However, based on the observations that type II cells cultured under these conditions begin to express some type I cell markers [Borok et al., 1998b; Campbell et al., 1999; Danto et al., 1995; Dobbs et al., 1985; Dobbs et al., 1988], an alternative hypothesis is that type II cells in vitro are transdifferentiating into type I cells. It remains an unanswered question how good a model system the dedifferentiated type II cell is for native type I cells.

Despite these caveats, the model system of cultured type II cells on TCP has been successfully employed for many years to study various functions of type II cells, particularly surfactant metabolism [Dobbs and Mason, 1978, 1979; Rooney et al., 1994; Wright and Dobbs, 1991; Wright and Youmans, 1993] and ion transport [reviewed in Matalon and O'Brodovich, 1999]. For studies of surfactant, cells are typically studied after culture for 20–24 h, at which time they are adherent to the substratum. Cells cultured for longer periods of time are routinely used for studies of ion transport; however, because of the changes in phenotypic expression that occur during culture, the interpretation of results obtained with these cells is not straightforward.

Using in vitro conditions similar to those that were developed to promote differentiation in primary cultures of mammary epithelial cells, several groups of investigators have devised tissue culture systems that preserve, to some extent, expression of the type II cell phenotype. Various factors, including extracellular matrix, cell shape, and soluble growth factors can prevent the loss of many type II cell differentiated characteristics. Cell culture conditions that have been reported to promote better preservation of expression of type II cell phenotypic characteristics include culturing cells on the laminin- and type IV-collagen rich EHS (Engelbreth-Holm-Swarm) matrix [Shannon et al., 1990], on floating collagen gels with irradiated feeder fibroblasts [Shannon et al., 1992], or on collagen gels with an apical surface exposed to air [Dobbs et al., 1997]. Adding soluble keratinocyte growth factor (KGF, FGF-7) to the culture medium [Sugahara et al., 1995, 1998] has similar effects. Interestingly, type II cells first cultured on TCP that have lost type II cell phenotypic characteristics, when transferred to a culture condition that promotes expression of the type II cell phenotype, begin to reexpress type II cell-specific markers [Borok et al., 1998a, 1998b; Danto et al., 1995; Dobbs et al., 1997]. Together, these results have generated the overall hypothesis that there is reversible transdifferentiation between the type I and the type II cell phenotypes, that is, that there is plasticity of the differentiated state. A corollary is that the expression of type I and type II cell phenotypic characteristics is inversely coregulated. This intriguing hypothesis is the subject of active investigation in a number of different laboratories.

The protocols outlined in Sections 2 and 3 of this chapter were current as of December 2000. We anticipate that improvements will continue to be made to the system of culturing type II cells to promote high levels of expression of type II cell phenotypic markers.

2. OVERVIEW OF CULTURE PROTOCOLS

The procedure for isolating type II cells that follows has evolved from progressive modifications of previously published methods [Dobbs et al., 1980, 1986]. In brief, lung cells are first dissociated by enzymatic digestion. Elastase is a key enzyme for this purpose, because under the correct conditions, it strips alveolar epithelial cells from the basal lamina without liberating many interstitial or endothelial cells. By virtue of this property and in contrast to other proteolytic enzymes such as trypsin or collagenase, elastase digestion provides an initial enrichment in type II cells. Once cells are dissociated, macrophages and lymphocytes are removed by differential adherence on IgG-coated plates. The resultant cells are ~85% type II cells by morphologic analysis. We usually obtain ~2×10^7 type II cells from one rat.

As the purity and viability of the isolated cells correlate inversely to the duration of the isolation procedure, it is recommended that, at first attempts, no more than one rat be used for each isolation. However, when the investigator becomes familiar with the technique, one person can easily isolate cells from two rats. If greater numbers of cells are required, two people working together, particularly during the surgical manipulations, will facilitate isolating cells from as many as six animals at one time.

3. PREPARATION OF REAGENTS AND MATERIALS

All containers up to the final culturing of type II cells should be disposable plastic containers that have not been coated for tissue culture (i.e., their surfaces should not be adhesive for living cells). It is best to avoid washing and reusing plastic ware because even traces of residual detergent may injure alveolar cells.

3.1. Preparation of Culture Dishes for "Panning" Cells

Coat polystyrene 100×15-mm sterile culture dishes with rat IgG as follows:

1. Filter a solution of rat IgG, 5 mg/10 ml 50 mM Tris buffer, pH 9.0 through a sterile 0.22-μm Millipore syringe filter under sterile conditions.
2. Add 5 ml of this solution to each dish, swirling to coat completely the bottom surface.
3. Remove the solution from the dishes after ~3 h.
4. Wash the plates 5× with PBSA (10–15 ml/dish) at room temperature, followed by two washes with DMEM. The DMEM used throughout this procedure is DMEM containing glucose, 1 g/l, and Na pyruvate, 2 mM.

3.2. Preparation of Buffers and Media

Buffers

All solutions are made with pyrogen-free, sterile, deionized water and are made fresh weekly.

Solution I

	g	mM
NaCl	8.0	136.9
$Na_2HPO_4 \cdot 7H_2O$	2.16	8.1
KH_2PO_4	0.2	1.5
KCl	0.2	2.7
EDTA-2Na	0.074	0.2
EGTA, free acid	0.076	0.2

Make up to 1 liter and adjust to pH 7.2.

Solution II

	g	mM
NaCl	8.0	136.9
$Na_2HPO_4 \cdot 7H_2O$	2.16	8.1
KH_2PO_4	0.2	1.5
KCl	0.2	2.7
$MgCl \cdot 6H_2O$	0.1	0.49
$CaCl_2 \cdot 2H_2O$	0.1	0.68

Make up to 1 liter and adjust to pH 7.2.

Solution III

RPMI 1640 medium buffered with HEPES, 25 mM, $NaHCO_3$, 2 g/l (24 mM), pH 7.4.

Solution IV (elastase)

Solution III containing lyophilized elastase, 1 mg/ml.

Prepare a volume of 40 ml for each rat and warm to 37°C.

Solution V (DNase)

Solution III containing DNase, 2 mg/ml.

Staining Solutions

Harris's hematoxylin. Use undiluted.
Lithium carbonate. Saturated solution.

Culture Media

For culture on tissue culture plastic: DMEM medium containing fetal bovine serum, 10%; gentamicin, 50 μg/ml; glutamine, 2 mM; penicillin G, 100 U/ml.

For culture on matrix to preserve differentiated characteristics: DMEM medium containing charcoal-stripped rat serum (CSRS), 1%, and gentamicin sulfate, 10 μg/ml; in addition, keratinocyte growth factor, 10 ng/ml, may be added (see below for details).

Charcoal-stripped rat serum (CSRS): Add 5 ml of rat serum (RS) to 0.5 g of activated charcoal and rotate end-over-end for 2 h at 4°C. Centrifuge at 3000 g for 20 min and filter through a 0.2-μm sterile filter.

4. ISOLATION OF TYPE II CELLS

4.1. Cell Dissociation and Purification

It is essential to use specific-pathogen-free rats. Rats that are not specific-pathogen-free are prone to murine pneumonia, which causes an increase in the number of pulmonary macrophages, which, in turn, makes it more difficult to obtain preparations of type II cells that are relatively pure. In addition, certain murine viral infections may adversely affect type II cell functions [Dobbs, unpublished observations]. We use male Sprague-Dawley specific-pathogen-free rats.

This procedure will be subject to animal experiment licensing in many countries. Please check with your animal usage committee, animal facility staff, or other appropriate authority.

Protocol 9.1. Isolation of Rat Lung Type II Alveolar Epithelial Cells

Reagents and Materials

Sterile

❏ Heparin solution, 1000 U/ml, containing pentobarbital, 50 mg/ml

❏ Syringe, 5 ml, and needle, 23 gauge, for injecting anesthetic

❏ Scissors, 6½ in., 4 in., Mueller scissors

❏ Luer stub adaptor, intramedic, 15 gauge (for tracheal cannulation)

- ❏ Plastic catheter, Angiocath, 20 gauge, connected to a perfusion bottle containing Solution I, 160 ml, elevated and clamped at a height of 20 cm
- ❏ Solution I at 37°C
- ❏ Solution II at 37°C
- ❏ Solution III at 37°C
- ❏ Solution IV (the elastase solution) at 37°C
- ❏ Beaker of sterile saline at 37°C
- ❏ Small plastic centrifuge tube containing Solution V (the DNase solution) and 10 ml FBS at room temperature
- ❏ Centrifuge tubes, "modified polystyrene" (Corning no. 25339-50)
- ❏ Erlenmeyer flask, 250 ml, plastic
- ❏ Cotton gauze, 1, 2, and 4 ply, 4 × 4 square. A ~1 internal diameter plastic tube holding ~10–15 ml of liquid (or a 20-ml plastic syringe barrel cut at ~15 ml mark will function well) is used as a support. A rubber band is used to secure tightly drawn mesh over the end of the tube.
- ❏ Nylon mesh, 150, 15, and 7 μm, is secured on supports as described previously for cotton gauze. In practice, it has not been found necessary to sterilize the nylon mesh, but, if problems with contamination are encountered, they may be sterilized with 70% EtOH and then rinsed in PBSA.

Nonsterile

- ❏ Sprague-Dawley rat, 180–200 g
- ❏ Water bath at 37°C
- ❏ Flask shaker

Protocol

(a) Anesthetize the rat with an i.p. injection of 0.3–0.5 ml heparin containing pentobarbital 200 mg/kg.

After the rat is well anesthetized, it is important to perform the following surgical procedures rapidly. Both adequate perfusion of the lungs and good cell viability are dependent on the rapidity with which the surgical maneuvers are performed. Ideally, the entire surgical procedure, from the time of the abdominal incision to removal of the perfused lungs, should ideally take no more than 4 min.

(b) Make an abdominal incision, cut the descending aorta, and make a small incision in the diaphragm to deflate the lungs.

(c)   Incise the neck, remove submandibular tissue and the thyroid gland, pass a suture under the trachea, and cannulate the trachea with a 15-gauge intramedic Luer stub adaptor, securing it with the suture.

(d)   Incise the chest wall along the entire length of the sternum and the anterior portions of the diaphragm, so that the chest is open.

(e)   Pull the rib cage laterally and horizontally to expose the heart and the lungs. The sharp cut edges of the ribs should not be close to the lungs, once they are inflated in subsequent steps.

(f)   Identify the pulmonary artery, pass a suture underneath it, nick the inferior portion of the right ventricle and cannulate the pulmonary artery with a 20-gauge plastic catheter (occluding the puncture site) connected to a perfusion bottle containing Solution 1 at 20 cm H_2O pressure. The perfusion buffer and length of tubing should be free of any bubbles before the perfusion is started (bubbles will lodge in the pulmonary capillary bed, obstructing perfusion).

(g)   Nick the left atrium to allow the perfusion fluid to exit the lungs.

(h)   During perfusion, inflate the lungs with air via the tracheal cannula to total lung capacity (8–10 ml) several times to perfuse the lungs completely and remove blood. If the heart is not spontaneously beating during the perfusion, it will be much more difficult to clear the lungs entirely of blood.

(i)   Carefully remove the lungs, trachea (still attached to the tracheal catheter), and heart from the chest cavity; trim off and discard the cardiac tissue.

(j)   Using the tracheal catheter to instill liquid, sequentially lavage the lungs to total lung capacity 10 times with Solution 1 at 37°C to remove macrophages.

(k)   Lavage once with Solution III and then lavage once with Solution IV (the elastase solution) at 37°C. Be careful not to over-inflate the lungs, which will cause pleural leaks.

(l)   Inflate the lungs to total lung capacity with Solution IV while the lungs are suspended in a beaker of saline in a 37°C water bath and then suspend the enzyme-filled lungs so that they float in the warm saline while additional enzyme is gradually instilled. We use a 3-ml plastic syringe taped to the side of the beaker and gradually add the remaining Solution IV by gravity over a 15-min period, for a total enzymatic digestion period of 20 min.

(m) Dissect the lung parenchyma away from the major airways (do not spend the time to do this meticulously) and add the lung pieces to a small plastic centrifuge tube containing Solution V (the DNase solution) and 10 ml of FBS.

(n) Quickly mince the lung pieces with a very sharp scissors to a final size of ~ 2 mm^3 (~ 150–200 scissor strokes, duration <1 min).

(o) Add additional Solution II to bring the final liquid volume to 20 ml (below the floating lung minced tissue) and transfer the lung minces and liquid to a 250-ml plastic Erlenmeyer flask.

(p) Shake the flask vigorously side-to-side at 130 cycles/min for 2 min. The goal of this step is to apply shear force to the lung minces, freeing the epithelial cells; the liquid in the flask should move in a back-and-forth fashion rather than swirling. If liquid starts to swirl in the flask, stop shaking until the swirling ceases.

(q) Filter the lung minces sequentially through filters prewetted with Solution II:
   i) cotton gauze, 1 ply
   ii) cotton gauze, 2 ply
   iii) cotton gauze, 4 ply
   iv) nylon mesh, 150 μm
   v) nylon mesh, 15 μm
   vi) nylon mesh, 7 μm.
   Let the filtering occur by gravity, using additional filters as needed when flow decreases because of filter clogging. We routinely use 2–4 separate filters of each size to prevent filter clogging. The filtering steps should take no more than 5 min.

(r) Remove 1 ml of the cell suspension in the final filtrate for a cell count, viability, and differential cell count. Refer to this step of the cell isolation as **STEP A**.

(s) Centrifuge the cell suspension at 150 g for 10 min.

All steps and procedures from this point are performed with sterile technique.

(t) Aspirate the supernatant liquid and resuspend the cells in 20 ml of DMEM at 37°C. Plate $\sim 5 \times 10^6$ cells in ~ 4 ml of medium on each of the rinsed, IgG-coated dishes.

(u) The next step requires careful observation and analysis by each individual who will be isolating cells. The goal of this step is to allow macrophages and lymphocytes to adhere to the IgG-coated plates but to remove the cell suspension before type II cells begin to adhere. Macrophages and lymphocytes will adhere before type II cells. A typical incubation time necessary to achieve this separation varies between 30 and 60 min at 37°C in an incubator containing 10% CO_2 in air at 100% humidity; the time will vary depending on the lot of rat IgG and the overall health of the cells. (Less healthy cells will take longer to adhere.)

(v) After the plates have incubated for 30 min, inspect them with an inverted microscope every 5–10 min. Macrophages can be easily recognized by their size ($\sim 2\times$ the cell diameter of type II cells) and because they rapidly spread and flatten on the IgG-coated surface. When smaller round cells start to adhere to the surface, the adherence step should be stopped. Determining the length of time for the adherence step requires the development of skills to distinguish macrophages and type II cells. By comparing the visual images with subsequent cytocentrifuge preparations, the investigator's ability to recognize optimal times of adherence will improve. The images shown in Fig. 9.2 can be used to recognize macrophages in various stages of adherence and to distinguish them from nonadherent type II cells.

(w) Remove the nonadherent cells with a sterile 10-ml pipette and place in a 50-ml sterile modified clear polystyrene centrifuge tube.

(x) Wash each plate with 5 ml of DMEM, tilting the plate to remove nonadherent cells and add these cells to the tube.

(y) Centrifuge the cells for 10 min at 150 g, aspirate the supernatant liquid, and resuspend pellet in 5 ml of culture media.

(z) Remove an aliquot for determination of cell number, viability, and differential cell counts. This step in the cell isolation procedure is referred to as **STEP B**.

4.2. Criteria for Identification of Cells

The development of the modified Papanicolaou stain by Kikkawa and co-workers was instrumental in modifying methods of isolating type II cells. Although a protocol for the stain has been described elsewhere [Dobbs, 1990; Kikkawa and Yoneda, 1974], we include the experimental details in this chapter. Images obtained from cells at both Steps A and B are shown in Fig. 9.3 and Plate 1. The protocol for the stain is as follows:

Protocol 9.2. Identification of Isolated Rat Type II Cells by Papanicolaou Staining

Reagents and Materials

Nonsterile

☐ Harris hematoxylin, filtered by gravity through Whatman #1 filter paper

☐ Lithium carbonate solution: made fresh before use by adding 2 ml of saturated solution of lithium carbonate to 158 ml of distilled water

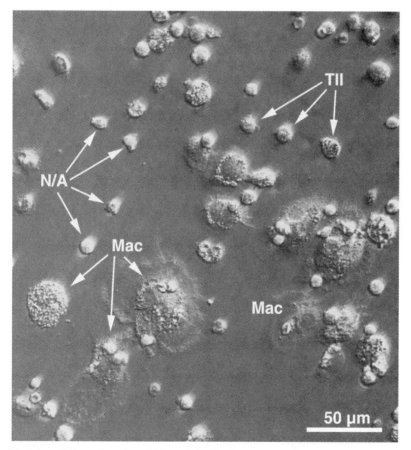

Fig 9.2. Cells undergoing differential adherence on IgG-coated plastic dishes. Hoffman modulation contrast visualization of cells undergoing adherence to IgG-coated dishes. Some examples of the different cell types are labeled. Macrophages (Mac) are attenuated and spreading on the surface. Type II cells (TII) are starting to adhere. Nonadherent cells (N/A) can be easily removed.

- ❏ Distilled water
- ❏ Dehydration and clearing reagents:
  - i) 50%, 80%, 95%, 100% ethanol
  - ii) xylene: ethanol, 1:1
  - iii) xylene
- ❏ Mountant: Permount
- ❏ Coverslips
- ❏ Cytocentrifuge

Fig 9.3. Modified Papanicolaou stain of cells at Step A (a) and Step B (b). Refractile bluish-purple inclusions are lamellar bodies, identifying type II cells. An asterisk (*) indicates representative type II cells. Macrophages (M) are larger than type II cells; these may have some smaller inclusions, which are more typically reddish-orange in appearance than blue/purple. Small round cells with scant cytoplasm are lymphocytes (L). Some cells cannot be identified (Unknown, UNK). Not all identifiable cells have been labeled. At Step A, ~40–50% of the cells are type II cells. At Step B, ~80–85% of the cells are type II cells.

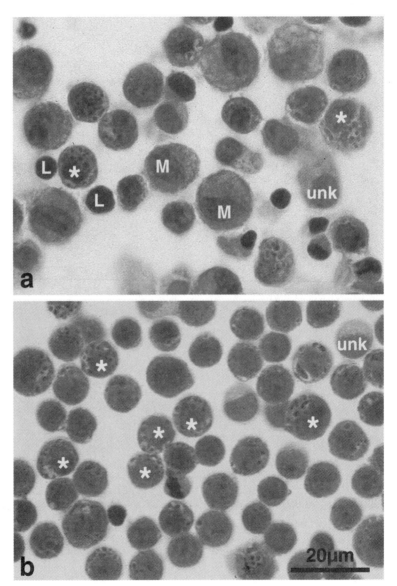

Protocol

(a) Cytocentrifuge cells (density 2×10^5 cells/ml) at 5–10 g for 5 min.

(b) Let slides dry for at least 12 h.

(c) Incubate slides in hematoxylin solution for 3–4 min. The length of the staining time correlates directly with the darkness of the blue color.

(d) Rinse 2–3× in distilled water.

(e) Incubate for 2 min in lithium carbonate solution.

(f) Rinse once

(g) Dehydrate by successive incubations:
   i)   50% ethanol for 1.5 min
   ii) 80% ethanol for 15 s
   iii) 95% ethanol for 15 s
   iv) 100% ethanol for 30 s
   v)   xylene:ethanol 1:1 for 30 s
   vi) xylene for 1 min

(h) Mount in Permount and coverslip.

(i) Inspect cells at 630–1000× magnification; count at least 400 cells to obtain % of type II cells.

The bluish-purple inclusions are lamellar bodies, which identify type II cells.

4.3. Troubleshooting Problems in Cell Isolation

We have found that it is essential to measure cell yields, purities, and viabilities at two steps in the isolation procedure. This should be performed in each and every cell isolation. The information to be learned by this analysis is as follows:

4.3.1. At STEP A (After Filtering Cell Suspension)

Typical ranges of yield, viability, and purity at this point should be: $4–8 \times 10^7$ cells/rat, >99% viability, and 40–50% type II cells. There should be no more than 10–15% macrophages at this step. Fewer cells, lower viabilities, and a lower-than-expected percentage of type II cells suggest problems with enzymatic digestion, mincing, shaking, or filtering. Fewer cells may be caused by poor lots of elastase or insufficient mincing and shaking. Low viabilities are often caused by either prolonged duration of surgery, over-mincing the lung tissue, or the use of dull scissors that shear tissue and cells. Low percentages of type II cells suggest problems with the elastase digestion, such as a poor lot of enzyme, inadequate warming of solutions before use, or inadequate filling of the lungs with the enzyme solution. An abnormally high number of macrophages suggests that the animals are infected; murine pulmonary infections are common and will result in lower yields, purities, and viabilities of type II cells.

4.3.2. At STEP B (After Adherence)

At this step, there should be $1.5–2.5 \times 10^7$ cells, >98% viability, and 80–92% type II cells. In comparison with the numbers in Step A, there should be an approximate doubling in the percentage of type II cells and a loss of an appropriate number of non-type II cells. If cell yield falls more than one would expect from comparing numbers and cell purities to Step A, the differential adherence step was carried out for too long a period of time and type II cells were lost. If cell purity was in the appropriate range at Step A but has not increased at Step B, then adherence should have been for a longer period of time. If viabilities are low, cell damage has occurred during the adherence. If this occurs, check the actual speed of the centrifuge, be careful to avoid shear forces when pipetting cells (use large-bore rather than small-bore pipettes), check media composition, measure the pH of the media in the incubator, and make sure that all containers and solutions are free of any traces of detergent.

5. CULTURE OF TYPE II CELLS

As reviewed in the Introduction, when type II cells are cultured on tissue culture plastic, they gradually lose the characteristics that are associated with type II cells in vivo. Various different investigators have developed conditions that promote, to a greater or lesser extent, these differentiated characteristics. When assessing how successful each set of conditions is in achieving this goal, it is essential to examine the full range of known differentially expressed morphologic, biochemical, and molecular markers and to compare quantitative expression of each marker to that of freshly isolated type II cells. Ideally, this type of assessment should include the following:

(i)   Analysis of the cells by transmission electron microscopy. Are the cells flattened or cuboid; do they contain typical lamellar bodies or merely autophagic vacuoles? An electron micrograph of a rat type II cell is shown in Fig. 9.1.

(ii) What are the levels of surfactant proteins (A, B, C, and D) expressed by the cells in comparison with freshly-isolated type II cells? Techniques of Western blotting [Hawgood et al., 1987; White et al., 1985] or ELISA [Greene et al., 1999] have been used to quantitate surfactant proteins.

(iii)   What are the levels of surfactant protein mRNAs (A, B, C, and D) in comparison with freshly isolated type II cells? Techniques of Northern blotting [Dobbs et al., 1997; Shannon et al., 1992] and ribonuclease protection [Paugam-Burtz et al., 2000; Shannon et al., 2001] have been used for quantification.

(iv)   Do cells synthesize and secrete appropriate phospholipids (high percentages of dipalmitoyl phosphatidylcholine and phosphatidylglycerol)? Fractionation of lipid classes has been performed by two-dimensional thin layer chromatography [Dobbs et al., 1985; Shannon et al., 1987].

(v)   Does material secreted by cultured cells have properties of surface activity similar to those of purified pulmonary surfactant? Methods used to measure surface tension have included the classical Wilhelmy balance [Goerke et al., 1970] and, more recently, bubble surfactometers [Schoel et al., 1994; Schürch et al., 1989], which have the advantage of using very small amounts of material.

Unfortunately, most published descriptions of culture conditions do not contain data addressing each of these criteria.

5.1. Culture on Tissue Culture Plastic

Type II cells have been cultured conventionally on tissue culture plastic in media containing fetal bovine serum. The plating density of cells will vary depending on the purpose of the experiment. For studies of surfactant secretion, cells are plated at low densities (~2.5–5×10^4 cells/cm^2) and for studies of ion transport, at higher densities ($\sim5 \times 10^5$ cells/cm^2).

5.2. Culture Conditions That Promote Expression of Differentiated Type II Cell Phenotype

Several of the methods referred to in the Introduction can be used to culture type II cells so that they maintain, at least in part, characteristics of the type II cell phenotype. These methods are continually undergoing modification and improvement, and we anticipate that this process will continue in the future.

We use modifications of the methods developed by Shannon and Mason [Shannon et al., 2001], which we believe currently provide the best overall conditions for promoting expression of proteins and lipids characteristic of the type II cell phenotype. The scientific foundations of this approach are in the work of Spooner [Spooner and Wessells, 1970] and Wessells [Wessells, 1970], who showed that mesenchyme has the capability of directing pulmonary epithelial cell determination in embryonic tissue. Similar paradigms apply to type II cells isolated from adult animals and maintained in culture [Dobbs et al., 1997; Shannon et al., 2001]. In the culture system described below, type II cells are cocultured with, but kept physically apart from, fibroblasts (see Protocol 9.3). Type II cells and fibroblasts are cultured on different extracellular matrices. At least two different methods can be used for coculture. Shannon [Shannon et al., 2001] embedded the fibroblasts in a gel of collagen (see Chapter 2) immobilized on a Nuclepore (polycarbonate, now Corning) filter "rafts" floating above cultures of type II cells grown on EHS matrix. We have found it somewhat easier to culture fibroblasts on the bottom of culture wells in a six-well culture dish. Type II cells are seeded on EHS matrix-coated Transwells (see also Chapter 4, Protocol 4.10), which are suspended in the media of the wells containing the fibroblasts.

We have prepared the fibroblasts by two separate methods; both yield similar results. In the first method, fibroblasts are cultured on a film of collagen adsorbed onto the surface of the well of the six-well dish; in the second method, fibroblasts are embedded in a collagen gel and this is polymerized on the bottom of the well.

Protocol 9.3. Coculture of Fibroblasts with Type II Cells

Reagents and Materials

Sterile

- ❏ Collagen, type I rat, tail, 100 µg/ml 50 mM acetic acid, pH 3.0
- ❏ Human lung fibroblasts (HLF cells) grown in DMEM with 10% FBS
- ❏ NaOH, 1 N
- ❏ UPW
- ❏ MEM, 10×, with Earle's salts and glutamine but without NaHCO₃
- ❏ DMEM, 1×, containing 1% CSRS and gentamicin sulfate, 10 µg/ml
- ❏ CSRS: charcoal-stripped rat serum
- ❏ EHS matrix (Matrigel; see also Chapter 11, Protocol 11.5)
- ❏ Centrifuge tube, 10–15 ml

❑ Multiwell plate, 6-well
❑ Transwell inserts, 24-mm diameter with a 0.4-μm pore size

Nonsterile

❑ Ice bath

Protocol

Method A: Culture of Fibroblasts on Preformed Adsorbed Collagen

(a) Incubate the solution of type I collagen on the bottom of the cluster wells for 3 h at 4°C.

(b) Plate HLF cells 0.25–0.5 × 10^6 cells/ml from active log-phase growth on the adsorbed collagen.

(c) After 24 h change the medium to CSRS and add the inserts containing type II cells (see below).

Method B: Culture of Fibroblasts Embedded within Gel

(a) Chill sterile solutions of 1 N NaOH, distilled water, and 10× DMEM to 4°C on ice

(b) Place a sterile tube submersed in the ice bath and add sequentially:
   i) collagen, 8 ml
   ii) 10× MEM, 1 ml
   iii) 1 N NaOH, 200 μl
   iv) UPW, 800 μl

(c) Adjust pH to pH 7.2 with additional NaOH

(d) Add approximately 5–10 × 10^6 HLF in 1 ml of 1× DMEM to the collagen mixture and mix thoroughly.

(e) Add 1 ml of this cell-containing gel slurry to the bottom of each well of a 6-well cluster well plate.

(f) Place the plate in a 10% CO_2 in air incubator at 37°C for at least 3 h to allow polymerization before adding medium.

Addition of Type II Cells

(a) Dilute EHS matrix 1:1 with 1× DMEM

(b) Add 0.5 ml of this solution to each of several Transwell inserts

(c) Allow to polymerize for 3–4 h at 37°C.

(d) Seed type II cells on the inserts coated with polymerized matrix.
   i) Suspend type II cells at a density of 1–1.5 × 10^6 cells/ml of DMEM containing 1% CSRS and 10 μg of gentamicin/ml.
   ii) Dispense 1 ml into each Transwell.

In general, when epithelial cells are cultured on EHS matrix, the cells reassociate after isolation and form spherules; this is also true for type II cells. The cells in the spherules are polarized, with apical surfaces pointed inward. The type II cells form lamellar bodies and secrete surfactant proteins and lipids into the internal lumina of the spherule [Shannon et al., 2001]. Shannon et al [Shannon et al., 2001] reported that, after 72 h in culture, the synthesis of surfactant proteins, their respective mRNAs, and appropriate surfactant lipids are all preserved, in comparison with type II cells cultured without fibroblasts, where they are not. These investigators also reported that keratinocyte growth factor (KGF, FGF-7; 10 ng/ml), which is produced by fibroblasts, mimicked the effects of coculture with fibroblasts on surfactant protein mRNA expression. We have observed similar results and also have noted continued improvements in expression of markers for the type II cell phenotype by culture for periods of time longer than 4 days [Gonzalez and Dobbs, unpublished observations).

5.3. Summary and Future Directions

Substantial progress has been made in developing methods of culturing type II cells that preserve expression of hallmark differentiated phenotypic characteristics; it is likely that additional progress will be made in the coming years. Questions that will be addressed include the following. Are both fibroblasts and KGF necessary to promote full expression of the type II cell phenotype? Can the type II cell phenotype be maintained by cells in monolayer culture as well as in the three-dimensional spherules? What is the optimal duration of culture? Does an apical surface exposed to air improve expression of type II cell phenotypic characteristics?

REFERENCES

Augustin-Voss HG, Schoon HA, Stockhofe N, Ueberschar S (1989): Isolation of bovine type II pneumocytes in high yield and purity. Lung 167: 1–10.

Borok Z, Danto SI, Lubman RL, Cao Y, Williams MC, Crandall ED (1998a): Modulation of t1α expression with alveolar epithelial cell phenotype in vitro. Am J Physiol 275: L155–L164.

Borok Z, Lubman RL, Danto SI, Zhang XL, Zabski SM, King LS, Lee DM, Agre P, Crandall ED (1998b): Keratinocyte growth factor modulates alveolar epithelial cell phenotype in vitro: expression of aquaporin 5. Am J Resp Cell Molec Biol 18: 554–561.

Campbell L, Hollins AJ, Al-Eid A, Newman GR, von Ruhland C, Gumbleton M (1999): Caveolin-1 expression and caveolae biogenesis during cell transdifferentiation in lung alveolar epithelial primary cultures. Biochem Biophys Res Commun 262: 744–751.

Corti M, Brody AR, and Harrison JH (1996): Isolation and primary culture of murine alveolar type II cells. Am J Respir Cell Mol Biol 14: 309–315.

Danto SI, Shannon JM, Borok Z, Zabski SM, Crandall ED (1995): Reversible transdifferentiation of alveolar epithelial cells. Am J Respir Cell Mol Biol 12: 497–502.

Diglio CA, Kikkawa Y (1977): The type II epithelial cells of the lung. IV. Adaptation and behavior of isolated type II cells in culture. Lab Invest 37: 622–631.

Dobbs LG (1990): Isolation and culture of alveolar type II cells. Am J Physiol 258: L134–L147.

Dobbs LG, Geppert EF, Williams MC, Greenleaf RD, Mason RJ (1980): Metabolic properties and ultrastructure of alveolar type II cells isolated with elastase. Biochim Biophys Acta 618: 510–523.

Dobbs LG, Gonzalez R, Williams MC (1986): An improved method for isolating type II cells in high yield and purity. Am Rev Resp Dis 134: 141–145.

Dobbs LG, Mason RJ (1978): Stimulation of secretion of disaturated phosphatidylcholine from isolated alveolar type II cells by 12-O-tetradecanoyl-13-phorbol acetate. Am Rev Respir Dis 118: 705–733.

Dobbs LG, Mason RJ (1979): Pulmonary alveolar type II cells isolated from rats. Release of phosphatidylcholine in response to beta-adrenergic stimulation. J Clin Invest 63: 378–387.

Dobbs LG, Pian M, Dumars S, Maglio M, Allen L (1997): Maintenance of the differentiated type II cell phenotype by culture with an apical air surface. Am J Physiol 273: L347–L354.

Dobbs LG, Williams MC, Brandt AE (1985): Changes in biochemical characteristics and pattern of lectin binding of alveolar type II cells with time in culture. Biochim Biophys Acta 846: 155–166.

Dobbs LG, Williams MC, Gonzalez R (1988): Monoclonal antibodies specific to apical surfaces of rat alveolar type I cells bind to surfaces of cultured, but not freshly isolated, type II cells. Biochim Biophys Acta 970: 146–156.

Douglas WH, Kaighn ME (1974): Clonal isolation of differentiated rat lung cells. In Vitro 10: 230–237.

Evans MJ, Cabral LJ, Stephens RJ, Freeman G (1975): Transformation of alveolar type 2 cells to type 1 cells following exposure to NO_2. Exp Mol Pathol 22: 142–150.

Folkesson HG, Matthay MA, Hasegawa H, Kheradmand F, Verkman AS (1994): Transcellular water transport in lung alveolar epithelium through mercurial-sensitive water channels. Proc Natl Acad Sci USA 91: 4970–4974.

Gazdar A, Linnoila RI, Oie HK, Mulshine JL, Clark JC, Whitsett JA (1990): Peripheral airway cell differentiation in human lung cancer cell lines. Cancer Res 50: 5481–5487.

Giard DJ, Aaronson SA, Todaro GJ, Arnstein P, Kersey JH, Dosik H, Parks WP (1973): In vitro cultivation of human tumors: Establishment of cell lines derived from a series of solid tumors. J Natl Cancer Inst 51: 1417–1423.

Goerke J, Harper H, Borowitz M (1970): In Blank M (ed): "Surface Chemistry of Biological Systems." New York: Plenum.

Goodman BE, Crandall ED (1982): Dome formation in primary cultured monolayers of alveolar epithelial cells. Am J Physiol 243: C96–C100.

Greene KE, Ye S, Mason RJ, Parsons PE (1999): Serum surfactant protein-A levels predict development of ARDS in at-risk patients. Chest 116: 90S–91S.

Hawgood S, Benson BJ, Schilling J, Damm D, Clements JA, White RT (1987): Nucleotide and amino acid sequences of pulmonary surfactant protein SP 18 and evidence for cooperation between SP 18 and SP 28–36 in surfactant lipid adsorption. Proc Natl Acad Sci USA 84: 66–70.

Kikkawa Y, Yoneda K (1974): The type II epithelial cell of the lung. I. Method of isolation. Lab Invest 30: 76–84.

Kikkawa Y, Yoneda K, Smith F, Packard B, Suzuki K (1975): The type II epithelial cells of the lung. II. Chemical composition and phospholipid synthesis. Lab Invest 32: 295–302.

Korst RJ, Bewig B, Crystal RG (1995): In vitro and in vivo transfer and expression of human surfactant SP-A- and SP-B-associated protein cDNAs mediated by replication-deficient, recombinant adenoviral vectors. Hum Gene Ther 6: 277–287.

Leslie CC, McCormick-Shannon K, Mason RJ, and Shannon JM (1993): Proliferation of rat alveolar epithelial cells in low density primary culture. Am J Respir Cell Mol Biol 9: 64–72.

Li J, Gao E, and Mendelson CR (1998): Cyclic AMP-responsive expression of the surfactant protein-A gene is mediated by increased DNA binding and transcriptional activity of thyroid transcription factor-1. J Biol Chem 273: 4592–4600.

Lieber M, Smith B, Szakal A, Nelson-Rees W, and Todaro G (1976): A continuous tumor-cell line from a human lung carcinoma with properties of type II alveolar epithelial cells. Int J Cancer 17: 62–70.

Mager E, Vanderbilt J, Dobbs L (1999): Differential gene expression by rat alveolar type I and type II cells determined by differential display-PCR. Am J Resp Crit Care Med 159: A175.

Mason RJ, Dobbs LG (1980): Synthesis of phosphatidylcholine and phosphatidylglycerol by alveolar type II cells in primary culture J Biol Chem 255: 5101–5107.

Mason RJ, Leslie CC, McCormick-Shannon K, Deterding RR, Nakamura T, Rubin JS, and Shannon JM (1994): Hepatocyte growth factor is a growth factor for rat alveolar type II cells. Am J Respir Cell Mol Biol 11: 561–567.

Mason RJ, Williams MC (1980): Phospholipid composition and ultrastructure of A549 cells and other cultured pulmonary epithelial cells of presumed type II cell origin. Biochim Biophys Acta 617: 36–50.

Mason RJ, Williams MC, Widdicombe JH, Sanders MJ, Misfeld DS, and Berry LCJ (1982): Transepithelial transport by pulmonary alveolar type II cells in primary culture. Proc Natl Acad Sci USA 79: 6033–6037.

Matalon S, O'Brodovich H (1999): Sodium channels in alveolar epithelial cells: molecular characterization, biophysical properties, and physiological significance. Annu Rev Physiol 61: 627–661.

Paine R, Rolfe MW, Standiford TJ, Burdick MD, Rollins BJ, Strieter RM (1993): MCP-1 expression by rat type II alveolar epithelial cells in primary culture. J Immunol 150: 4561–4570.

Paugam-Burtz C, Molliex S, Lardeux B, Rolland C, Aubier M, Desmonts JM, Crestani B (2000): Differential effects of halothane and thiopental on surfactant protein C messenger RNA in vivo and in vitro in rats. Anesthesiology 93: 805–810.

Pfleger RC (1977): Type II epithelial cells from the lung of Syrian hamsters: isolation and metabolism. Exp Mol Pathol 27: 152–166.

Robinson PC, Voelker DR, Mason RJ (1984): Isolation and culture of human alveolar type II epithelial cells. Am Rev Respir Dis 130: 1156–1160.

Rooney SA, Young SL, Mendelson CR (1994): Molecular and cellular processing of lung surfactant. FASEB J 8: 957–967.

Schneeberger EE (1978): Structural basis for some permeability properties of the air-blood barrier. Fed Proc 37: 2471–2478.

Schoel WM, Schürch S, Goerke J (1994): The captive bubble method for the evaluation of pulmonary surfactant: surface tension, area, and volume calculations. Biochim Biophys Acta 1200: 281–290.

Schürch S, Bachofen H, Goerke J, Possmayer F (1989): A captive bubble method reproduces the in situ behavior of lung surfactant monolayers. J Appl Physiol 67: 2389–2396.

Shannon JM, Emrie PA, Fisher JH, Kuroki Y, Jennings SD, Mason RJ (1990): Effect of a reconstituted basement membrane on expression of surfactant apoproteins in cultured adult rat alveolar type II cells. Am J Respir Cell Mol Biol 2: 183–192.

Shannon JM, Jennings SD, Nielsen LD (1992): Modulation of alveolar type II cell differentiated function in vitro. Am J Physiol 262: L427–L436.

Shannon JM, Mason RJ, Jennings SD (1987): Functional differentiation of alveolar type II epithelial cells in vitro: Effects of cell shape, cell-matrix interactions and cell-cell interactions. Biochim Biophys Acta 931: 143–156.

Shannon JM, Pan T, Nielsen LD, Edeen KE, Mason RJ (2001): Lung fibroblasts improve differentiation of rat alveolar type II cells in primary culture. Am J Respir Cell Mol Biol, 24: 235–44.

Sikpi MO, Nair CR, Johns AE, Das SK (1986): Metabolic and ultrastructural characterization of guinea pig alveolar type II cells isolated by centrifugal elutriation. Biochim Biophys Acta 877: 20–30.

Spooner BS, Wessells NK (1970): Mammalian lung development: Interactions in primordium formation and bronchial morphogenesis. J Exp Zool 175: 445–454.

Stone KC, Mercer RR, Gehr P, Stockstill B, and Crapo JD (1992): Allometric relationships of cell numbers and size in the mammalian lung. Am J Respir Cell Mol Biol 6: 235–243.

Sugahara K Mason RJ, Shannon JM (1998): Effects of soluble factors and extracellular matrix on DNA synthesis and surfactant gene expression in primary cultures of rat alveolar type II cells. Cell Tissue Res 291: 295–303.

Sugahara K, Rubin JS, Mason RJ, Aronsen EL, Shannon JM (1995): Keratinocyte growth factor increases mRNAs for SP-A and SP-B in adult rat alveolar type II cells in culture. Am J Physiol 269: L344–L350.

Wessells NK (1970): Mammalian lung development: Interactions in formation and morphogenesis of tracheal buds. J Exp Zool 175: 455–466.

White RT, Damm D, Miller J, Spratt K, Schilling J, Hawgood S, Benson B, and Cordell B (1985): Isolation and characterization of the human pulmonary surfactant apoprotein gene. Nature 317: 361–363.

Wikenheiser KA, Vorbroker DK, Rice WR, Clark JC, Bachurski CJ, Oie HK, Whitsett JA (1993): Production of immortalized distal respiratory cell lines from surfactant protein C/simian virus 40 large tumor antigen transgenic mice. Proc Natl Acad Sci USA 90: 11029–11033.

Wright JR, Dobbs LG (1991): Regulation of pulmonary surfactant secretion and clearance. Annu Rev Physiol 53: 395–414.

Wright JR, Youmans DC (1993): Pulmonary surfactant protein A stimulates chemotaxis of alveolar macrophage. Am J Physiol 264: L338–L344.

APPENDIX: SOURCES OF MATERIALS

Material	Catalog No.	Supplier
Activated charcoal	C9157	Sigma
Angiocath (plastic catheter) 20 gauge	2816	Becton Dickinson
Centrifuge tubes	15 ml: 540055 50 ml: 2533950	Corning
Centrifuge tubes, modified	25339-50	Corning
Collagen, type I, rat tail	40236	Becton Dickinson
Cotton gauze	4 × 4 size: 2733	Kendall
Culture dishes, polystyrene, 100 × 15 mm sterile	08-757-13	Fisher
Cytocentrifuge		Bayer (Miles), IEC, Shandon
DMEM "low glucose"	11885	GIBCO
DNase: Deoxyribonuclease I	D-5025	Sigma
EHS matrix (Matrigel)	40234	Becton Dickinson
Elastase	100 909	Roche (Boehringer Mannheim)
Fetal bovine serum (FBS)	16000-044	GIBCO
Gentamicin sulfate	G1397	Sigma
Glutamine, 200 mM	15032	GIBCO
Harris hematoxylin	SH26-5000	Fisher
Heparin	2440-42	Elkins-Sinn
HEPES, 1 M solution	15630	GIBCO
HLF cells	AG02262	Coriell Institute for Medical Research
IgG, rat	I-4131	Sigma
KGF, human recombinant	251-KG-050	R&D
Lithium carbonate	L4283	Sigma
Luer stub adaptor, intramedic, 15 gauge, Clay Adams	427560	Becton Dickinson
MEM, 10×	11435-039	GIBCO
Nylon mesh 150 μm 15 μm 7 μm	03-150/38 03-15/10 03-7/2	Tekto

Appendix continues

Material	Catalog No.	Supplier
PBSA (Ca^{2+}- and Mg^{2+}-free PBS)	14190	GIBCO
Penicillin G	P3414	Sigma
Pentobarbital	0074-3778-04	Abbott
Permount mounting medium	SP 15-1000	Fisher
Rat serum	36126-1	Pel-Freeze, Rogers, AK
RPMI 1640 medium	52400	GIBCO
Scissors	Mueller	ROBOZ Surgical Instruments
Sprague-Dawley specific-pathogen-free rats		Charles River
Transwell inserts	3450	Corning

10

Isolation and Culture of Intestinal Epithelial Cells

Catherine Booth[1] and Julie A. O'Shea

EpiStem Ltd., Incubator Building, Grafton St., Manchester, M13 9XX, UK.
[1]Corresponding Author; email: *Cbooth@epistem.co.uk*

1. INTRODUCTION

The adult intestinal epithelium lines the small and large bowel, covering both luminal protrusions (villi) and invaginations (crypts) (Fig. 10.1). The epithelium is simple, being a monolayer, although each cell is polarized, with a basal and apical surface (the latter possessing many membrane protrusions or microvilli). There is also a polarity associated with the maturation of each cell along the crypt-villus axis. The cells on the small intestinal villi or in the upper positions of colonic crypt are the most mature or differentiated and cannot proliferate. These differentiated cells are continuously lost into the lumen from either the top of the villi (small intestine) or the top of the crypt (large intestine, which does not possess villi), that is, the apical pole of the tissue. Massive levels of proliferation in the mid-crypt generate replacements for these shed cells, with the cells ultimately responsible for cellular repopulation, the stem cells, located toward the base of the small intestinal crypt or at the very base of a colonic crypt. The maturation gradient has the most immature cells, that is, those with the greatest proliferative potential, located at the lower positions within the crypt. It is these immature cells that are essential for the long-term culture of this tissue. (In some species, including mouse and human, the cells at the very base of the small intestinal crypt are populated by Paneth cells, differentiated cells with no proliferative capacity.)

When isolating intestinal epithelium for tissue culture, it is essential that the cells with the greatest proliferative potential are used and that this potential is maintained ex vivo. Not only do the differentiated phenotypes fail to proliferate, their products (mucus, lysozyme, etc) can compromise the culture of the immature cell types.

Successful crypt isolation can be easily achieved by incubation with chelating agents that release cells from their calcium- and magnesium-dependent interactions with the basement membrane and stromal cell types (Fig. 10.1). Epithelial cell-cell attachment is maintained, at least in the short term, causing the epithelium to be released from the underlying tissue in large units. Villi (probably less strongly attached to the underlying tissue for a variety

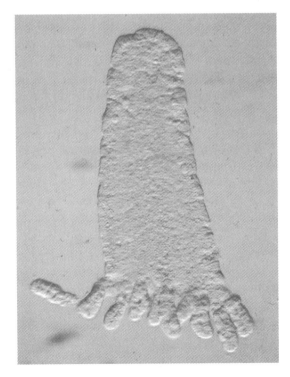

Fig 10.1. A small intestinal villus unit with its associated crypts, released by incubation in the chelating agent buffer described in text (see Section 2.4). Each villus is served by a number of smaller crypts. Objective magnification: 10×.

of biological reasons) are the first to be released, followed by the individual crypts. Preparations enriched for each type of unit can therefore be prepared. Incorporation of agents such as dithiothreitol minimizes any problems caused by mucous release. However, although such protocols can release macroscopically intact units suitable for short-term ex vivo maintenance, immunohistochemistry, or protein isolation, the severe disruption of the cell-cell contacts caused by the high levels of chelating agents inhibits long-term cell survival, with crypts gradually dying via apoptosis over the next 24 h. The problem of isolating viable crypt cells has, until recent years, restricted epithelial culture models. A variety of techniques modifying the levels of mechanical disruption, chelating agent concentrations, or using various enzymes have been published, with varying degrees of success. Frequently scientists have resorted to established adenocarcinoma, fetal, or neonatal cell lines. However, in addition to the problems arising from their origin, these cell lines have been selected and adapted for tissue culture. They have little resemblance to normal adult intestine in terms of growth factor responses, susceptibility to apoptosis, gene expression, and differentiation.

Over the last 10 years the more successful attempts at primary culture techniques have relied on enzymatic procedures, aided by some form of mechanical disruption to produce fragments of tissue small enough to limit the length of time the tissue is exposed to the enzyme. Crypts isolated in this manner appear to maintain their structure and, crucially, their proliferative capacity. One significant advance in this methodology was that of Evans et al. [1992]. Their paper described the culture of neonatal rat small intestine isolated using a number of techniques and plated on various substrata and concluded that digestion in a mixture of collagenase and dispase followed by growth on collagen produced the most successful long-term cultures. We have subsequently adapted this technique to the adult tissue [Booth et al., 1995, 1999]. Grafting techniques have shown that both methods appear to isolate and maintain functional stem cells [Tait et al., 1994a,b; Booth, 1999].

Recently, a technique originally based on lower levels of chelating agent has been adapted to include enzymatic steps, a crucial inclusion in this procedure being pancreatin [Whitehead et al., 1999]. This technique involves culturing individual cells as opposed to intact crypts and has been reported to ultimately result in a colony-forming assay, the first described for this tissue. The cells are plated out onto nutrient agar and grown for 2–3 wk until they form small colonies. Agents can be added to the growth media to examine their effects on colony-forming ability. This is the first report of a successful technique based on single cells— previously maintenance of crypt cell-cell contacts had always been regarded as essential for successful primary culture.

In this chapter we describe the procedures for both the isolation and culture of intestinal crypt cells and a brief description of the ways in which these cultures can be characterized. Each is followed by a discussion of the various alternative approaches and their limitations.

2. PREPARATION OF REAGENTS AND MEDIA

All solutions should be prepared in a laminar flow hood and filter sterilized where necessary before use.

N.B. Water quality is crucially important when preparing tissue culture reagents. Throughout this chapter, ultrapure water (UPW) is assumed.

2.1. Media

2.1.1. Hanks' Balanced Salt Solution (HBSS)

This is used to maintain and wash the tissue. It can be purchased ready to use or made from a $10\times$ concentrate or powder, with the pH appropriately adjusted using sodium bicarbonate. Add antibiotics at the following concentrations:

Benzyl penicillin	100 U/ml
Streptomycin sulfate	30 μg/ml
Gentamicin	25 μg/ml

2.1.2. Growth Medium

		Final conc.
DMEM, pyruvate free		500 ml
Glucose (as in high-glucose DMEM)	4.5 g/l	25 mM
Sodium pyruvate, 7.5% (0.68 M)	5 ml	6.8 mM
Fetal bovine serum	12.5 ml	2.5%
Insulin		0.25 U/ml

Antibiotics at the same concentrations as in Section 2.1.1, above.

EGF (for human cultures)	50 ng/ml	8.3 nM

Equilibrate with $NaHCO_3$ to pH 7.4 under 7.5% CO_2.

2.1.3. S-DMEM

Growth medium + 2% sorbitol (S-DMEM) is used in the sedimentation step of the isolation.

		Final conc.
D-Sorbitol	10 g	0.11 M
Growth medium	500 ml	

Add the sorbitol powder to the DMEM and shake to dissolve. Sterilize by filtration.

2.2. Collagenase/Dispase Enzyme Digestion Mix

This digestion mix is used to release the crypts from the underlying connective tissue. It consists of:

	Mouse		Human	
	Amount	Final conc.	Amount	Final conc.
Collagenase Type XI	2250 units	75 U/ml	4500 units	150 U/ml
Dispase neutral protease	600 μg	20 μg/ml	1.2 mg	40 μg/ml
FBS	0.3 ml	1%	0.3 ml	1%
DMEM to	30 ml		30 ml	

Thirty milliliters is sufficient for one isolation.

A stock 10× supply of collagenase and dispase can be made up in HBSS or DMEM and stored as frozen aliquots at −20°C. These can be diluted in DMEM with 1% FCS to produce the working enzyme concentration. However, the activity of the enzyme appears to be reduced over time when stored in frozen aliquots, and hence a maximum storage period of 2 wk is recommended.

2.3. Preparation of Collagen-Coated Plates

Vitrogen is the routine coating for tissue culture plastic. Prepare as follows:

1. Dilute stock 10× in UPW.
2. Sterilize by filtration.
3. Add 0.5 ml to each well of the 24-well plates.
4. Leave at room temperature for at least 3 h.
5. Remove the excess Vitrogen.
6. Leave the plates to air dry in a laminar flow hood.

7. Wrap any plates that are not used immediately in cling film (Saran Wrap) and store at 4°C for a period of up to 1 wk.

Others have reported increased cellular attachment if all of the Vitrogen is left in the wells within the hood overnight, such that all the liquid evaporates. The acid within the coated surface is then neutralized by 2–3 washes with HBSS.

2.4. Chelating Solution

Generally, a 5× or 10× stock of the chelating solution can be prepared and stored at 4°C (or −20°C if stored for long periods). This can then be diluted as and when required. The recipe for one liter of 5× stock is:

		mM	
	g/l	5× Stock	Final
Na$_2$HPO$_4$	3.95	28	5.6
KH$_2$PO$_4$	5.45	40	8.0
NaCl	28.1	480	96.2
KCl	0.6	8	1.6
Sucrose	75	220	43.4
D-Sorbitol	50	274	54.9
DL-Dithiothreitol	0.4	2.6	0.5

Dilute 5× stock to working strength with UPW and add:

EDTA	2		5
EGTA	2		5

Adjust to pH 7.3. Sterilize by filtration.

2.5. Reagents for Clonogenic Assay (Protocol 10.7)

2.5.1. EDTA-DTT

EDTA, 3 mM, dithiothreitol (DTT), 0.5 mM, in PBSA, sterilized by filtration.

2.5.2. Pancreatin

Pancreatin, 0.3% in PBSA, sterilized by filtration.

2.5.3. Agar

1%, in UPW, sterilized by autoclaving.

2.5.4. Agarose

Agarose, 0.8%, in UPW, sterilized by autoclaving.

2.5.5. RPMI 1640 Medium

RPMI 1640, $2\times$, prepared from $10\times$ concentrate or powder using half the recommended UPW.

2.5.6. Sodium Hypochlorite

NaOCl, 0.04% (5 mM), in deionized water.

3. ISOLATION AND PRIMARY CULTURE OF ADULT MOUSE COLONIC EPITHELIUM

Protocol 10.1. Isolation of Crypts from Mouse Colon

Reagents and Materials

Sterile (All media should be at 37°C)
- ❑ HBSS (see Section 2.1.1)
- ❑ Digestion mix (see Section 2.2, *Mouse*, above)
- ❑ Petri dishes, 9 cm
- ❑ Flasks, 25 cm²
- ❑ Scalpels, holder #4, blade #22
- ❑ Syringe, 10 ml
- ❑ Needles, 21 gauge
- ❑ Movette pipette (or similar wide-bore plastic pipette)

Nonsterile
- ❑ Mice

Protocol

(a) Remove the colons and place in HBSS immediately on excision.

(b) Place the tissue into a plastic Petri dish and flush out the contents of the colon with HBSS using a 21-gauge needle and a 10-ml syringe.

(c) Transfer the tissue to a clean Petri dish.

(d) Slice the colons down the center and then into small pieces with a scalpel.

(e) Wash the tissue by transferring it to a 25-cm² flask containing 20 ml HBSS and agitate by pipetting up and down using a Movette pipette.

(f) Allow contents of the flask to settle and remove HBSS.

(h) Repeat the process until the HBSS remains almost clear. This usually takes about 5 repeats of the washing process.

(h) Remove any excess HBSS and place the tissue in a Petri dish.

(i) Chop the tissue with the scalpel until it has the consistency of a smooth paste and transfer to a 25-cm^2 flask with a wide-bore pipette (ensure that the inside of the pipette is already wet with HBSS to prevent pieces sticking).

(j) Allow pieces to settle and remove excess HBSS.

(k) Add 25–30 ml of the digestion mix.

(l) Incubate at 37°C in a water bath for 2–3 h (to minimize contamination from the water bath, the flask should be placed in a beaker of sterile water previously equilibrated to 37°C; the level of the water should be well below the neck of the flask, which should be wrapped in Parafilm).

(m) After 1 h, agitate the flask and return it to the water bath, checking the tissue every 15–30 min thereafter to ensure crypts do not become over-digested (Fig. 10.2a). The isolation is ready when approximately 70–80% of the crypts have become liberated as individual free crypts.

N.B. Do not wait until all crypts are liberated, because those that detached at an earlier stage will be over-digested by the enzyme. The final isolation will be a compromise between viability and yield.

The next step is to remove any undigested material, bacteria, and single cells from the crypt preparation.

Protocol 10.2. Sedimentation Protocol for Mouse Colonic Crypts

Reagents and Materials

Sterile

❑ Growth medium (see Section 2.1.2, above)
❑ S-DMEM (see Section 2.1.3, above)
   All media should be at 37°C.
❑ Universal containers, 30 ml (clear-walled 30-ml plastic tubes)
❑ Plates, 24 well, collagen coated (see Section 2.3, above)

Protocol

(a) Divide the contents of the digestion flask between two 30-ml sterile universal containers and label "Set 1."

(b) Top up to 25 ml with S-DMEM.

(c) Allow the contents of the tubes to settle for a period of 1 min to allow any undigested matter to sediment.

(d) Gently remove the supernatant suspension from the tubes and transfer it to two clean tubes; label "Set 2."

(e) Let the suspensions in Set 2 settle for 30 s.

(f) Transfer the supernatant suspension from Set 2 to a further set of clean tubes; label "Set 3."

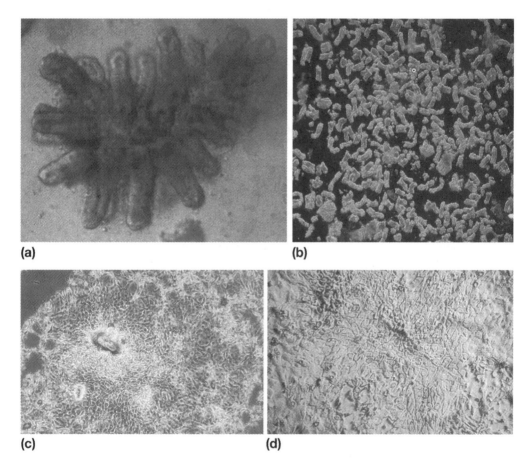

(a)   (b)

(c)   (d)

Fig 10.2. Isolation and culture of mouse colonic epithelial cells. During incubation in collagenase and dispase the mesenchymal tissue surrounding the crypts is gradually digested, leaving intact crypts that often remain connected at the luminal surface (plateau region) (a). Further digestion and mechanical agitation releases the individual crypts that can be purified by centrifugation (b). When plated onto collagen-coated plastic the epithelial cells within the crypt spread and proliferate (c, d). Objective magnification: (a) 25×, (b, c), 10×, (d) 20×.

(g) Top up the Set 3 tubes with S-DMEM.

(h) Centrifuge at 200–300 g for 4 min. (The slowest speed on a standard bench top centrifuge is usually about right.)

(i) Discard the supernatant.

(j) Disperse the pellet by flicking/tapping the base of the tube.

(k) Resuspend the crypts once more with S-DMEM and repeat the centrifugation step. This S-DMEM washing/centrifugation step must be repeated about five times, or until the supernatant is clear (Fig. 10.2b).

(l) The debris left behind in Set 1 and 2 tubes should be examined microscopically for the presence of crypts. If a high proportion of crypts remain, the material can be agitated and the initial sedimentation step repeated. If only undigested material remains, this can be discarded.

(m) The crypts are ready to be plated out when the supernatant appears clear. A critical plating density is required for good culture growth. Generally, the crypts appear to grow best when plated at a density of 800–1000 crypts/ml/well in a 24-well plate. To determine the number of crypts isolated:
   i) Resuspend the isolation in 10 ml of growth medium and agitate.
   ii) Remove 100 μl and add to 900 μl growth medium.
   iii) Take 100-μl sample from this and count the number of crypts present.
   No. of crypts/ml = No. of crypts counted $\times$ 100

(n) Incubate the plates at 37°C in 7.5% CO_2 and allow the cells to attach for 2 days.

(o) Remove the medium, containing all unattached material, from the plates and replace with fresh medium.

(p) Supplement the medium at 5-day intervals with 0.5 ml fresh medium.

The cultures will generally grow happily for a period of up to 15 days, but this can be extended to 20–30 days when the crypts are grown in the presence of a 3T3 feeder layer (see Chapters 2 and 5). Culture growth can be increased by the inclusion of EGF (10 ng/ml, $\sim$2 $\times$ 10^{-9} M) and transferrin (5 μg/ml, 6 $\times$ 10^{-8} M) in the medium (see Chapters 3, 4, and 5), if appropriate for the experimental assay (Fig. 10.2c,d).

Crypts will be released with some pericryptal fibroblasts, and hence the cultures will not be pure epithelial preparations (Fig. 10.3). However, the sedimentation steps should remove all other mesenchymal material. The low serum concentration (2.5%) in

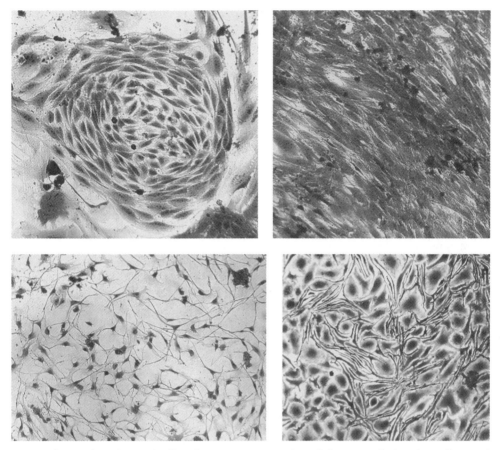

Fig 10.3. Incomplete enzymatic digestion or poor separation of the crypts during the sedimentation steps often results in cultures that contain other contaminating cell types (fibroblasts and other mesenchymal cells of various morphologies). Objective magnification: 32×.

the growth media minimizes fibroblast growth, but it is also advisable to batch test serum for epithelial versus fibroblast growth promotion.

4. ADAPTATIONS TO THE ISOLATION PROCEDURE

4.1. Small Intestine

Viable colonic crypts are much more easily isolated than their small intestinal counterparts. Although the reasons for this remain to be conclusively demonstrated, contributing factors are likely to be:

(i)   The colonic epithelium produces far fewer endogenous proteases (which are likely to contribute to the enzymatic digestion process in a nonspecific uncontrolled manner in the small bowel isolation process).

(ii) There are no villi in the colon. Early release of this epithelium in the small bowel and the subsequent exposure of the nuclear material as the cells lyse in the digestion mix can cause serious clumping of the cells. To reduce this problem DNase, 50 μg/ml, should be included in the digestion mix, and this should be changed part way through to remove the cells released early in the digestion.

(iii) The colonic stem cells are themselves much more resistant to apoptosis than their small intestinal equivalents [Potten, 1977; reviewed in Potten et al., 1997].

4.2. Neonatal Intestine

Isolating viable tissue from neonatal intestine uses essentially the same principle except that lower concentrations of collagenase and dispase are used and the digestion process is carried out at room temperature with constant agitation (on an orbital shaker). This less well-developed tissue can be released in just 20 min, and the same sorbitol sedimentation procedure can be used to purify the released epithelium. This adaptation is that of Evans et al. [1992], which was designed for small intestine from 6-day-old rats, an age at which the animals possess small villi but no true crypt invaginations—the epithelium undulates with the proliferative cells clustered at the base of the undulations. At this age it is believed that many of these proliferative cells possess stem cell attributes. Others have described different techniques for isolating and culturing neonatal epithelium [e.g., Yeh and Chopra, 1980; Fukamachi 1992].

4.3. Tumors

Intestinal epithelium can be isolated from adenomatous tissue in both mouse and human. One example of a source of the former is the Min +/− mouse, which has a pathology equivalent to human FAP (familial adenomatous polyposis) [Moser et al., 1992]. The abnormal tissue in these animals can appear as hyperplastic elongated crypts, "cystic" crypts (early adenoma), or typical adenoma. All can be isolated using the standard collagenase-dispase method. Further descriptions of the techniques involved in the growth of intestinal tumors can be found in Hague and Paraskeva [1997].

4.4. Preparation and Use of 3T3 Feeder Layers

The presence of a 3T3 cell feeder layer generally improves epithelial cell survival and growth. However, whether it is an appropriate coculture system for this tissue remains to be seen (one would assume that a pericryptal fibroblast cell line would be the best system). There are two approaches that can be used to reproductively sterilize feeder cells, mitomycin C treatment or γ-irradiation. Both will prevent the cells from dividing but allow the cells to retain the ability to attach and release growth factors into the culture media. The irradiation protocol is described below.

Protocol 10.3. Preparation of 3T3 Feeder Layers for Intestinal Epithelium (*See also Protocols 5.2, 5.3, and 5.4*)

Reagents and Materials

☐ 3T3 cells: Swiss 3T3 (ATCC CCL92), or L1 (ATCC CCL173) strains, maintained subconfluent at all times and replenished regularly from frozen stocks.

☐ Growth medium: DMEM with 5% FBS and 100 U/ml penicillin and 100 μg/ml streptomycin

☐ Trypsin/EDTA: 0.25% trypsin, 0.3 mM EDTA, in PBSA

Protocol

(a) Trypsinize 3T3 cells at 60% confluence using trypsin/EDTA.

(b) Resuspend the cells in fresh medium and irradiate with 60 Gy using a γ-irradiation source.

(c) Once cells are irradiated, recentrifuge the cells, resuspend them in fresh medium, and determine the total cell number.

(d) Plate out at 2.5 × 10^4/ml/well in a 24-well plate and incubate at 37°C in 7.5% CO_2 for 24 h before the addition of crypts (alternatively, cells can be stored at 10^6/ml at 4°C for up to 1 wk).

4.5. Adult Human Colonic Epithelium

This is an adaptation of the murine procedure.

△*Safety note.* All work should be carried out wearing suitable protective clothing (lab coat, gloves, and safety spectacles) and carried out on a disposable plastic tray. A disinfectant solution such as Virkon should be readily available to decontaminate equipment and any spillages, and waste products should be disposed of in accordance with health and safety regulations.

Human intestine, particularly the large bowel, has a much thicker muscle layer than that in the mouse. As much of this as possible should be removed with a scalpel blade (to improve enzyme access), and then the tissue should be cut into small pieces and washed as previously described. Although there is likely to be little fecal contamination (because patients are starved before surgery), there will be heavy mucous contamination because of the large number of goblet cells. The tissue is much more difficult to mince than the mouse colon and therefore may take longer to prepare. However, it is advisable to persist, because a coarser preparation will take longer to digest in the enzyme and is likely to be less viable.

Protocol 10.4. Isolation of Crypts from Human Colon

Reagents and Materials

Sterile

- ❏ HBSS (see Section 2.1.1)
- ❏ Digestion mix (see Section 2.2, *Human*)
- ❏ Growth medium (see Section 2.1.2, with 50 ng/ml EGF as specified for human cells)
- ❏ All media should be at 37°C.
- ❏ Petri dishes, 9 cm
- ❏ Flasks, 25 cm^2
- ❏ Scalpels, #4 holder , #22 blade
- ❏ Movette pipette (or similar wide-bore plastic pipette)

Protocol

(a) Tissue for culture should be placed in DMEM as soon as possible after excision from the patient. Preliminary studies indicate that as long as the tissue is quickly placed into DMEM it will withstand a short period (up to 2 h) at 4°C, although a longer period is not advisable.

(b) Wash the intact tissue twice in 1× HBSS to remove any contaminating factors.

(c) Transfer the tissue to a clean Petri dish with fresh HBSS.

(d) Remove as much muscle as possible and chop the tissue into pieces with two opposed scalpels.

(e) Wash the chopped tissue pieces by transferring them to a 25-cm^2 flask containing 20 ml HBSS and pipette up and down using a Movette pipette.

(f) Allow contents of the flask to settle and remove the HBSS.

(g) Repeat the process until the HBSS remains almost clear. This usually takes about 5 repeats of the washing process.

(h) Transfer the tissue to a Petri dish and remove any excess HBSS.

(i) Chop the tissue with the scalpels until it has a fairly smooth consistency. Because of the nature of the tissue it is impracticable to produce the smooth pastelike consistency that is attainable with mouse colon. Transfer the chopped tissue to a 25-cm flask with a wide-bore pipette (ensure that the inside of the pipette is already wet with HBSS to prevent sticking).

(j) Allow pieces to settle and remove excess HBSS.

(k) Add 25–30 ml of the digestion mix.

(l) Incubate at 37°C for 1 h.

(m) Replace the digestion mix:

    i) Allow the tissue to settle.

    ii) Carefully remove the digestion mix from the flask and discard it (being sure not to remove any undigested tissue in the process).

    iii) Add fresh digestion mix and continue incubation at 37°C for a further 1–2 h.

    iv) Check the tissue every 15–30 min to ensure that crypts do not become over-digested (*cf.* Fig. 10.2a). The isolation is ready when approximately 70–80% of the crypts have become liberated as individual free crypts.

N.B. As in the case of the mouse primary cultures, do not wait until all crypts are liberated as this may result in a reduction in yield caused by over-digestion.

Protocol 10.5. Sedimentation Protocol for Human Colonic Crypts

Released crypts are purified using sorbitol sedimentation as described previously. You may find that large aggregates of fatty/mesenchymal tissue rise to the top of the sedimentation tube; these should be discarded in the first steps because they may cause problems during the sedimentation process.

Reagents and Materials

Sterile

❑ Growth medium (see Section 2.1.2, with 50 ng/ml EGF as specified for human cells)

❑ S-DMEM (see Section 2.1.3)

Booth and O'Shea

- ❏ All media should be at 37°C
- ❏ Universal containers, 30 ml (clear-walled 30-ml plastic tubes)
- ❏ Plates, 24 well, collagen coated (see Section 2.3)

Protocol

(a) Divide the contents of the digestion flask between two 30-ml sterile universal containers and label "Set 1."

(b) Top up to 25 ml with S-DMEM and remove any floating fatty or other mesenchymal tissue.

(c) Allow the contents of the tubes to settle for a period of 1 min to allow any undigested matter to sediment.

(d) Discard any fatty material floating on the surface and then gently remove the supernatant suspension from the tubes and transfer two clean tubes; label "Set 2."

(e) Let the solution settle for 30 s.

(f) Transfer the contents to a further set of clean tubes; label "Set 3."

(g) Top up with S-DMEM.

(h) Centrifuge Set 3 tubes at 200–300 g for 4 min. (The slowest speed on a standard bench top centrifuge is usually about right.)

(i) Discard the supernatant.

(j) Disperse the pellet by flicking/tapping the base of the tube.

(k) Resuspend the crypts once more with S-DMEM and repeat the centrifugation step. This S-DMEM washing/centrifugation step must be repeated about 5 times, or until the supernatant is clear (Fig. 10.2b).

(l) The debris left behind in Set 1 and 2 tubes should be examined microscopically for the presence of crypts. If a high proportion of crypts remain, the material can be agitated and the initial sedimentation step repeated. If only undigested material remains, this can be discarded.

(m) The crypts are ready to be plated out when the supernatant appears clear. A critical plating density is required for good culture growth. Generally, the crypts appear to grow best when plated at a density of 800–1000 crypts/ml/well in a 24-well plate. To determine the number of crypts isolated:

    i) Resuspend the isolation in 10 ml of growth medium and agitate.

    ii) Remove 100 μl and add to 900 μl growth medium.

    iii) Take 100-μl sample from this and count the number of crypts present.

    No. of crypts/ml = No. of crypts counted × 100

(n) Incubate the plates at 37°C in 7.5% CO_2 and allow the cells to attach for 2 days.

(o) Remove the medium, containing all unattached material, from the plates and replace with fresh medium.

(p) Supplement the medium at 5-days intervals with 0.5 ml fresh medium.

Crypts can be plated out on either collagen-coated plates or a 3T3 feeder layer. This method will allow routine culture for a period of about 1 wk. After this period the epithelial cells deteriorate and the contaminating fibroblasts become prevalent. The cultures do not subculture well. Various cell recovery agents have been utilized, but so far we have had limited success subculturing intestinal epithelial cells. Not surprisingly, fibroblasts can be quite easily subcultured and are a potential source of feeder layer cells.

There are a number of problems associated with obtaining useful human material, the first being that biopsy samples are too small. In addition to containing too few crypts, most do not sample the entire crypt, that is, the bottom of the crypt is often missed and therefore the progenitor cells necessary for long-term culture are not present. Larger biopsies are possible, but the yield is still very small. Samples from tumor resections are often the best source of material. However, although tumor tissue is readily available, and grows easily using the collagenase-dispase isolation method, the opportunities for getting normal tissue that has not been anoxic for a long period during surgery are rare.

Tissue samples are often also provided from patients having surgery for inflammatory conditions such as Crohn disease. In such situations, it may be difficult to determine whether the tissue, even if taken from disease margins, can really be classified as normal.

Finally, the age of the patient is often a concern. Patients undergoing surgery are often of an older age and hence it is possible that the capacity of the tissue to survive and regenerate is somewhat limited. Such age-related differences have been reported for other tissues. Ideally, tissue from a younger adult is required, but such samples are few and far between.

The differences associated with any of these parameters, in addition to those introduced by the culture procedure itself, all tend to make human primary cultures quite variable. Any assays must be performed within a single run (from a single sample), and a degree of caution must be employed when comparing different runs.

4.6. Chelating Agent Isolations

This method has been the basis of many attempts at intestinal primary culture. Although the crypts are isolated in high yield, they generally have a reduced viability. Such preparations, however, may be useful for short-term functional studies and three-dimensional structural and positional studies. For example, we have fixed such isolations in 4% formol saline and used immunohistochemistry and confocal microscopy to examine the three-dimensional distribution of proliferation markers. The most widely used approach is that first described by Weiser [1973] but since adapted by Flint et al. [1991, 1994] to separate crypt and villus fractions for measuring mRNA or protein expression levels in the two sites.

Protocol 10.6. Isolation of Intestinal Epithelium by Chelating Agents

Reagents and Materials

Nonsterile if for short-term examination but sterile if prolonged culture is attempted

- ❑ HBSS (see Section 2.1.1)
- ❑ Growth medium (see Section 2.1.2, with 50 ng/ml EGF as specified for human cells)
- ❑ Petri dishes, 9 cm
- ❑ Flasks, 25 cm^2
- ❑ Syringe, 10 ml
- ❑ Needles, 21 gauge
- ❑ Glass rod or rigid plastic tube, #3 mm $\times$ 150 mm (the refill from a ballpoint pen can be used)
- ❑ Movette pipette (or similar wide-bore plastic pipette)

Protocol

(a) Remove small or large intestine and flush out the luminal contents with HBSS using a needle and syringe.

(b) Expose the luminal surface by slicing the intestine longitudinally, although for rodent tissue the 5- to 10-cm lengths may be inverted.

(c) Mouse intestine is most easily inverted by threading the glass rod, tube, or pen refill through the lumen. One end of the intestine can be secured in place using cotton thread and the remaining intestine eased over the secured site so that it turns "inside out" over the attached site. The inverted tissue can then be eased off the support. It is possible to tie the inverted tissue at one end and then inflate it with liquid at various stages during incubation, so that any loosened crypts "pop" out as the tissue inflates. However, we have found this awkward and unnecessary.

(d) Wash the material in 2 changes of HBSS and then place in a 25-cm^2 flask with the chelating agent solution at 4°C for 1 h.

(e) The solution containing released debris is then replaced with fresh HBSS and the flask is vigorously shaken by hand. The contents of the flask are then examined under an inverted microscope to see whether any epithelium has been liberated. Continue the incubation at 4°C, checking at 15-min intervals. Generally, crypts will be released after about 2 h.

(f) Villi will be released before crypts, with adenomatous tissue last. If it is necessary to separate these fractions, the tissue should be incubated at 4°C in the chelating agent for just 30 min. Any loosened material will be released by shaking (the first stage is generally debris and single cells from the villus). By replacing the solution every 5–10 min and shaking each time, successive fractions will contain first villi, then villi with attached crypts, then crypts, then adenomatous tissue (Fig. 10.4).

(g) If large, intact sheets of tissue are required, use a longer incubation time (about 2–3 h) with no shaking during this period. Agitation at the end of this period will release larger sheets of material.

(h) Remove the released epithelium from the chelating agent to prevent further disruption into a single-cell suspension.

(i) Using a refrigerated bench top centrifuge, gently pellet the tissue using the slowest speed possible ($\sim$100–300 g). The supernatant can be discarded and the pellet suspended in the appropriate medium, solution, or fixative.

The same protocol can be used for small or large bowel from mouse or human. The length of time required to release the intact crypts may vary if the crypts are long, for example, from the human large bowel. Generally, tumors are released after most of the normal tissue.

5. CLONOGENIC ASSAYS

Clonogenic assays measure the number and long-term proliferative potential of the clonogenic cells within the epithelium. They can form standard assays for the quantification of cytotoxic injury and regeneration potential of the tissues ex vivo. Although such assays are well established for the progenitor cells of the bone marrow and to some extent for the epidermis, robust assays remain elusive for the intestinal epithelium. Two methods are cur-

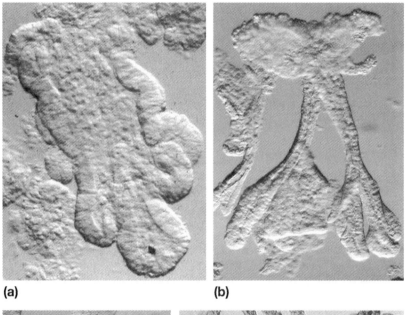

(a)   (b)

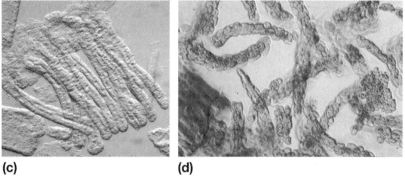

(c)   (d)

Fig 10.4. Chelating agents can release intact units of epithelial tissue with a maintained 3-D structure. In addition to normal small intestinal epithelium as in Fig. 1, irradiated regenerating small intestinal tissue (a), hyperplastic crypts (from a Min +/− mouse) (b, c), and epithelium from other tissues can be released (d, stomach). These will survive in the short term but are best used for expression analysis. Objective magnification: (a) 25×, (b) 16×, (c) 25×, (d) 16×.

rently available that can be optimized for this kind of assay. The first was developed by ourselves and is better termed a colony-forming assay rather than a clonogenic assay, because it is a measurement of the colony derived from each crypt (which may contain varying numbers of clonogenic cells depending on the status of the tissue). The second is a recently published method developed by Whitehead et al. [1999], in which small numbers of colonies originate from single cells, and is therefore a more typical clonogenic assay.

5.1. Intestinal Crypt Colony-Forming Assay

This is an extension of the standard primary culture procedure and measures colony-forming ability, that is, crypt survival, after various treatments.

Protocol 10.7. Colony-Forming Assay for Intestinal Crypt Survival

Reagents and Materials

Sterile or Aseptically Prepared

- ❑ 3T3 feeder cells (see Section 4.4, above, and Protocols 5.2 and 5.4)
- ❑ 3T3 growth medium: DMEM with 5% donor calf/newborn bovine serum (NBS), 100 U/ml penicillin, and 30 μg/ml streptomycin
- ❑ Growth medium for crypt cells (see Section 2.1.2)
- ❑ Multiwell plates, 24 well, collagen coated (see Section 2.3, above)

Protocol

(a) Plate out 3T3 feeder cells at 2.5×10^4 cells per ml in each well of a 24-well plate and leave to attach for 24 h.

(b) Isolate the crypts using the standard primary culture protocol (collagenase and dispase) as described in Protocols 10.1 and 10.2, above, and dilute the crypts to 50, 100, 200, and 500 crypts/ml in growth medium.

(c) Remove the medium from the feeder layer and replace with the various concentrations of crypts in fresh growth medium.

(d) Incubate at 37°C in 7.5% CO_2 for 30 days, fixing a control plate 2 days after seeding (to measure initial attachment and colony number) and on days 10, 20, and 30 (or as appropriate for the individual experiment). A complete media change should occur on day 2, with 0.5-ml supplements at successive 5-day intervals.

(e) Fixed colonies can be visualized using histologic stains such as 0.1% crystal violet (Fig. 10.5).

(f) The number and size of the colonies formed can then be determined. Proliferation can be measured using an S phase marker such as [^{3}H]thymidine or bromodeoxyuridine and the labeled cells can be counted. Scintillation or "whole culture" measurements should be avoided because these will not discriminate between proliferation in epithelial cells and gut-derived fibroblasts.

The cultures may be treated with various factors or the crypts themselves derived from pretreated animals. Similarly, factors can be added to the culture media at the time of plating or after manipulation, for example, cytotoxic insult.

5.2. Clonogenic Assay

One clonogenic assay that utilizes a mixture of both enzymatic and chelating agents is that described by Whitehead [1999]. This technique is based on disaggregating intact crypts to produce a single-cell suspension and can be used to test the ability of various growth factors to alter the colony size (cell proliferation capacity) and number (survival rate).

Protocol 10.8. Clonogenic Assay for Murine Intestinal Crypt Epithelium

Reagents and Materials

Sterile

❏ PBSA
❏ Growth medium: RPMI 1640 with 10% FBS
❏ EDTA-DTT (see Section 2.5.1)
❏ Pancreatin in PBSA, 0.3% (see Section 2.5.2)
❏ Agar 1% (see Section 2.5.3)
❏ Agarose, 0.8% in UPW (see Section 2.5.4)
❏ RPMI 1640, 2×, with 10% FBS (see Section 2.5.5)

Nonsterile

- ☐ Sodium hypochlorite, 0.04% (5 mM) (see Section 2.5.6)
- ☐ Mice

Protocol

Agar-Coated Plate Preparation

(a) Melt both the agars and return to 40°C.

(b) Warm the 2× RPMI 1640 to 37°C.

(c) Mix equal volumes of the 2× RPMI 1640 and the 1% agar and add 2 ml to each well of a 6-well plate to produce an underlay. When dealing with the agar solutions, pipette slowly to avoid bubble formation. Leave at room temperature to set.

Disaggregation and Cloning of Colonic Epithelium

(d) Sacrifice mice and remove colons.

(e) Slice open and wash in 3 changes of sterile PBSA.

(f) Place in 0.04% sodium hypochlorite at room temperature for 20 min to reduce bacterial contamination.

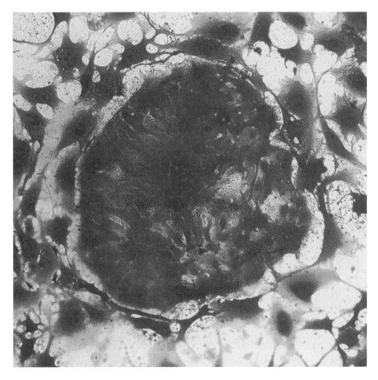

Fig 10.5. A colony derived from a single crypt, grown on a 3T3 feeder layer. Colonies remain as discrete entities that can be scored. Objective magnification: 25×.

(g) Rinse in PBSA and transfer to the EDTA-DTT solution and incubate at room temperature for 90 min.

(h) Remove the solution and replace with sterile PBSA.

(i) Shake the tube vigorously for 30 s and collect the supernatant.

(j) Repeat three times, collecting the supernatant each time.

(k) Pellet the cells at 400 rpm.

(l) Place the pellet in the 0.3% pancreatin and incubate at room temperature for 90 min.

(m) Dilute the solution with an equal volume of sterile PBSA and centrifuge at 1000 rpm for 5 min.

(n) Carefully remove the supernatant and resuspend the pellet in the EDTA-DTT solution.

(o) Centrifuge at 1000 rpm for 5 min.

(p) Resuspend the pellet in growth medium.

Cloning

(q) Examine the suspension microscopically to check whether a single-cell suspension has been achieved. If not, gently pass the suspension three times through an 18-G needle and then three times through a 21-G needle. If small clumps of cells are still present, it may be necessary to filter the suspension through a cotton wool plug in a Pasteur pipette, although this can result in considerable cell loss.

(r) Count the cells and dilute in equal volumes of 0.8% agarose and 2× RPMI to produce a cell concentration of 50,000 cells/ml.

(s) Add any test factors at this stage.

(t) Aliquot into the wells of the agar-coated plate(s).

(u) Cool the plates at 4°C for 5 min to set the agarose and then place the plates in a sealed container holding a small volume of H_2O to humidify the atmosphere and incubate at 37°C for 3–4 wk. The plates can then be examined and the colonies counted. Whitehead et al. [1999] decreed a colony to be 30 cells or more, whereas 15 cells or more was named a cluster. Colonies can be removed with a Pasteur pipette and disaggregated for subcloning and examination of their long-term proliferative potential, that is, stem cell characteristics.

6. QUANTIFICATION AND ANALYSIS

The growth of primary cultures can be analyzed by various means. Examples include proliferation measurements (e.g.

[^{3}H]thymidine labeling), cell number measurements (e.g., crystal violet dye binding) or cellular metabolism measurements (e.g., MTT). Each has advantages and disadvantages, and therefore the appropriate assay must be chosen for each culture application.

6.1. Thymidine Labeling

Tritiated thymidine labeling of cultures followed by autoradiography, rather than measurement of total uptake by scintillation counting, allows the visualization of the proliferating cells present. The labeled nuclei can be counted and cell types discriminated, ensuring that the results only reflect the epithelial cell population (Fig. 10.6a). Bromodeoxyuridine labels the same population of cells, but these are visualized by immunohistochemical rather than radioactive techniques.

Protocol 10.9. Measurement of Labeling Index in Intestinal Epithelium

Reagents and Materials

Sterile

❑ [^{3}H]thymidine, 6.7 Ci/mmol (250 GBq/mmol), 250 μCi/ml ($\sim$10 MBq/ml)

Nonsterile

❑ Ethanol, 70%
❑ Ethanol, absolute
❑ Trichloracetic acid, 0.3 M (5%)
❑ Materials for autoradiography: radiosensitive emulsion, photographic developer, and fixer [see Freshney, 2000]

Protocol

(a) Add 74 kBq (2 μCi) [^{3}H]thymidine to each 1 ml of culture medium and incubate for 3 h.
(b) Remove the medium and fix the cells in 70% ethanol.
(c) Remove the unincorporated thymidine by incubating the plates in cold 0.3 M TCA for 10 min.
(d) Wash twice in absolute alcohol.
(e) After the plates are thoroughly air dried, the cells can be processed for autoradiography [Freshney, 2000]. This involves coating the plates with a thin layer of photographic

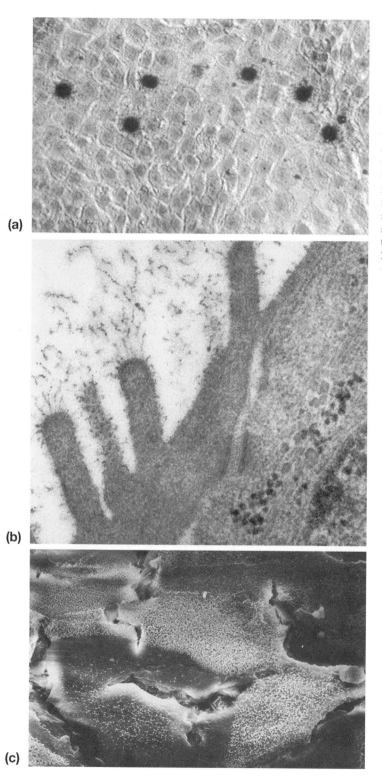

Fig 10.6. Characterization of epithelial cells in culture. Cells undergoing proliferation can be visualized via treatment with [³H]thymidine and autoradiography (a). Information regarding their junctional complexes and differentiation state can be obtained from ultrastructural analysis. Functional microvilli (b, c) and desmosomes (b) can often be seen and used as epithelial specific markers. Objective magnification: (a) 20×, (b) 98,000×, (c) ~5000×.

(a)

(b)

(c)

Isolation and Culture of Intestinal Epithelial Cells

emulsion; the plates are then dried, incubated at 4°C for 5 days, and then developed (all autoradiography must take place under safe light conditions in a dark room). Once developed the plates can be counterstained with hematoxylin (nuclei only) or Giemsa (polychromatic, stains nuclei and cytoplasm), allowing the visualization of the labeled, and hence proliferating, cells.

6.2. Crystal Violet Assay

The standard crystal violet assay is a useful quick method of estimating the total cell number. The intensity of the solubilized stain can be considered as being proportional to the number of cells present. For intestinal cultures, however, there is a problem associated with measuring the total numbers of cells present. In general, these cultures do not grow as pure epithelial isolations but also contain contaminating fibroblasts. With any dye binding technique the cells should therefore always be examined microscopically before releasing the dye, to determine the cell types present and the relative uptake of the dye by the different cell types. If on examination there appears to be little mesenchymal contamination, the assay may then be considered as an index of epithelial cell number.

With crystal violet this problem of the fibroblasts influencing the outcome of the assay can be overcome by lowering the pH of the dye. It has been shown that at pH 2.8 the epithelial specificity of the stain increases, giving a more accurate analysis of epithelial cell number [Booth et al., 1995].

Protocol 10.10. Estimating Epithelial Cell Number by Crystal Violet Staining

Reagents and Materials

Nonsterile

☐ Glutaraldehyde, 2% (0.2 M), or 4% (1.3 M) formaldehyde
☐ Crystal violet, 0.1%, made up in distilled water
☐ Sodium deoxycholate, 2% in distilled water
☐ Ethanol, 70%
☐ Microtitration plate, 96 well

Protocol

(a) Fix cultures (in a fume cupboard) for 2 h in a 2% (0.2 M) glutaraldehyde or 4% (1.3 M) formaldehyde solution made up in HBSS.

(b) Remove fixative and rinse down the fume hood sink.

(c) Wash the plates in two changes of 70% alcohol and allow to air dry.

(d) Add 0.5 ml of crystal violet to each well of the 24-well plate and leave for 5 min.

(e) Remove the excess stain by washing in distilled water and air dry the plates. Stained cells can be examined microscopically at this stage.

(f) Solubilize the stain in a 2% solution of sodium deoxycholate:
   i)   Add 400 μl to each well of the plate and leave until the stain has dissolved.
   ii) Transfer 200 μl from each well to a 96-well plate.

(g) Read optical density (absorbance) at 595 nm on an ELISA plate reader. The values obtained can then be considered as an accurate index of cell number [Potten et al., 1993].

Other cell viability assays, such as MTT, have also been successfully used on intestinal primary cultures although, again, these do not distinguish between the cell types present or the metabolic effects of any treatment on each cell type.

7. CHARACTERIZING CULTURED INTESTINAL EPITHELIAL CELLS

Primary epithelial cells gradually change their properties in vitro, often because of the inability to differentiate. As a result, the use of any single intracellular marker can be difficult to interpret. For example, cells may lose desmosomal interactions (and associated protein expression) and change their pattern of (or even lose) cytokeratin and brush border enzyme expression. At the moment there is no effective solution to this problem, and a combination of immunohistochemical, PCR, and ultrastructural evidence (Fig. 10.6b,c) tends to be used. For example, the presence of cytokeratins 8 and 18 and desmosomal or tight junctions may positively identify epithelial cells whereas vimentin may identify a fibroblast. The major problem, however, is characterizing cells that are negative for these markers—are they fibroblasts or actually derived from the epithelium?

7.1. Measuring Stem Cell Function

Sustained proliferation, as measured in a clonogenic assay, is one property of a stem cell. Using such assays it is theoretically possible to distinguish between true stem cells and their daughters (the shorter-lived transit-amplifying cells). However, stem cells must also be capable of producing differentiated progeny and, to date, the current culture models of normal tissue have been unable to conclusively demonstrate differentiation into the various epithelial lineages. This is probably due to the limitations of the current techniques. The media and substrata constituents (in terms of extracellular matrices, growth factor production, and three-dimensional organization) that control differentiation remain to be determined.

To circumvent this problem we have assayed stem cell function by taking either isolated crypts or primary cultures and grafting them subcutaneously in Matrigel into immunocompromised animals [Booth et al., 1999]. This simply involves mixing crypts or cultured cells with 50% Matrigel, injecting 0.1 ml in each flank of a mouse, and allowing the grafts to grow for 2–16 wk. The greatest problem with such a technique is removing viable, functional cells from the tissue culture dish. As in subculturing, simple trypsin-based methods do not appear to yield viable cells. We have found that digestion with collagenase and dispase or incubation with Acutase (TCS/Upstate Biotechnology) provides the best yield of viable cells.

8. LIMITATIONS AND FUTURE PERSPECTIVES

There are a huge number of applications for intestinal epithelial primary cultures. The most exciting involve using the system to elucidate the factors controlling stem cell renewal and differentiation along the various lineages, similar to the in vitro models already developed for the hematopoietic system. If the current culture protocols can be adapted for such purposes, a variety of new clinical opportunities will arise:

(i) The factors that control differentiation along the different lineages will be identified. Differentiation-inducing factors, and their synthetic analogs, will be potential anticancer agents.

(ii) The identification of the factors that induce stem cell amplification in vitro will aid mucosal transplantation (both as an ulceration therapy and for gene therapy approaches, such as for the treatment of cystic fibrosis where the introduction of the CFTR gene into a stem cell may regenerate a permanently expressing tissue).

(iii) The identification of the factors that induce such stem cell amplification will also provide novel targets for anticancer drugs.

Improvement of the human intestinal culture models is currently limited by the quality and quantity of tissue available from surgical resections. Adaptation of the current protocols to use single (or very few) crypts would enable biopsy samples to be a feasible assay material. These are much more frequently available and can be placed into the appropriate medium immediately after excision from the patient. This would enable the effects of various agents to be monitored directly on human tissue. Although cytotoxicity assays can be performed routinely using the techniques described above, the ability to predict an individual person's normal tissue response to different chemotherapy agents, for example, would be an invaluable tool when designing therapy regimes.

Current studies of transport through the epithelial monolayer and of brush border enzyme regulation rely almost exclusively on cell lines or organ cultures. Confluent layers of polarized primary cultures, able to undergo controlled differentiation, will again provide a valuable investigative tool.

ACKNOWLEDGMENTS

This work was carried out at the Paterson Institute For Cancer Research and funded by the UK Cancer Research Campaign. We also thank Christopher Potten (Manchester), Gareth Evans (Sheffield), Robert Whitehead (Melbourne and Nashville), and the various members of the Epithelial Biology Department who have contributed to this work over the years.

REFERENCES

Booth C, Patel S, Bennion GR, Potten CS (1995): The isolation and culture of adult mouse colonic epithelium. Epithelial Cell Biol 4: 76–86.

Booth C, O'Shea JA, Potten CS (1999): Maintenance of functional stem cells in isolated and cultured intestinal epithelium. Exp Cell Res 249: 359–366.

Evans GS, Flint N, Somers AS, Eyden B, Potten CS (1992): The development of a method for the preparation of rat intestinal epithelial cell primary cultures. J Cell Sci 101: 219–231.

Flint N, Cove FL, Evans GS (1991): A low-temperature method for the isolation of small-intestinal epithelium along the crypt-villus axis. Biochem J 280: 331–334.

Flint N, Pemberton PW, Lobley RW, Evans GS (1994): Cytokeratin expression in epithelial cells isolated from the crypt and villus regions of the rodent small intestine. Epithelial Cell Biol 3: 16–23.

Freshney RI (2000): "Microautoradiography. In Culture of Animal Cells, 2nd ed." New York: John Wiley & Sons, pp 424–429.

Fukamachi H (1992): Proliferation and differentiation of foetal rat intestinal epithelial cells in primary serum free culture. J Cell Sci 103: 511–519.

Hague A, Paraskeva C, (1997): Primary/established cultures of human adenocarcinoma cells. In Doyle A, Griffiths JB, Newall DG (eds): "Cell & Tissue Culture: Laboratory Procedures." New York: John Wiley & Sons, 1: 12C: 1.1–1.9.

Kedinger M, Simon-Assmann P, Lacroix B, Marxer A, Hauri HP, Haffen K (1986): Fetal gut mesenchyme induces differentiation of cultured intestinal endodermal and crypt cells. Dev Biol 113: 474–483.

Moser AR, Dove WF, Roth KA, Gordon JI (1992): The *Min* (multiple intestinal neoplasia) mutation: Its effect on gut epithelial cell differentiation and interaction with a modifier system. J Cell Biol 116: 1517–1526.

Patel HR, Tait, IS, Evans GS, Campbell FC (1996): Influence of cell interactions in a novel model of postnatal mucosal regeneration. Gut 38: 679–686.

Potten CS (1977): Extreme sensitivity of some intestinal crypt cells to X and γ irradiation. Nature 269: 518–521.

Potten CS, Booth C, Chadwick CA, Evans GS (1993): A potent stimulator of small intestinal cell proliferation extracted by simple diffusion from intact irradiated intestine: in vitro studies. Growth Factors 10: 53–61.

Potten CS, Booth C, Pritchard DM (1997): The intestinal epithelial stem cell: The mucosal governor. Int J Exp Pathol 78: 219–243.

Tait IS, Evans GS, Kedinger M, Flint N, Potten CS, Campbell FC (1994a): Progressive morphogenesis in vivo after transplantation of cultured small bowel epithelium. Cell Transplantation 3: 33–40.

Tait IS, Flint N, Campbell FC, Evans GS (1994b): Generation of neomucosa in vivo by transplantation of dissociated rat postnatal small intestinal epithelium. Differentiation 56: 91–100.

Weiser MM (1973): Intestinal epithelial cell surface membrane glycoprotein synthesis. J Biol Chem 248: 2536–2541.

Whitehead RH, Demmler K, Rockman SP, Watson NK (1999): Clonogenic growth of epithelial cells from normal colonic mucosa from both mice and humans. Gastroenterology 117: 858–865.

Yeh KY, Chopra DP (1980): Epithelial cultures derived from the colon of the suckling rat. In Vitro Cell Dev Biol 16: 976–986.

APPENDIX: SOURCES OF MATERIALS

Material	Catalog No.	Supplier
Acutase	AT104	TCS/Upstate Biotechnology
Agar, Bacto	—	Difco (Becton Dickinson)
Agarose, type VII	A9045	Sigma
Collagenase type XI	C9407	Sigma
Crystal Violet	BDH 340245L	Merck
Disodium hydrogen orthophosphate	BDH 30158	Merck
Dispase neutral protease	1284 908	Roche
Dithiothreitol	D5545	Sigma
DMEM, pyruvate free	41965-039	Life Technologies
EDTA	BDH 28026 3E	Merck
EGF	E-4127	Sigma
EGTA	E-0396	Sigma
FBS	Cf018	TCS
Formaldehyde	F1635	Sigma
Gentamicin	G1397	Sigma
Glutaraldehyde	G/0518/pb08	Fisher Scientific
Insulin	Hypurin	CP Pharmaceuticals
Movette pipette	S-40673	GIBCO
NaCl	S7653	Sigma
Pancreatin	P1500	Sigma
Potassium dihydrogen orthophosphate	BDH 10203	Merck
RPMI 1640 medium, 10×	22511	GIBCO
Sodium deoxycholate	D6750	Sigma
Sodium pyruvate	S8636	Sigma
Sorbitol	S1876	Sigma
Streptomycin sulfate	S0890	Sigma
Sucrose	S9378	Sigma
[^{3}H]thymidine	Net 027	NEN Life Sciences
Virkon	cle1554	Scientific Laboratory Supplies
Vitrogen (Bovine dermal collagen)	—	Cohesion

11

Isolation and Culture of Animal and Human Hepatocytes

Christiane Guguen-Guillouzo

INSERM U522, Régulations des Equilibres Fonctionnels du Foie normal et Pathologique, Hôpital Pontchaillou, 35033 Rennes, France.
christiane.guillouzo@rennes.inserm.fr

I. INTRODUCTION

The liver plays a critical role in the organism. It performs numerous important metabolic functions, mainly the regulation of glucose metabolism, the production of plasma proteins including clotting proteins, and the detoxification of endogenous and exogenous compounds. Hence, hepatocyte culture represents (a) a cell model for analyzing the molecular mechanisms involved in common and liver-specific gene regulation of differentiated cells, (b) a simple model system for studying liver diseases, (c) a tool for measuring hepatotoxicity and metabolism of drugs, and (d) a source of cells for therapy and hepatic supplementation.

The liver is a unique organ in its differentiation and proliferation characteristics. During development the liver differentiates in gradual and sequential steps in a process that covers all the periods before and after birth up to weaning and is linked directly to the physiologic needs of organisms [Greengard, 1977]. Another characteristic is that hepatic cells, when they mature, are highly stable and remain alive, in contrast to various other cell types, such as keratinocytes, lipocytes, or enterocytes, that undergo terminal differentiation and die. This results in a low rate of cell renewal that does not exceed 5% of the whole population at the adult stage. However, the main characteristic is the remarkable property of actively producing new cells for restoring the tissue mass after surgical removal or cell loss caused by toxic agents. This cell supply can originate from two main sources, mainly from simple duplication of the remaining hepatocytes or from division and differentiation of stem cells located in the liver [Diehl and Rai, 1996; Lazaro et al., 1998] or outside the liver in peripheral organs [Lagasse et al., 2000; Lamy et al., 2000]. This regenerating process involves distinct environmental signals that induce phenotypic changes in the remaining cells, many genes of which are regulated by complex cellular mechanisms, often reciprocally controlled, such as the genes involved in proliferation, differentiation, and cell death [Thorgeirsson, 1996]. The understanding of these molecular control mechanisms has greatly progressed in the last 10 years. This unique in vivo behavior of liver cells must be considered when establishment or analysis of ex vivo model systems is attempted.

Conditions are currently known, and can be selected appropriately, that allow culture systems to mimic either cell proliferation or highly stable, quiescent mature hepatocyte populations as found in vivo. The other main advance in the recent past concerns the elucidation of the hepatic cell lineage and the possible contribution of stem cells from bone marrow, even at the adult stage, to the liver regeneration program [Fausto, 2000; Theise et al., 2000]. Regardless of cellular origin, these different hepatic lineages converge and fundamental transduction signals are induced in individual cells, which respond by developing cell death or survival programs and then undergoing proliferation or differentiation through activation of cascades of transducing pathways that are common to all cell members constituting the multicellular organ. This emphasizes some hypotheses about the origins of continuous hepatic cell lines. Furthermore, it highlights new strategies for establishing and selecting new cell lines and opens new applications for tissue engineering and cell therapy for treating acute and chronic liver diseases.

This chapter presents protocols and updates data, derived from studies in primary cultures and cell lines, that contribute to the improvement of our understanding of the regulatory processes that control hepatocyte behavior in vitro, enabling these systems to be more representative of the liver in vivo.

2. PREPARATION OF MEDIA AND REAGENTS

2.1. HEPES-Buffered Saline (HBS)

NaCl	160.8 mM
KCl	3.15 mM
$NaHPO_4 \cdot 12H_2O$	0.7 mM
HEPES	33 mM

Adjust to pH 7.65 and sterilize by autoclaving or filtration.

2.2. Collagenase

Collagenase	0.025% (rat liver)
	0.05% (human liver)
$CaCl_2 \cdot 2H_2O$	5 mM

In HBS (see Section 2.1).

Sterilize by filtration and store at $-20°C$.

2.3. Leibowitz L-15 with Bovine Serum Albumin (L-15/BSA)

Leibowitz L-15 medium containing 0.2% bovine serum albumin.

2.4. Hepatocyte Minimal Medium (HMM)

Eagle's MEM   67.5%
Medium 199   22.5%

(or 90% Williams E in place of MEM and medium 199)

FBS   10%
Bovine insulin   5 μg/ml
BSA   1 mg/ml
Pyruvate   20 mM
Penicillin   100 U/ml
Streptomycin   100 μg/ml

2.5. Tris-Buffered Saline (TBS)

	M
NaCl	3.4
Tris·HCl	0.05
EDTA	0.004
N-ethylmaleimide	0.002

Adjust to pH 7.4. When required sterile, sterilize by filtration.

2.6. Buffered Urea

	M
Urea	2.0
Tris·HCl	0.05
NaCl	0.15

Adjust to pH 7.4

2.7. HEPES-Buffered Trypsin (HBT)

Trypsin, 1:250 2.5% in HBS (see Section 2.1)

Adjust to pH 7.65 and sterilize by autoclaving or filtration.

3. CELL PREPARATION AND SUBPOPULATION ISOLATION

In the liver, hepatocytes represent 90% of the whole tissue volume but correspond to only 70% of the total cell population. This cellular heterogeneity has led investigators to devise techniques for obtaining purified hepatocyte populations. However, both short-term survival and poor functional stability have characterized these pure cell populations.

3.1. Liver Dissociation

The two-step in situ collagenase perfusion technique is widely used for disaggregation of the adult rat liver. The method applied in our laboratory is based on that of Seglen [1976] with modifications [Guguen-Guillouzo et al., 1982, 1986].

Protocol 11.1. Disaggregation of Rat Liver by Collagenase Perfusion

Reagents and Materials

Sterile

- ❑ Nembutal
- ❑ Heparin
- ❑ HBS: HEPES-buffered saline, calcium-free (see Section 2.1)
- ❑ Collagenase, 0.025% in HBS containing 5 mM CaCl$_2$ (see Section 2.2)
- ❑ L-15/BSA (see Section 2.3)
- ❑ Growth medium (see Sections 2.4 and 4.1)
- ❑ Winged infusion set syringes
- ❑ Needle, winged infusion set (0.9-mm diam.), connected via silicone tubing to the outlet of a two-way valve, one inlet connected to a reservoir of HBS (see Section 2.1) and the other to collagenase in HBS (see Section 2.2)
- ❑ Gauze: Scrynel NYHC nylon, 60–100 μm (or equivalent Cell-Strainer)

Nonsterile

- ❑ Rats: male, Sprague-Dawley, 150–200 g
- ❑ EtOH, 70%

Protocol

(a) Anesthetize rats by intraperitoneal injection of Nembutal (1.5 ml/kg).
(b) Inject heparin (1000 IU) into the femoral vein.
(c) Swab the underside of the rat with 70% EtOH.

(d) Open the abdomen.

(e) Cannulate the liver via the portal vein and flush with HBS for 15 min at 37°C at a flow rate of 30 ml/min.

(f) Perfuse with collagenase for 15 min at 37°C at a flow rate of 20 ml/min.

(g) At the end of the perfusion, excise the liver and disperse the cells in L-15/BSA.

(h) Allow the disaggregate to sediment at unit gravity for 20 min.

(i) Filter the supernatant cell suspension through gauze.

(j) Wash the filtrate twice with HBS by centrifugation at 50 g for 45 s to remove cell debris, damaged cells, and non-parenchymal cells.

(k) Wash once [by centrifugation as in step (j)] with the culture medium to be used for cell seeding (see Section 4.1).

(l) Check cell yield and viability with trypan blue in a hemocytometer counting chamber. Cell yields range from 4×10^8 to 6×10^8 hepatocytes with a viability often greater than 95%. Very few nonparenchymal cells remain in the final suspension.

This basic two-step perfusion procedure can be used for obtaining viable hepatocytes from various other rodents, including mouse, rabbit, woodchuck, guinea pig, and hamster, as well as from domestic hen, fish, dog, baboon, and human. Livers from the small rodent species such as mouse and hamster, or from 2-week-old rat, are perfused through the portal vein with the washing buffer at a flow rate of 3 ml/min for 10 min and with the collagenase solution (0.025%) at 2 ml/min for 15 min. Cell yields range from 1×10^8 to 1.5×10^8 hepatocytes. For fish like trout or carp, a flow rate of 11–12 ml/min for 30 min at 15°C is used for the first perfusion step and a flow rate of 11–12 ml/min at 20°C for 20 min for the second step with a 0.075% collagenase solution. For the other species mentioned above, the conditions of liver perfusion are the same as those used for human liver and described below.

Well-established techniques have been developed that enable isolation of viable adult human hepatocytes by perfusion either of a lobe of the whole liver or of biopsies [Guguen-Guillouzo et al., 1982]. Whole organs are obtained from kidney donors, whereas liver pieces are resected from patients undergoing partial hepatectomy. In the first case the left lobe is selected, preferentially, and perfusion is generally confined to part of this lobe.

Protocol 11.2. Disaggregation of Human Liver by Collagenase Perfusion

Reagents and Materials

Sterile

- ☐ HBS (see Section 2.1)
- ☐ Collagenase, 0.05% in HBS (see Section 2.2)
- ☐ Pediatric catheter, silicone, 0.5–1.0 mm in diameter
- ☐ Hemostats

Protocol

(a) Immediately after resection, cannulate biopsies through the largest vein with a silicone pediatric catheter and perfuse at a flow rate of 10–20 ml/min, depending on the size of liver pieces. To increase the well-perfused area, insert several catheters so that perfusion goes through several vessels at the same time [Strom et al., 1982].

(b) Wash the liver by perfusing with HBS at 75 ml/min at 37°C for 20 min.

(c) Perfuse with HBS containing 0.05% collagenase and 5 mM $CaCl_2$ at 50 ml/min for 20 min.

(d) Dissociation is improved by clamping the largest vascular orifices.

Cell viability obtained averages 70–90%.

3.2. Separation of Centrilobular and Periportal Hepatocytes

The metabolic heterogeneity of the lobule, closely related to the microcirculatory unit of the liver, results in heterogeneous intralobular distribution of various enzymes including those involved in drug metabolism. To study the basis for the consequences of such metabolic zoning, partial separation of periportal and perivenous hepatocytes has been achieved by careful high-resolution density-gradient centrifugation. By using 15–40% Ficoll density gradients, two types of hepatocytes were separated. The lighter cells were considered to correspond to centrilobular cells and the heavier hepatocytes to cells located in the other regions of the lobule. Problems caused by high osmolality and viscosity that occur with Ficoll can be at least partly overcome by using metrizamide gradients [Bengtsson et al., 1981].

A much better separation of hepatocyte subpopulations according to their intralobular distribution was achieved by Lindros and Penttilä [1985], who developed a high-yield method based on initial selective destruction of one acinar region followed by isolation of the cells from the intact part. This method consists of a selective destruction of periportal or perivenous cells by antegrade or retrograde infusion of digitonin, a cholesterol-complexing agent previously used to destroy plasma membranes for isolation of subcellular organelles. The infusion of digitonin solution (7 mM) is performed at a low infusion rate of 2 ml/min for 75–105 s in antegrade or retrograde direction. After the digitonin solution is washed out in the opposite direction, the dissociation of the intact tissue is always carried out by antegrade perfusion for 10–20 min. The subsequent steps are performed as described for normal liver cell preparation. The combination of a digitonin perfusion and the classic two-step collagenase perfusion results in high-yield production of periportal and perivenous hepatocytes characterized by differences in marker enzyme activities [Schrode et al., 1990] and carbohydrate metabolism [Agius et al., 1990].

Centrifugal elutriation has also been used to separate isolated hepatocytes into subpopulations, for example, according to the degree of ploidy [Le Rumeur et al., 1983].

3.3. Functional Characteristics of Isolated Hepatocytes

3.3.1. Induction of Entry to G_1 Phase and Activation of Cell Death Program

Washing the liver with a Ca^{2+}-free buffer followed by a collagenase treatment results in disruption of cell-cell communications and cell isolation. In 1988, the Guguen-Guillouzo group proposed the hypothesis that hepatocytes undergo the G_0/G_1 transition during the isolation process [Etienne et al., 1988]. This transition is correlated with a sequential expression of immediate-early protooncogenes associated with cell entry into the cell cycle. Expression of *c-fos*, *c-jun*, and *jun-B* is undetectable in normal liver, but rapid induction occurs after a few minutes of washing, increases during collagenase perfusion, and reaches a maximum in freshly isolated cells, whereas *jun-D* and *c*-myc start to be expressed and remains detectable up to attachment and spreading. This transition is now clearly established.

Paralleling these events, one fraction of cells dies during liver perfusion followed by a second fraction during centrifugations while the major part of the remaining population of the suspension gradually progresses to cell death in 4–5 h. It is increasingly evident that most mammalian cell types require complex and ill-defined survival signals to override their natural tendency to undergo programmed cell death [Evan and Littlewood, 1998; Taub, 1998]. Among them, interactions between heterologous cell types appear to be critical. These signals are lost when the architecture of the tissue in vivo is destroyed during collagenase perfusion and when pure hepatocyte populations are selected.

Meanwhile, liver-specific functions expressed by cells at the time of perfusion are present in isolated cells but decline thereafter. The transcription levels of liver-specific genes are representative of those in cells in vivo if cells are collected and analyzed rapidly. The amounts of corresponding mRNAs are very close to those in vivo for around 1 h. Besides protooncogenes, some transcription factors such as c/EBPβ are induced whereas others, like c/EBPα, are extinguished [Greenbaum et al., 1998; Hanson, 1998α.

3.3.2. Similarities with Early Steps of Liver Regeneration

This G_0/G_1 transition mimics well the entry to G_1 of hepatocytes *in vivo* after partial hepatectomy, corresponding to the "priming step" in regeneration [DuBois, 1990; Webber et al., 1994; Fausto, 2000]. Indeed, one hypothesis is that this process of G_1 transition is the consequence of metabolic changes associated with alterations in cell-cell interactions and loss of signals related to the disruption of the extracellular matrix. Liu et al [1994] have shown that the partial degradation of the extracellular matrix in vivo could trigger the G_0/G_1 transition. Moreover, the loss of these signals, which in turn modifies cell survival potency, constitutes a stress.

In addition, this G_0/G_1 transition is controlled by a release of cytokines, mainly tumor necrosis factor (TNF)-α and IL-6 [Diehl et al., 1994; Diehl and Rai, 1996]. TNF-α is promptly produced by liver cells after partial hepatectomy in vivo. A release during liver perfusion is observed as well. It has been reported that after partial hepatectomy, TNF-α activates NF-κB, a transcription factor inactive in quiescent hepatocytes in vivo [FitzGerald et al., 1995] which results in a cascade of induction and translocation to the nucleus that both cause induction of early protooncogenes and entry in G_1.

3.4. Tissue Preservation and Cell Cryopreservation

From these previous observations the need to protect the cells from stress conditions that induce them to rapidly undergo a death program is evident. Cell preservation is important both before perfusion and after isolation. Applications include organs for transplantation and hepatocyte collections for hepatic supplementation.

3.4.1. Liver Preservation

The number of human livers suitable for transplantation or for metabolism research has long been limited by the lack of conditions for extended preservation of the organs from ischemia during storage. Recently, successful transplantations of canine and human livers after 20 h or more of storage in a new solution known as the University of Wisconsin (UW) solution were reported. The UW solution contains lactobionate and raffinose, which are thought to be effective impermeants and to suppress ischemia-induced cellular lesions. The effects of long-term hypothermic storage in UW solution on specific hepatic functions have been further evaluated in our laboratory using rat livers [Guyomard et al., 1990]. Perfusion at 10 ml/min and storage of rat livers for 48 h in cold UW solution before collagenase dissociation showed no major effect of storage on cell viability and functional activities. Studies with human livers have shown that high yields of isolated hepatocytes can also be obtained from organs hypothermically preserved for 10–20 h in UW solution. Such hypothermic storage should reduce, at least in part, individual variations from one donor to another that are due to liver damage.

It is important to note that it is also possible to store cells in UW solution at 0–5°C for a few days after isolation. Unexpectedly, although the UW solution can be successfully used for human hepatocyte storage, cell viability and capacity for further attachment decline faster when isolated rat hepatocytes are stored in cold UW rather than in a culture medium such as Leibovitz L-15 medium [Poullain et al., 1992].

3.4.2. Hepatocyte Cryopreservation

Hepatocytes from UW-preserved or unstored organs can be cryopreserved and further cultured. The protocol established for rat hepatocytes can also be applied to human cells. The choice of the cryoprotectant is critical. DMSO appears to be the most potent cryoprotectant at concentrations ranging between 10 and 20%.

Protocol 11.3. Cryopreservation of Hepatocytes

Reagents and Materials

Sterile

- ❏ L-15/BSA (see Section 2.3)
- ❏ Dimethyl sulfoxide (DMSO)
- ❏ Fetal bovine serum (FBS)
- ❏ Cryopreservation medium: L-15/BSA containing 32% DMSO and 20% FBS
- ❏ L-15 medium containing 0.6 mM L-glucose
- ❏ Cryopreservation vials

Protocol

(a) Suspend cells at 1×10^7/ml in L-15/BSA.

(b) Add an equal volume of cryopreservation medium to give the final concentrations of 16% DMSO and 10% FBS and 5×10^6 cells/ml.

(c) Dispense into 1.2-ml cryopreservation vials.

(d) Keep vials for 20 min at room temperature and then for 15 min at $-20°C$.

(e) Transfer to $-70°C$ for a further 2 h.

(f) Transfer to liquid N_2.

△ *Safety note.* Wear cryoprotective gloves, a face mask, and a closed lab coat when working with liquid nitrogen. Make sure the room is well ventilated to avoid asphyxiation from evaporated nitrogen.

(g) Thawing:

△ *Safety note.* An ampoule that has been stored in liquid nitrogen can inspire liquid nitrogen if not properly sealed. The ampoule will then explode violently when warmed. To protect from potential explosion of ampoules, thaw in a covered container, such as a large plastic bucket with a lid, or store in the vapor phase. Wear gloves, a face mask, and a closed lab coat.

  i) Remove from liquid nitrogen and place at 37°C

  ii) Dilute the cell suspension from one vial in 10 ml L-15 medium containing 0.6 mM L-glucose.

iii) Centrifuge at 100 g for 2–5 min.

iv) Resuspend the pellet in growth medium and seed culture vessel.

Under these conditions 50–60% of the cells survive.

Great improvement has been obtained by immobilizing the cells on microcarriers, by culture on gelatin, or by culturing between two layers of collagen before freezing. Alginate-entrapped human or rat hepatocytes incubated in a culture medium used for suspended cells are currently used by the Guillouzo laboratory for cryopreservation [Guyomard et al., 1996].

It is important to note that in all cases the percentage of viable cells can be greatly improved by using a Percoll cushion. Five milliliters of a cell suspension are layered onto fifteen milliliters of 30% Percoll solution in PBSA and centrifuged at 1000 rpm for 5 min at 4°C. Viable cells are pelleted at the bottom, whereas dead cells are collected at the interface and upper phase.

4. ADVANCES IN EXTENDED PURE HEPATOCYTE CULTURE

4.1. Choice of Basal Medium

Basal media such as RPMI 1640, Eagle's BME, Ham's F12, and Williams E are commonly used. Comparing cell survival and albumin secretion of hepatocytes maintained in RPMI 1640 or Williams E, or in 75% MEM and 25% medium 199, (a medium generally used in our laboratory), only few differences result from choice of the basal medium. However, several indications show that hepatocytes have individual nutrient requirements that greatly influence their behavior in culture, and enrichment of medium with a cocktail of such nutrients and hormonal factors may change cell survival and functions. In that respect, the use of the Landford medium is spectacular [Ferrini et al., 1997]. However, defining unequivocally the role of each component is complex because they act variously on survival, proliferation, or differentiation signals and these signals are reciprocally controlled [Fraser and Evan, 1996; Hueber and Evan, 1998]. In addition, their individual role depends on combination with other nutrients. It is clear that the effects of one amino acid, for instance, depend on the combination of other amino acids present [Li et al., 1995]. Macronutrients such as carbohydrates and amino acids may play a critical role: inclusion of glucose (11 mM), with or without galactose

(11 mM), is important to support growth [Block et al., 1996; Cable and Isom, 1997]. Supplementation with proline (0.26 mM) and glutamine (5 mM), and ornithine (0.6 mM) in addition to the arginine already present, is critical when cells stimulated to proliferate lose part of their differentiated functions, including specific metabolic enzymes such as urea cycle enzymes [Block et al., 1996]. Serum albumin is generally added to the basal medium, and addition of pyruvate significantly increases total protein and DNA syntheses [McGowan et al., 1983].

Trace metal requirements have also been examined. They include Zn^{2+}, Cu^{2+}, and Fe^{2+}. In the presence of EGF and DMSO, they induce quiescent hepatocytes to proliferate, suggesting that these metal ions have a key role in supporting growth [Block et al., 1996; Cable and Isom, 1997]. Conversely, iron depletion in the medium by chelation mediators inhibits DNA synthesis and favors apoptosis [Chenoufi et al., 1998].

Alterations in NaCl and $NaHCO_3$ concentrations can also prolong hepatocyte survival and differentiation. Thus a concentration of bicarbonate decreased from 40 mM to 5 mM significantly reduces cell spreading while favoring cell viability. The whole cell population can be maintained alive for 10–12 days instead of 5 days. Increasing osmolality by adding 50–100 mM additional NaCl also promotes cell survival.

Other factors are important in that they prevent the loss of enzymes involved in drug metabolism. In parallel, they all significantly favor cell viability in keeping the whole population alive at least for 5 days. They include sodium phenobarbital (2–3 mM) [Miyazaki et al., 1998; Morel et al., 1990], clofibrate (0.5–1 mM), isonicotinamide (7.5 mM), and nicotinamide (10–20 mM) [Morel et al., 1990; Mitaka et al., 1996; Paine, 2001]. When added early in culture and at appropriate concentrations, these compounds were found to maintain 75% of the initial P-450 content of hepatocytes cultured for 24 h in Williams E medium. In addition, when added with EGF, nicotinamide sustains DNA synthesis beyond an initial round of replication. Nicotinamide has been found to be an important component in the HGM of Block et al. [Block et al., 1996], where it contributes to sustained division of "proliferating hepatocytes." It seems to be important in facilitating transition from mature to "small" or "proliferating" hepatocytes [Mitaka et al., 1992; Block et al., 1996].

DMSO, a dipolar solvent, is probably one of the most powerful modulators of hepatocyte behavior in vitro. When added at a final concentration of 1.5% or 2% to a serum-free medium on day 1 of culture, in newly established primary cultures, DMSO prolongs hepatocyte survival and greatly preserves cellular functions for more than 1 month [Isom et al., 1987]. Most of the liver-specific functions are well preserved, and the cells remain cuboid and form numerous bile canaliculi. An increased rate of transcription parallels the steady-state mRNA levels. In parallel, it is clearly a growth-inhibitory factor [Mitaka et al., 1993; Cable and Isom, 1997]. However, DMSO now appears to provide one way of sustaining hepatocyte longer-term survival and growth [Mitaka et al., 1993; Tateno and Yoshizato, 1996]. The Michalopoulos group has shown that 2% DMSO reversibly inhibits DNA synthesis in hepatocytes stimulated by EGF or HGF [Kost and Michalopoulos, 1991] and that cycles of DMSO addition and removal in presence of growth factor result in multiple cycles of DNA synthesis. Isom's laboratory also demonstrates a burst of DNA synthesis when DMSO is removed from nonproliferating cultures maintained long term in the presence of DMSO and EGF [Cable and Isom, 1997]. Furthermore, early inclusion of Zn^{2+}, Cu^{2+}, and Fe^{2+} to their medium allows slow proliferation activity over a long period. Therefore, according to the combination of factors and nutrients in the medium, DMSO appears to greatly favor hepatocyte differentiation and survival without totally blocking their proliferation potency.

Another area of study in the last decade has been the involvement of nitric oxide (NO) in the acute-phase response to inflammatory stimuli in culture systems [Curran et al., 1991]. These signals, acting through multiple postreceptor and gene regulatory mechanisms, modulate plasma protein synthesis. NO inhibits the production of the proteins albumin and fibrinogen by limiting protein translation without influencing the quantity of mRNAs. These signals have revealed an intimate association with the modulation of apoptosis and, consequently, with the cell survival potency.

Insulin was found to be beneficial in increasing the percentage of seeded cells that survive and attach, in inducing total de novo protein synthesis, and in regulating many specific functions, particularly lipid and carbohydrate metabolism [Agius et al., 1990]. Insulin has a direct effect on glycogen storage, and this effect is an almost linear function of glucose concentration [Agius and Peak, 1993]. Using distinct signaling pathways and in the absence of other hormones, insulin also causes a transient and monophasic increase of Ca^{2+}. This effect of insulin on cell Ca^{2+} is dependent on the extracellular Ca^{2+} concentration. Its physiologic significance is poorly known and has been associated with the activation of the

MEK/ERK kinase pathway [Benzeroual et al., 1997]. Bovine insulin is generally used at concentrations ranging from 1×10^{-7} to 1×10^{-6} M. HMM contains 5 μg/ml insulin (see Section 2.4).

Corticosteroids have been known for many years to have a dose-dependent beneficial effect on hepatocyte survival and function in vitro [Guguen-Guillouzo, 1986]. They also favor deposition of a fibronectin network that plays a positive role on cell adhesion and spreading. Hydrocortisone hemisuccinate at 1×10^{-7} M induces a permissive effect to, for example, the response to growth factors, whereas, when added alone after cell attachment at a concentration up to 1×10^{-5} M, it greatly improves viability, formation of bile canaliculi, and maintenance of specific functions [Baffet et al., 1982]. Dexamethasone is 10 times more active and, consequently, is used at $1 \times 10^{-7} - 1 \times 10^{-6}$ M.

Protocol 11.4. Extended Primary Culture of Hepatocytes

Reagents and Materials

Sterile

❑ Hepatocyte minimal medium (HMM). (see Section 2.4)
❑ HMM/SF: serum-free HMM supplemented with 1×10^{-5} M hydrocortisone hemisuccinate

Protocol

(a) Suspend isolated hepatocytes in HMM.
(b) After 2–3 h, living cells will attach to plastic and begin to spread. Remove the dead cells with the supernatant medium.
(c) After cell attachment, FBS can be removed, so replace medium with fresh HMM/SF supplemented with hydrocortisone and renew every day thereafter.

When appropriate biomatrix components are used for coating the dish, FBS addition can be avoided completely (see Section 6.3).

4.2. Hepatocyte Behavior

Hepatocytes, seeded on plastic and maintained in pure populations with HMM containing 1×10^{-5} M hydrocortisone, survive for only 1 wk as nonreplicating cell monolayers and contain differentiated hepatocytes as characterized by both morphologic and functional properties. They form typical trabeculae of granular cuboid cells and possess one or two regular rounded nuclei with one or two dark, well-delineated nucleoli. After 1 day, formations of typical bile canaliculi, partly induced by corticosteroids, are easily recognized. However, after 3–4 days, the cells are widespread and lose their characteristic features.

The functional capacities of freshly isolated hepatocytes closely resemble those of in vivo hepatocytes. They are used as references for in vitro analyses. The production of plasma proteins and the expression of specific enzymes involved either in drug metabolism or in glyconeogenesis and/or glycolysis are routinely used as markers. Expression of all these specific properties drastically decreases within the first 3 days of culture [Steward et al., 1985; Guguen-Guillouzo, 1986]. This observation correlates well with the general assumption that liver-specific gene transcription drops following cell isolation [Clayton and Darnell, 1983] and is not restored after hepatocyte aggregation and spreading in culture. Even in the presence of glucocorticoids and insulin, transcription of specific genes fell to 3–10% of that found in vivo, suggesting that these hormones are mainly involved in stabilization of liver-specific mRNAs [Jefferson et al., 1984; Fraslin et al., 1985]. However, their permissive effects when used in combination with other factors makes them crucial for hepatocyte behavior modulation. In the same way, drug metabolism is altered. Cytochrome P-450 (CYP450) levels decrease by approximately 50% during the first 48 h in rodent hepatocytes. In parallel with this decrease of liver-specific functions, fetal CYP isozymes, as well as fetal glutathione-S-transferase (GST) isoforms, multidrug resistance gene products, or fetal isoforms of enzymes involved in glucose metabolism like pyruvate kinase or aldolase, are all significantly increased [Guguen-Guillouzo, 1986; Morel et al., 1990; Fardel et al., 1992; Paine, 2001]. These changes are associated with a shift in transcription factors: decrease of C/EBPα and increase of C/EBPβ [Hanson, 1998; Soriano et al., 1998] and induction of Id1 and Id2 [Le Jossic et al., 1994].

These factors all contribute to modify the differentiation status in close correlation with promotion of responsiveness to growth signals. Cells that have entered G1 during hepatocyte isolation, as mentioned above, do not return to the quiescent G0 status but progress in G1 as indicated by the maintenance of expression of protooncogenes like *myc* and the appearance of Ras, and later, of p53 that confirms location in mid-G1 [Loyer et al., 1996]. However, hepatocyte growth is totally dependent on addition of growth factors.

5. MODULATING FACTORS OF HEPATOCYTE REPLICATION

5.1. Main Growth-Regulating Substances

Growth-regulating substances may act on, or depend on, a variety of synergistic interactions. A great deal has been learned in recent years about the actions and interactions of growth factors and hormones in the stimulation of hepatocyte DNA synthesis. Growth factors such as epidermal growth factor (EGF, 25–50 ng/ml), hepatocyte growth factor (HGF, 10–40 ng/ml), and transforming growth factor (TGF)-α (20 ng/ml) are able to induce the initial round of DNA synthesis. However, maximal activity is reached when they act synergistically with one comitogenic factor [Block et al., 1996, Ilyin et al., 2000]. Thus EGF requires insulin or angiotensin II for maximal DNA synthesis stimulation (about 8-fold instead of 2-fold). Numerous factors are secreted by the nonparenchymal cells present in the liver. This paracrine mechanism can be further studied in vitro by using purified populations of nonparenchymal cells seeded in filter wells.

The role of intermediary metabolites in promoting hepatocyte DNA synthesis has also been widely demonstrated. Supplementation with 20 mM pyruvate enhances, by a factor of two, the growth-stimulating activity of HMM containing EGF. It also promotes the synthesis of specific proteins like albumin. Lactate is as active as pyruvate in stimulating hepatocyte DNA synthesis.

Growth factors other than EGF, HGF, and TGF-α have been shown to stimulate hepatocyte DNA synthesis; these include cytokines such as IL-6 and TNF-α [Webber et al., 1998]. As mentioned above, such factors "prime" cells to enter G1. Recent work suggests that TNF-α, for instance, may be mitogenic only in combination with serum or growth factors.

5.2. Early Antagonism Between Growth Signals and Apoptotic Reaction

Hepatocytes cultured in HMM cannot wait more than 2–3 days without a mitogenic signal provided by addition of growth factor. Indeed, this growth factor also provides survival signals without which cells soon undergo programmed cell death. This death program is associated with early activation of apical caspases and later with induction and activation of executioner caspases such as caspase 3 [Feldmann, 1997].

The short life span of cells in absence of growth factor could, at least in part, be explained by the "dual signal" hypothesis

[Evan and Littlewood, 1998]. This proposes that proliferation and cell death are coupled and that the apoptotic program, unless forestalled by a survival signal, precipitates cell suicide. Substantial evidence from other models suggests that different genes including c-*myc*, *ras*, and p53 can participate in this dual control. The Evan group's observations support the conclusion that expression of *ras*, for instance, located in mid-G1 may antagonize the apoptotic signal mediated by the MYC protein [Hueber and Evan, 1998]. Interestingly, these two genes are expressed in G1 in cultured hepatocytes [Loyer et al., 1996].

Intriguingly, in the absence of growth factor, hepatocytes are able to spread and then to progress up to the restriction point (R-point) at which they remain blocked and die [Loyer et al., 1996]. In the presence of growth factor, additional and distinct morphogenic changes occur. The Guguen-Guillouzo group has recently shown that EGF plays a double role in regulation that strikingly controls the decision of cells to progress to S phase in a sequential manner [Rescan et al., 2001]. One role is related to a morphogen signal located in early G1 that regulates changes of cell shape. Unexpectedly, this morphogen signal also induces a cell survival signal through reciprocal regulating mechanisms. They result in inducing specific transduction signals mainly mediating the MEK/ERK signaling pathway but also the PI3 kinase pathway, which never appear without mitogen. The other role in regulation is related to the mitogen signal that controls cell progression to late G1 at the R-point located in mid-late G1 [Talarmin et al., 1999]. In this respect, hepatocytes share similarities with many other cell types. In addition, this mitogenic signal also appears to induce another survival signal after the R-point, partly through a distinct transducing pathway [Rescan et al., 2001], allowing the living cells to progress further up to the transition G1/S.

5.3. Overriding the R-Point, Progression up to Mitosis, and Completion of the Cell Cycle

The mitogen-dependent MAP kinase pathway activation also occurs in vivo 10–12 h after partial hepatectomy in rats [Talarmin et al., 1999]. Interestingly, hepatocytes isolated from rats early after partial hepatectomy, that is, before 10–12 h after the operation, corresponding to the R-point, cannot undergo DNA synthesis without addition of EGF to the cultures, whereas cells isolated after 12 h after the operation are becoming independent of any growth factor and spontaneously progress to DNA synthesis. This clearly illustrates the crucial role of the MEK/ERK kinase pathway activation in overriding the R-point in mid-late G1.

A large number of proteins involved in the cell cycle have been identified. Of those characterized to date, the cyclin-dependent serine/threonine kinases (CDKs) and their cyclin partners play a crucial role in controlling the progression through a series of checkpoints during the cell cycle. Cyclin D1 is a cyclin that acts in mid-late G1. Its accumulation after growth factor stimulation is mainly mediated by the induction of the MEK/ERK kinase pathway. This cyclin is essential. However, recent data have shown that its presence is not sufficient to irreversibly program hepatocytes to S phase [Rescan et al., 2001].

Cyclin A is a cell cycle regulatory protein that acts in S and mitotic phases. Inhibition of its expression blocks cell cycle progression, whereas over-expression advances entry to S phase in hepatocytes [Zindy et al., 1992]. As a characteristic of these cells, CDK1 induction strictly correlates with cyclin A induction at the G1/S transition, making CDK1 a specific marker of entry to S phase in these cells in vitro as well as in vivo [Loyer et al., 1994].

Hepatocytes with different ploidy status (diploid, binuclear, and tetraploid cells) are present in cultures from rat and human. For example, after EGF stimulation, one-half of the mitoses are of the binucleated type in cultures from rat, causing one-third of the postmitotic cells to become binuclear. Furthermore, morphologic observations of 1-wk-old rat hepatocytes reveals a significant fraction of multinuclear cells. This increased ploidy level in culture could account for the limited growth capacity of hepatocytes [Mitaka et al., 1992; Seglen et al., 1997]. The mechanism that controls this ploidy is poorly understood at present and is likely to involve a deregulation of mitosis control molecules such as polo-like kinases [Nigg, 1998] and/or cytokinesis regulators, which may account for hepatocyte growth arrest.

5.4. Modulation of Growth Activity

Because of their gradual progression up to mid-late G1 and their dependence on the environment providing survival signals, growth activity of hepatocytes is clearly associated with the time at which the growth factor is added to the medium. There is a "window" covering approximately the first half of G1, during which cells may wait for survival signals and after which they have irreversibly engaged a cell death program [Ilyin et al., 2000]. In addition, it may be expected that providing growth factor early to newly established primary cultures would induce survival signals through specific transduction pathways that would irreversibly program the cells to continue their progression through the cell cycle when blocking signals are raised and conditions are appropriate. This would explain the modulation of growth arrest and activation obtained in long-term cultured hepatocytes after addition and removal of DMSO in the presence of a growth factor [Kost and Michalopoulos, 1991]. Another example is provided by the low proliferation activity observed in hepatocytes cultured in the collagen-sandwich configuration in the continuous presence of growth factor [Hansen and Albrecht, 1999], although late addition of the mitogen to this model system fails to induce cell growth and instead causes cell death [De Smet et al., 2001]. Addition of inhibitory factors such as TGF-β (5 ng/ml), TNF-α, used alone, or interferon (IFN)-γ may exert a negative effect on hepatocyte growth [Bour et al., 1996; Kano et al., 1997; Nishikawa et al., 1998].

Finally, it is important to note that plating density may also modulate hepatocyte responsiveness to growth factors. The nature of the regulating mechanisms is probably complex. Indeed, the importance of cell plating at low density has been demonstrated by many authors [Nakamura et al., 1983; Mesnil et al., 1987]. However, plating at moderate density instead of low density has been reported to be better, suggesting that cell-cell contacts might be important. In culture systems involving more complex combinations of hepatocytes, nonparenchymal cells, and extracellular matrix, hepatocytes can proliferate to form multilayers where close contact between cells does not block growth [Michalopoulos et al., 1999]. Furthermore, the combination of nutrients in the medium of these systems adds another level of complexity [Greuet et al., 1997].

6. MODULATION OF HEPATOCYTE DIFFERENTIATION

Except for DMSO, no soluble factor has been found to be sufficient to maintain well-differentiated hepatocytes beyond a few days. This implies a role for environmental factors, such as cell and matrix interaction, in the preservation of the hepatocyte-differentiated phenotype in vitro [Ben-Ze'ev et al., 1985]. Participation of proximal and/or contacting cells in the control of development and differentiation of various tissues, including liver, is now well established. The role of different types of cells, particularly mesodermal cells, on epithelial cell maturation has been widely demonstrated for many tissues including liver [Houssaint,

1980]. These interactions can process through the production of extracellular matrix components, and this property has been successfully used in culture.

6.1. Role of Soluble Factors in Differentiation

DMSO is one of the most efficient differentiation factors. Added at the concentration of 1.5–2% to newly established primary cultures, DMSO induces a long-term stability (several weeks) of nearly complete differentiation potential. In particular, detoxification metabolism, which involves several specific isoenzymes, is very well maintained. However, in parallel, DMSO induces a high level of protection against apoptosis that may mask, as in vivo, the effects of toxic agents [Bruck et al., 1999]. In the course of this induction, proliferation is reversibly blocked [Isom et al., 1987; Tateno and Yoshizato, 1996]. As mentioned above, DMSO does not totally block proliferation of large or small hepatocytes present in primary cultures, given the presence of an appropriate combination of growth factors and nutrients [Cable and Isom, 1997; Kost and Michalopoulos, 1991]. This clearly illustrates the reciprocal controls between proliferation, differentiation, and death.

Sodium butyrate (5 mM) also induces differentiation in rat hepatocyte cultures. Prevention of the increase in γ-glutamyl transpeptidase with time in culture has been reported. Various cytokines may influence the expression of CYP isoforms [Abdel-Razzak et al., 1993]. However, supplementation of the culture medium or modification of the substratum, reported by several groups to prevent the loss of the different CYP forms content, may only retard this loss of total hepatic CYP content but never maintain their concentration at the same level as found in the initial tissue [Paine, 2001].

6.2. Hepatocytes on Extracellular Matrix Components

Various matrix components are found in the liver. They include several collagens (types I, III, IV, V, and VI), noncollagenous glycoproteins (e.g., fibronectin and laminin), and heparan sulfate proteoglycan [Clement et al., 1986]. This probably explains why these different components influence hepatocytes in culture [Bissell et al., 1987; Spray et al., 1987; Caron, 1990]. When the cells are plated in plastic dishes coated with a collagen or fibronectin film, attachment efficiency, cell spreading, and survival of the cultures are all significantly increased. However, these conditions do not markedly delay the occurrence of phenotypic changes. In contrast, the fundamental observation that functional potencies are closely related to the preservation of the cuboid cell shape has led investigators to define conditions that limit cell spreading and restore the specific compartments of the plasma membranes. Assays done by culturing hepatocytes between two layers of type I collagen have shown that in such a sandwich configuration hepatocytes restore their polarity and maintain a high albumin secretion for a prolonged period [Dunn et al., 1989] and enhanced hepatocyte function [Lee et al., 1993]. Interestingly, we have recently shown that, in this system, hepatocytes are blocked in G1 and express the MYC protein (De Smet et al., 2001).

A complex connective tissue biomatrix, isolated from the liver and used with a cocktail of hormones, has also been used to prolong the functional stability of hepatocytes in culture [Enat et al., 1984]. However, probably the main advance in the field was the use of a laminin-rich gel matrix called Matrigel, obtained from the solid EHS sarcoma tumor (see Section 6.3), as a substrate [Bissell et al., 1987]. The cells plated on this gel retain a spherical shape and mimic reconstruction of matrix geometry by organizing cell aggregates. They exhibit remarkably enhanced expression of many liver-specific functions for several weeks. These include plasma proteins but also enzymes involved in drug metabolism and glycogen metabolism with activation of the transcriptional machinery that occurs in parallel [Guzelian et al., 1988; Caron, 1990]. Meanwhile, the mitogenic response to growth factors is blocked [Gardner et al., 1996], illustrating the reciprocal control of growth and differentiation. The adequacy of this model has been illustrated for long-term studies of physiologic processes such as the acute-phase response [Bader et al., 1992]. Data argue for a critical role of laminin [Caron, 1990]. However, it is important to note that although Matrigel is very rich in laminin, it contains other extracellular components such as collagen IV and heparan sulfate proteoglycan. Moreover, growth factors might also be present, particularly TGF-β. This heterogeneity, to some extent, hampers rapid progress in the understanding of the mechanisms involved in the induction effect [Vukicevic et al., 1992].

6.3. Protocols for Preparation and Strategy for Use of Matrix Components

6.3.1. Preparation of Biomatrix Components

Fibronectin is prepared from human plasma by affinity chromatography on a gelatin Sepharose-4B column, using the high affinity of this protein to gelatin (40 mg gelatin bind 20 mg fibronectin). Collagens can be prepared in either native or truncated forms. Their biological properties may vary accordingly. The following protocols only concern extraction of native molecules. Collagens I and IV are routinely prepared at the concentration of approximately 500 μg/ml in 0.5 M acetic acid either from rat tails (type I) or from placenta and Matrigel (type IV). Collagen IV is extracted with 2 M guanidinium/HCl and 0.002 M dithiothreitol in the saline buffer, followed by purification on a DEAE-cellulose column in 2 M urea. Matrigel is prepared from the Engelbreth-Holm-Swarm (EHS) sarcoma tumor propagated into C57 BL/6 mice [Orkin et al., 1977].

Protocol 11.5. Preparation of Matrigel-like Extract from EHS Sarcoma

Reagents and Materials

Sterile

❑ TBS (see Section 2.5)
❑ PBSA

Nonsterile

❑ TBS
❑ Chloroform
❑ Buffered urea (see Section 2.6)

Protocol

(a) Extract the tumor by homogenization in TBS
(b) Centrifuge at 10,000 g for 30 min at 4°C.
(c) Wash pellet twice in TBS by centrifugation.
(d) Extract matrix by two overnight incubations in 2 M urea prepared in buffered urea.
(e) Centrifuge the extract at 10,000 g for 10 min.
(f) Dialyze the supernatant extract against TBS.
(g) Sterilize the extract with chloroform (0.5%).
(h) Dialyze extensively against sterile TBS.
(i) Dialyze against sterile PBSA.
(j) EHS matrix contains ~10 mg of proteins per 1 ml.
(k) Store at −20°C.

Collagen IV, laminin-entactin, and heparan sulfate proteoglycan can be extracted from EHS tumor matrix.

6.3.2. Matrix Coating with EHS Matrix Extracts and Other Matrix Constituents

Protocol 11.6. Matrix Coating for Hepatocytes

Depending on the strategy selected, these different extracellular matrix components can be used either as a thick gel film for coating dishes or in solution. When they are chosen only for their properties as adhesion factors, to favor attachment and establishment of cells in culture, thick-coating gels are preferred.

Protocol

Fibronectin gel

(a) Add fibronectin to dish at a final concentration of 40–50 μg/ml and allow to stick to the plastic.
(b) After 2 h, remove the buffer gently and allow the dish to dry.
(c) A dry film is obtained within 2 h.
(d) Wash three times in PBSA.
(e) Sterilize under UV.

Collagen gel [adapted from Dunn et al., 1989]

(a) Increase molarity with 10-fold dilution of 10× MEM or RPMI 1640 enriched with 1 mg/ml BSA and adjust the pH of the solution (~pH 4.0 as prepared) to 7.4 with 1 N NaOH. For Petri dishes of 10-cm diameter, mix 5 ml of the collagen solution with 1.4 ml of 10× medium solution containing 0.34 M NaOH at pH 8.5.
(b) Transfer to the dish.
(c) Formation of the gel occurs at room temperature, but it is faster at 37°C. A dry film is obtained within 4–6 h.
(d) Wash three times with culture medium before use.

EHS Matrix or Matrigel™

(a) Use 400–500 μg of EHS matrix or Matrigel to coat 3.5-cm dishes. Coating is performed at 4°C to delay gel formation.
(b) Incubate for 30-min at 37°C to produce a dry film ready for cell seeding. It is very important to note that regular addition of EHS matrix or Matrigel to the culture medium is needed to keep a high level of cellular functional activity after 1 wk of culture.

Protocol 11.7. Extracellular Matrix Components Used in Solution

Another strategy is to use the different extracellular matrix components to analyze their role in hepatocyte behavior and to study their mechanisms of action. For this purpose they are added at low concentrations and in solution.

Protocol

(a) Seed hepatocytes in serum-free defined medium (e.g., HMM/SF) in untreated bacterial grade plastic dishes precoated with either a thin gel of EHS matrix or Matrigel (see Protocol 11.6) or any of the purified components according to the purpose of the experiment.

(b) Prepare a wet gel of EHS matrix or Matrigel:
  i) Add 2 μg/ml EHS matrix or Matrigel, or other purified matrix components, to HMM/SF medium.
  ii) Incubate in a water-saturated atmosphere for 2 h at 37°C.
  iii) Incubate the gel for 30 min with 3% BSA to lower the risks of nonspecific reactions. For the same reason, the culture medium subsequently used also contains 0.02% bovine albumin.

(c) Add the factors under study daily thereafter at the appropriate concentrations. A maximum effect is generally observed at ~2 μg/ml of protein.

7. ROLE OF CELL COMMUNICATION

The advantages of coculturing hepatocytes with other cell types are obvious. Besides the fact that it represents a means for getting highly stable long-term hepatocyte cultures, it offers the capacity to mimic a more physiologic environment that should make possible a better understanding of the role of cell-cell interactions in differentiation of liver tissue. Major progress was made by using untransformed epithelial cells presumably derived from primitive biliary cells [Williams et al., 1971; Tsao et al., 1984; Guguen-Guillouzo et al., 1983, 1986]. This model system requires that the epithelial cells are untransformed. This has led some workers to study the suitability of using permanent nonhepatic cell lines, which are easy to grow and stable in their phenotype, including 3T3 cells [Kuri-Harcuch and Mendoza-Figueroa, 1989; Donato et al., 1990].

7.1. Hepatocytes in Coculture with Rat Liver Epithelial Cells (RLEC)

When cocultured with RLEC, hepatocytes from various species including human, and from adult or fetus [Fraslin et al., 1985;

Guguen-Guillouzo, 1986], survive for several weeks and retain high functional capacities. Among the functions preserved are production of plasma proteins, CYP-450 content, metabolism of drugs by phase I and phase II reactions [Vandenberghe et al., 1990; Akrawi et al., 1993], taurocholate uptake, and metabolism of glycogen [Agius, 1988]. Furthermore, the reappearance of fetal-like functions is observed, although DNA synthesis is almost absent throughout the culture period. In contrast to the functioning of hepatocytes maintained in a serum-free hormonally defined medium, hepatocytes cocultured with RLEC retain the capability of transcribing specific genes at a rate identical to that found in DMSO-treated cells and in cells seeded on Matrigel [Fraslin et al., 1985]. In addition, the coculture system with RLEC possesses specific characteristics [Corlu et al., 1997]:

(i) It provides direct cell-cell contacts and thus represents a useful tool for analyzing intercellular communication.

(ii) It involves contacts between parenchymal and nonparenchymal cells through the mediation of recognition signals among which a plasma membrane protein, LRP, plays a critical role [Corlu et al., 1991].

(iii) There is a spontaneous early production and deposition of extracellular matrix components that reflects the composition of the hepatic extracellular matrix, including collagens I, III, and IV, fibronectin, laminin, and heparan sulfate proteoglycan.

(iv) Addition of corticosteroids to the culture medium is required to obtain the "coculture effect," indicating that some soluble factors are also essential in this model [Baffet et al., 1982].

Protocol 11.8. Isolation of Rat Liver Epithelial Cells (RLEC)

RLEC are isolated by trypsinization of 10-day-old rat livers according to Williams et al. [1971].

Reagents and Materials

Sterile

❑ HEPES-buffered trypsin solution (0.25%) (HBT, see Section 2.7)
❑ PBSA
❑ Williams E medium

Protocol

(a) Incubate finely chopped fragments of liver for 15 min in HBT.
(b) Wash twice in PBSA.
(c) Eliminate contaminating fibroblastic cells by taking advantage of their faster attachment to the plastic dish:
  i) Seed dish
  ii) Collect the supernatant with unattached cells 20 min after seeding and seed into another dish.
  iii) Repeat step (ii) three times so that the third and fourth dishes mainly contain epithelial cells.
(d) Feed with Williams E medium supplemented with 5–10% FBS. This medium is essential for active epithelial cell growth; the cells are maintained by serial subcultures in this medium.

It is important to note that these cells are very sensitive to culture conditions, particularly to different serum batches. When carefully cultivated they are stable for up to 100 passages. Otherwise, they spontaneously undergo transformation associated with a gradual loss of cell contact inhibition at confluence and a change of adhesion properties (increased sensitivity to calcium), both of which hamper further use in coculture.

Protocol 11.9. Establishment of Cocultures of Hepatocytes with RLEC

Reagents and Materials

Sterile

❑ Serum-supplemented HMM (see Section 2.4)
❑ Petri dishes, 3.5 cm

Protocol

(a) Plate 8×10^5 hepatocytes in 2 ml 10% serum-supplemented HMM in 3.5-cm Petri dishes.
(b) Remove the medium containing unattached cells 3 h later.
(c) Seed 1×10^6 RLEC per dish in fresh medium to reach confluence with hepatocyte colonies within 24 h. RLEC stop dividing when they reach confluence with hepatocytes.
(d) At confluence, renew the medium with HMM supplemented with 3.5×10^{-6} M hydrocortisone hemisuccinate, with or without FBS, and replace every day.

It is also possible to seed hepatocytes onto a preexisting confluent epithelial cell monolayer. For biochemical assays, hepatocytes must be selectively detached from RLEC by incubation in a calcium-free HEPES-buffered collagenase solution (0.075%) (pH 7.6) for 10 min at 37°C followed by energetic pipetting.

7.2. Hepatocytes in Coculture with Nonepithelial Types of Liver Cells (NPC)

The influence of purified sinusoidal endothelial cells on hepatocyte functional stability, in the presence of corticoids, has been demonstrated, and Ito cells have been found to cooperate with hepatocytes in the deposition of an extracellular matrix [Loreal et al., 1993].

An interesting model [Landry et al., 1985] is the spheroidal aggregate culture of rat liver cells. Construction of hepatic organoids by rat small hepatocytes and hepatic nonparenchymal cells has also been described more recently [Mitaka et al., 1999]. In these systems, hepatocytes, which are mixed with different types of liver cells, preserve their typical organization, secrete an extracellular matrix, and maintain high functional stability. Although very complex, these model systems are useful for analyzing the critical role of interactions of various types of liver cells on hepatocyte differentiation under three-dimensional culture conditions.

Block and colleagues have reported focal growth of fibroblastic cells that favors differentiation of adjacent hepatocytes [Block et al., 1996]. The Bissell group had previously demonstrated that these cells mostly derive from hepatic stellate cells present in the initial population [Mahler et al., 1988]. There is presumably a major contribution of these stellate cells and other cells to deposition of extracellular matrix and also production of cytokines that play a critical role on growth and differentiation [Tateno and Yoshizato, 1998].

Matrigel overlay favors hepatocyte differentiation and growth arrest. However, in the more complex three-dimensional model used by the Michalopoulos group [Michalopoulos et al., 1999] in which hepatocytes and nonparenchymal cells are mixed and synthesize an extracellular biomatrix network, active proliferation can be observed even when Matrigel is added to the culture.

7.3. Coculture with Nonhepatic Fibroblastic Cells

Another approach has been to analyze the suitability of using permanent nonhepatic cell lines. Cocultures of hepatocytes with mouse fibroblastic 3T3 cells have been successfully tested [Kuri-Harcuch and Mendoza-Figueroa, 1989]. Both NIH 3T3 cells and 3T3-J2 cells, used as a feeder layer for keratinocytes, induce a coculture effect, and we have verified that the latter cells are much more efficient (unpublished data). Fibroblastic cells from C_3H mice have also been reported to support cocultures of hepatocytes [Donato et al., 1990]. A very interesting observation is the possibility of efficiently coculturing hepatocytes on a layer of stromal cells coming from bone marrow or thymus [Corlu et al., 1997]. This observation has been associated with the expression of the LRP protein, also involved in the RLEC coculture system.

Although these systems are potentially interesting, they suffer at the present time from two major limitations: one is the overgrowth of the cells that gradually cover the hepatocyte colonies after 4–5 days of culture; the second is the great difficulty encountered in selectively collecting hepatocytes from the feeder cells, which is obviously a prerequisite for all biochemical and molecular studies requiring quantitative measurements.

8. PERMANENT DIFFERENTIATED HEPATIC CELL LINES

An alternative to primary culture systems, which all fail to support hepatocyte stability longer than 1 or 2 months, is the use of permanent cell lines. Hepatoma cell lines from primitive tumors are very useful when they constitutively express specific markers. Two main categories can be distinguished: (i) cell lines derived from tumors and (ii) experimentally immortalized cell lines obtained by gene transfer.

8.1. Cell Lines Derived from Tumors

8.1.1. Numerous Variations from One Line to the Other

Several lines derived from hepatocarcinoma have been reported. The population is generally composed of epithelioid cells at confluence, characterized by (i) abnormal karyotype with few or numerous genetic disorders, (ii) a high capacity to proliferate compared to normal hepatocytes, and (iii) ability or inability to undergo a process of differentiation in a few days after reaching confluence. The choice of using one line should take account of these characteristics and, principally, the ability to perform a complete differentiation program. In that respect, three main categories of lines can be distinguished:

(i) *Lines that fail to express at least one liver specific marker.* Cell lines such as BRL-1, RLEC [Williams et al., 1971], HTC [Martin and Tomkins, 1970], and WB-F344 [Tsao et al., 1984] from rat but also PLC/PRFs or Alexander line [Marion et al., 1979] from human origin can be placed in this category;

(ii) *Lines that differentiate at confluence but rapidly detach.* Most lines belong to this category. They express albumin, transferrin, and α-fetoprotein particularly in lines derived from hepatoblastoma, such as HepG2 [Knowles et al., 1980], Hep3B, or HuH7 [Nakabayashi et al., 1984]. Functions that are maintained in only a few lines are those generally occurring in late stages during liver maturation program in vivo [Greengard, 1977]. They include expression of specific CYP isoforms and isozymes characteristic of the hepatic metabolism of glucose, lipids, and drugs. Because cells continuously detach, part of the population is dividing and most cells have no time to undergo a complete differentiation program. FAO cells from rat or HuH7 from human origin belong to this category;

(iii) *The few lines that are able to undergo a high level of differentiation.* These are characterized by a long-term survival and functional stability at confluence, allowing them to express numerous hepatocyte functions including drug metabolism. This differentiated status is accompanied by important morphologic changes leading the cells to restore a polarity corresponding to the reorganization of functional bile canaliculi. The clones Faza 967 and Fu55 from the Reuber rat hepatoma [Deschatrette and Weiss, 1974; Pitot et al., 1964] and the clones BC1 and BC2 from the HBG line belong to this category [Glaise et al., 1998; Le Jossic et al., 1996; Gomez-Lechon et al., 2001].

8.1.2. Diversity of the Origin of the Cells and Selection Methods

The origin and the functional status of the cells from which a line has derived greatly determine the physiologic characteristics of this line. For instance, the lines derived from hepatoblastoma express fetal markers at a higher frequency than the others. In general, differences from one line to another are due to the genetic accidents responsible for the development of the tumor, to the stage in the tumor progression at the time of surgical operation and cell collection, and to the cell selection method. Complexity is increased by the fact that possible hepatocyte precursors are not very well established [Thorgeirsson, 1996; Lazaro et al., 1998]. Schematically, it may be postulated that the lines belonging to the first group described above could derive from "stemlike" oval cells. Indeed, they sometimes are able to undergo differentiation when injected into syngeneic animals [Coleman et al., 1993]. In contrast, highly differentiated cell lines could derive from cells already engaged in the hepatocytic differentiation lineage, that is, from hepatoblasts [Kitten and Ferry, 1998].

It is important to note that maintenance of the differentiation potential of a line is not easy and requires regular cell recloning by using selective medium and/or unicellular dilution. Improvement of the functional stability can be obtained by culturing the cells in the presence of hormones and nutrients known to favor differentiation of normal hepatocytes. Although abnormal, these cells provide extremely interesting models for studying hepatocyte biology, mainly the molecular regulation of the successive cycles of differentiation and proliferation and reversibility of these phenomena. They often represent unique tools for studying hepatic diseases related to carcinogenesis, parasitology, and virology. They are also very useful in pharmacology for selecting new drugs.

8.2. Strategies for Establishing New Immortalized Cell Lines

Several technical approaches have been tested. The following are among those most frequently used:

(i) *Hybridization between normal and transformed cells.* Hybrids have been obtained between mouse hepatocytes and fibroblasts [Szpirer et al., 1980] and between human fibroblasts and rat hepatoma cells. The WIF-B9 obtained by this protocol is particularly interesting because of the biliary polarity restored in these cells [Decaens et al., 1996].

(ii) *Infection of hepatocytes by viruses such as SV40 or transfection of genes coding viral proteins such as SV40 LT [Pfeifer et al., 1993].* A high immortalization efficacy is observed. However, the selected lines are generally poorly differentiated and extremely unstable.

(iii) *Creation of transgenic animals that harbor transgene constructs often carrying oncogenes and chosen for targeting their expression in the liver, thus leading to hepatocarcinoma development [Paul et al., 1988].* The limits of this approach include (a) poor stability of the lines, except when cells are derived early from young animals before carcinoma development, (b) the uncertainty in the origin of the selected cells, and (c) the inability to apply this technique for establishing human cell lines.

(iv) New strategies are in progress to immortalize normal hepatocytes by targeting genes that play critical roles in cell death or proliferation programs and by using constructs allowing reversible stimulation of these target genes. Such a strategy has been used efficiently for immortalizing human fibroblasts [Littlewood et al., 1995; Hahn et al., 1999].

Obtaining untransformed proliferating hepatocytes should provide a source of subnormal cells for expansion in bioreactors that would be useful for several applications.

9. CONCLUSIONS

Although this review cannot cover all the developments related to hepatic cells in vitro, it does show the richness and the diversity of the models of normal and immortalized hepatocytes existing today. In addition, it illustrates the substantial progress, acquired over the last few years, in the understanding of hepatocyte behavior in vitro. This owes much to the improvement in our understanding of the mechanisms that control the biological events essential for the choice between cell death or survival and between proliferation or differentiation (Fig. 11.1), including the reciprocal induction or inhibition of transducing pathways related to these signals. Two main consequences may be listed:

(i) The development of model systems in which normal hepatocytes are able to undergo several rounds of division separated by periods of quiescence; these models are immediately available. This opens new fields of investigation for establishing improved hepatocytic models with higher capacity of proliferation by combining the appropriate inducers.

(ii) The possibility to make the most appropriate choice between the different models according to the expected applications.

Furthermore, new perspectives can be drawn for the near future, mainly, the development and selection of new lines of immortalized hepatocytes by using more appropriate and powerful selective controls and differentiating agents and/or the development of

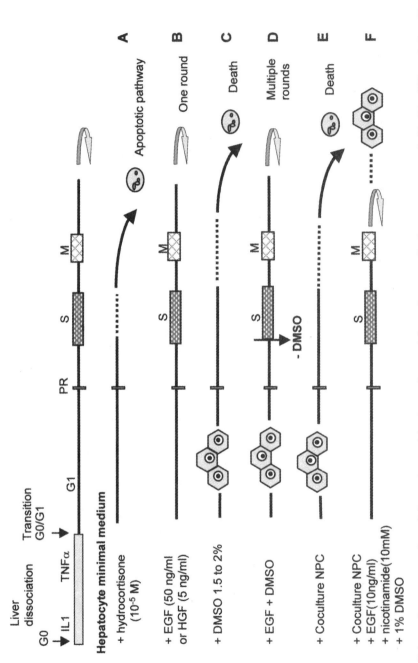

Fig 11.1. Schematic representation of the main combinations of essential requirements for hepatocyte growth (B, D), differentiation (A, C, E), or growth and differentiation (D, F) on simple substrata conditions. NPC, nonparenchymal liver cells.

human immortalized hepatocytes by stably and reversibly transfecting target genes for proliferation and survival. All these new differentiating lines would be useful not only for applications in pharmacology and toxicology but also in virology and development of new cancer therapies. They might well represent a major interest as tools for setting large-scale screenings of new target gene products and/or new drugs.

However, the main challenges for the next few years are certainly associated with hematopoietic stem cells. In 1998, Corlu provided evidence that culturing hepatocytes in an environment of bone marrow stromal cells and, conversely, coculturing hematopoietic progenitors with an hepatic parenchymal cell layer resulted in induction of hematopoietic and hepatic maturation, respectively [Corlu et al., 1998; Lamy et al., 1997; Rialland et al., 2000]. Several recent exciting demonstrations have reported the ability of hematopoietic stem cells from bone marrow to differentiate into hepatocytes and to repopulate the liver [Lagasse et al., 2000; Theise et al., 2000], suggesting a potential role for circulating hematopoietic progenitor cells in liver tissue homeostasis. This opens promising future prospects such as ex vivo liver organogenesis from embryonic stem cells and/or a source of human hepatocytes from hematopoietic stem cells. Expertise in manipulating these models will be very useful for several applications, many related to cell therapy, particularly for treating hepatocellular insufficiencies or metabolic disorders.

REFERENCES

Abdel-Razzak Z, Loyer P, Fautrel A, Gautier JC, Corcos L, Turlin B, Beaune P, Guillouzo A (1993): Cytokines down-regulate expression of major cytochrome P-450 enzyme in adult human hepatocytes in primary culture. Mol Pharmacol 44: 707–715.

Agius L (1988): Metabolic interactions of parenchymal hepatocytes and dividing epithelial cells in co-culture. Biochem J 252: 23–28.

Agius L, Peak M, Alberti KG (1990): Regulation of glycogen synthesis from glucose and gluconeogenic precursors by insulin in periportal and perivenous rat hepatocytes. Biochem J 266: 91–102.

Agius L, Peak M (1993): Intracellular binding of glucokinase in hepatocytes and translocation by glucose, fructose and insulin. Biochem J 296: 785–796.

Akrawi M, Rogiers V, Vandenberghe Y, Palmer CN, Vercruysse A, Shephard EA, Phillips IR (1993): Maintenance and induction in co-cultured rat hepatocytes of components of the cytochrome P450-mediated mono-oxygenase. Biochem Pharmacol 45: 1583–1591.

Bader A, Rinkes IH, Closs EI, Ryan CM, Toner M, Cunningham JM, Tompkins RG, Yarmush ML (1992): A stable long-term hepatocyte culture system for studies of physiologic processes: Cytokine stimulation of the acute phase response in rat and human hepatocytes. Biotechnol Prog 8: 219–225.

Baffet G, Clement B, Glaise D, Guillouzo A, Guguen-Guillouzo C (1982): Hydrocortisone modulates the production of extracellular material and albumin in long-term cocultures of adult rat hepatocytes with other liver epithelial cells. Biochem Biophys Res Commun 109: 507–512.

Ben-Ze'ev A, Robinson GS, Bucher NLR, Farmer SR (1985): Cell- and cell-matrix interactions differentially regulate the expression of hepatic and cytoskeletal genes in primary cultures of rat hepatocytes. Proc Natl Acad Sci USA 85: 2894–2898.

Bengtsson BG, Kiessling KH, Smith-Kielland A, Morland J (1981): Partial separation and biochemical characteristics of periportal and perivenous hepatocytes from rat liver. Eur J Biochem 118: 591–597.

Benzeroual K, van de Werve G, Meloche S, Mathe L, Romanelli A, Haddad P (1997): Insulin induces Ca^{2+} influx into isolated rat hepatocyte couplets. Am J Physiol 272: G1425-G1432.

Bissell DM, Arenson DM, Maher JJ, Roll FJ (1987): Support of cultured hepatocytes by a laminin-rich gel. Evidence for a functionally significant subendothelial matrix in normal rat liver. J Clin Invest 79: 801–812.

Block GD, Locker J, Bowen WC, Petersen BE, Katyal S, Strom SC, Riley T, Howard TA, Michalopoulos GK (1996): Population expansion, clonal growth, and specific differentiation patterns in primary cultures of hepatocytes induced by HGF/SF, EGF and TGF alpha in a chemically defined (HGM) medium. J Cell Biol 132: 1133–1149.

Bour ES, Ward LK, Cornman GA, Isom HC (1996): Tumor necrosis factor-alpha-induced apoptosis in hepatocytes in long-term culture. Am J Pathol 148: 485–495.

Bruck R, Aeed H, Shirin H, Matas Z, Zaidel L, Avni Y, Halpern Z (1999): The hydroxyl radical scavengers dimethylsulfoxide and dimethylthiourea protect rats against thioacetamide-induced fulminant hepatic failure. J Hepatol 31: 27–38.

Cable EE, Isom HC (1997): Exposure of primary rat hepatocytes in long-term DMSO culture to selected transition metals induces hepatocyte proliferation and formation of duct-like structures. Hepatology 26: 1444–1457.

Caron JM (1990): Induction of albumin gene transcription in hepatocytes by extracellular matrix proteins. Mol Cell Biol 10: 1239–1243.

Chenoufi N, Baffet G, Drenou B, Cariou S, Desille M, Clement B, Brissot P, Lescoat G, Loreal O (1998): Deferoxamine arrests in vitro the proliferation of porcine hepatocyte in G1 phase of the cell cycle. Liver 18: 60–66.

Clayton DF, Darnell JE (1983): Changes in liver-specific compared to common gene transcription during primary culture of mouse hepatocytes. Mol Cell Biol 3: 1552–1561.

Clement B., Grimaud JA, Campion JP, Deugnier Y, Guillouzo, A (1986) Cell types involved in collagen and fibronectin production in normal and fibrotic human liver. Hepatology 6: 225–234.

Coleman WB, Wennerberg AE, Smith GJ, Grisham JW (1993): Regulation of the differentiation of diploid and some aneuploid rat liver epithelial (stemlike) cells by the hepatic microenvironment. Am J Pathol 142: 1373–1382.

Corlu A, Kneip B, Lhadi C, Leray G, Glaise D, Baffet G, Bourel D, Guguen-Guillouzo C (1991): A plasma membrane protein is involved in cell contact-mediated regulation of tissue-specific genes in adult hepatocytes. J Cell Biol 115: 505–515.

Corlu A, Ilyin G, Cariou S, Lamy I, Loyer P, Guguen-Guillouzo C (1997): The coculture: a system for studying the regulation of liver differentiation/proliferation activity and its control. Cell Biol Toxicol 13: 235–242.

Corlu A, Lamy I, Ilyin GP, Fardel O, Kneip B, Le Jossic C, Guguen-Guillouzo C (1998): Hematopoiesis-promoting activity of rat liver biliary epithelial cells: involvement of a cell surface molecule, liver-regulating protein. Exp Hematol 26: 382–394.

Curran RD, Ferrari FK, Kispert PH, Stadler J, Stuehr DJ, Simmons RL, Billiar TR (1991): Nitric oxide and nitric oxide-generating compounds inhibit hepatocyte protein synthesis. FASEB J 5: 2085–2092.

De Smet K, Loyer P, Gilot D, Vercruysse A, Rogiers V, Guguen-Guillouzo C (2001): Effects of epidermal growth factor on CYP inducibility by xenobiotics, DNA replication and caspase activations in collagen I gel sandwich cultures of rat hepatocytes. Biochem Pharmacol. 61:1293–303.

Decaens C, Rodriguez P, Bouchaud C, Cassio D (1996): Establishment of hepatic cell polarity in the rat hepatoma-human fibroblast hybrid WIF-B9. A biphasic phenomenon going from a simple epithelial polarized phenotype to an hepatic polarized one. J Cell Sci 109: 1623–1635.

Deschatrette J, Weiss MC (1974): Characterization of differentiated and dedifferentiated clones from a rat hepatoma. Biochimie 56: 1603–1611.

Diehl AM, Yin M, Fleckenstein J, Yang SQ, Lin HZ, Brenner DA, Westwick J, Bagby G, Nelson S (1994): Tumor necrosis factor-α induces c-jun during the regenerative response to liver injury. Am J Physiol 267: G552–G561.

Diehl AM, Rai RM (1996): Liver regeneration 3: Regulation of signal transduction during liver regeneration. FASEB J 10: 215–227.

Donato MT, Gomez-Lechon MJ, Castell JV (1990): Drug metabolizing enzymes in rat hepatocytes co-cultured with cell lines. In Vitro Cell Dev Biol 26: 1057–1062.

DuBois RD (1990): Early changes in gene expression during liver regeneration: What do they mean? Hepatology 11: 1079–1082.

Dunn JC, Yarmush ML, Koebe HG, Tompkins RG (1989): Hepatocyte function and extracellular matrix geometry: Long-term culture in a sandwich configuration. FASEB J 3: 174–177.

Enat R, Jefferson DM, Ruiz-Opazo N, Gatmaitan Z, Leinwand LA, Reid LM (1984): Hepatocyte proliferation in vitro: Its dependence on the use of serum-free hormonally defined medium and substrata of extracellular matrix. Proc Natl Acad Sci USA 81: 1411–1415.

Etienne PL, Baffet G, Desvergne B, Boisnard-Rissel M, Glaise D, Guguen-Guillouzo C (1988): Transient expression of c-fos and constant expression of c-myc in freshly isolated and cultured normal adult rat hepatocytes. Oncogene Res 3: 255–262.

Evan G, Littlewood T (1998): A matter of life and cell death. Science 281: 1317–1322.

Fardel O, Ratanasavanh D, Loyer P, Ketterer B, Guillouzo A (1992): Overexpression of the multidrug resistance gene product in adult rat hepatocytes during primary culture. Eur J Biochem 205: 847–852.

Fausto N (2000): Liver regeneration. J Hepatol 32: 19–31.

Feldmann G (1997): Liver apoptosis. J Hepatol 26: 1–11.

Ferrini JB, Pichard L, Domergue J, Maurel P (1997): Long-term primary cultures of adult human hepatocytes. Chem Biol Interact 107: 31–45.

FitzGerald MJ, Webber EM, Donovan JR, Fausto N (1995): Rapid DNA binding by nuclear factor kappa B in hepatocytes at the start of liver regeneration. Cell Growth Differ 6: 417–427.

Fraser A, Evan G (1996): A license to kill. Cell 85: 781–784.

Fraslin JM, Kneip B, Vaulont S, Glaise D, Munnich A, Guguen-Guillouzo C (1985): Dependence of hepatocyte-specific gene expression on cell-cell interactions in primary culture. EMBO J 4: 2487–2491.

Gardner MJ, Fletcher K, Pogson CI, Strain AJ (1996): The mitogenic response to EGF of rat hepatocytes cultured on laminin-rich gels (EHS) is blocked downstream of receptor tyrosine-phosphorylation. Biochem Biophys Res Commun 228: 238–245.

Glaise D, Ilyin GP, Loyer P, Cariou S, Bilodeau M, Lucas J, Puisieux A, Ozturk M, Guguen-Guillouzo C (1998): Cell cycle gene regulation in reversibly differentiated new human hepatoma cell lines. Cell Growth Differ 9: 165–176.

Gomez-Lechon MJ, Donato T, Jover R, Rodriguez C, Ponsoda X, Glaise D, Castell JV, Guguen-Guillouzo C (2001): Expression and induction of a large set of drug-metabolizing enzymes by the highly differentiated human hepatoma cell line BC2. Eur J Biochem 268: 1448–1459.

Greenbaum LE, Li W, Cressman DE, Peng Y, Ciliberto G, Poli V, Taub R (1998): CCAAT enhancer-binding protein beta is required for normal hepatocyte proliferation in mice after partial hepatectomy. J Clin Invest 102: 996–1007.

Greengard O (1977): Enzymic differentiation of human liver: Comparison with the rat model. Pediatr Res 11: 669–676.

Greuet J, Pichard L, Ourlin JC, Bonfils C, Domergue J, Le Treut P, Maurel P (1997): Effect of cell density and epidermal growth factor on the inducible expression of CYP3A and CYP1A genes in human hepatocytes in primary culture. Hepatology 25: 1166–1175.

Guguen-Guillouzo C, Campion JP, Brissot P, Glaise D, Launois B, Bourel M, Guillouzo A (1982): High yield preparation of isolated human adult hepatocytes by enzymatic perfusion of the liver. Cell Biol Int Rep 6: 625–628.

Guguen-Guillouzo C, Clement B, Baffet G, Beaumont C, Morel-Chany E, Glaise D, Guillouzo A (1983): Maintenance and reversibility of active albumin secretion by adult rat hepatocytes co-cultured with another liver epithelial cell type. Exp Cell Res 143: 47–54.

Guguen-Guillouzo C (1986): Role of homotypic and heterotypic cell interactions in expression of specific functions by cultured hepatocytes. In Guillouzo A, Guguen-Guillouzo C (eds.): "Isolated and Cultured Hepatocytes." Paris: Les Editions INSERM and John Libbey, Eurotext, pp 259–283.

Guyomard C, Chesne C, Meunier B, Fautrel A, Clerc C, Morel F, Rissel M, Campion JP, Guillouzo A (1990): Primary culture of adult rat hepatocytes after 48-hour preservation of the liver with cold UW solution. Hepatology 12: 1329–1336.

Guyomard C, Rialland L, Fremond B, Chesne C, Guillouzo A (1996): Influence of alginate gel entrapment and cryopreservation on survival and xenobiotic metabolism capacity of rat hepatocytes. Toxicol Appl Pharmacol 141: 349–356.

Guzelian PS, Li D, Schuetz EG, Thomas P, Levin W, Mode A, Gustafsson JA (1988): Sex change in cytochrome P-450 phenotype by growth hormone treatment of adult rat hepatocytes maintained in a culture system on Matrigel. Proc Natl Acad Sci USA 85: 9783–9787.

Hahn WC, Counter CM, Lundberg AS, Beijersbergen RL, Brooks MW, Weinberg RA (1999): Creation of human tumour cells with defined genetic elements. Nature 400: 464–468.

Hansen LK, Albrecht JH (1999): Regulation of the hepatocyte cell cycle by type I collagen matrix: Role of cyclin D1. J Cell Sci 112: 2971–2981.

Hanson RW (1998): Biological role of the isoforms of C/EBP. J Biol Chem 273: 28543.

Houssaint E (1980): Differentiation of the mouse hepatic primordium. I. An analysis of tissue interactions in hepatocyte differentiation. Cell Differ 9: 269–279.

Hueber AO, Evan GI (1998): Traps to catch unwary oncogenes. Trends Genet 14: 364–367.

Ilyin G, Rialland M, Rescan C, Loyer P, Baffet G, Guguen-Guillouzo C (2000): Growth control and cell cycle progression in cultured hepatocytes. In Berry MN, Edwards AM (eds.): "The Hepatocyte Review." Dordrecht: Kluwer Academic, pp 263–280.

Isom I, Georgoff I, Salditt-Georgieff M, Darnell JE Jr. (1987): Persistence of liver-specific messenger RNA in cultured hepatocytes: Different regulatory events for different genes. J Cell Biol 105: 2877–2885.

Jefferson DM, Clayton DF, Darnell JE Jr., Reid LM (1984): Posttranscriptional modulation of gene expression in cultured rat hepatocytes. Mol Cell Biol 4: 1929–1934.

Kano A, Watanabe Y, Takeda N, Aizawa S, Akaike T (1997): Analysis of IFN-gamma-induced cell cycle arrest and cell death in hepatocytes. J Biochem (Tokyo) 121: 677–683.

Kitten O, Ferry N (1998): Mature hepatocytes actively divide and express gamma-glutamyl transpeptidase after D-galactosamine liver injury. Liver 18: 398–404.

Knowles BB, Howe CC, Aden DP (1980): Human hepatocellular carcinoma cell lines secrete the major plasma proteins and hepatitis B surface antigen. Science 209: 497–499.

Kost DP, Michalopoulos GK (1991): Effect of 2% dimethyl sulfoxide on the mitogenic properties of epidermal growth factor and hepatocyte growth factor in primary hepatocyte culture. J Cell Physiol 147: 274–280.

Kuri-Harcuch W, Mendoza-Figueroa T (1989): Cultivation of adult rat hepatocytes on 3T3 cells: Expression of various liver differentiated functions. Differentiation 41: 148–157.

Lagasse E, Connors H, Al-Dhalimy M, Reitsma M, Dohse M, Osborne L, Wang X, Finegold M, Weissman IL, Grompe M (2000): Purified hematopoietic stem cells can differentiate into hepatocytes in vivo. Nat Med 6: 1229–1234.

Lamy I, Corlu A, Fardel O, Gandemer V, Rialland M, Leberre C, le Prise PY, Fauchet R, Coulombel L, Guguen-Guillouzo C (1997): Rat liver biliary epithelial cells support long-term production of haemopoietic progenitors from human CD34 cells. Br J Haematol 98: 560–568.

Landry J, Bernier D, Ouellet C, Goyette R, Marceau N (1985): Spheroidal aggregate culture of rat liver cells: histotypic reorganization, biomatrix deposition, and maintenance of functional activities. J Cell Biol 101: 914–923.

Lazaro CA, Rhim JA, Yamada Y, Fausto N (1998): Generation of hepatocytes from oval cell precursors in culture. Cancer Res 58: 5514–5522.

Le Jossic C, Ilyin GP, Loyer P, Glaise D, Cariou S, Guguen-Guillouzo C (1994): Expression of helix-loop-helix factor Id-1 is dependent on the hepatocyte proliferation and differentiation status in rat liver and in primary culture. Cancer Res 54: 6065–6068.

Le Jossic C, Glaise D, Corcos L, Diot C, Dezier JF, Fautrel A, Guguen-Guillouzo C (1996): trans-Acting factors, detoxication enzymes and hepatitis B virus replication in a novel set of human hepatoma cell lines. Eur J Biochem 238: 400–409.

Le Rumeur E, Guguen-Guillouzo C, Beaumont C, Saunier A, Guillouzo A (1983): Albumin secretion and protein synthesis by cultured diploid and tetraploid rat hepatocytes separated by elutriation. Exp Cell Res 147: 247–254.

Lee J, Morgan JR, Tompkins RG, Yarmush ML (1993): Proline-mediated enhancement of hepatocyte function in a collagen gel sandwich culture configuration. FASEB J 7: 586–591.

Li Y, Sattler GL, Pitot HC (1995): The effect of amino acid composition of serum-free medium on DNA synthesis in primary hepatocyte cultures in the presence of epidermal growth factor. In Vitro Cell Dev Biol Anim 31: 867–870.

Lindros KO, Penttila KE (1985): Digitonin-collagenase perfusion for efficient separation of periportal or perivenous hepatocytes. Biochem J 228: 757–760.

Littlewood TD, Hancock DC, Danielian PS, Parker MG, Evan GI (1995): A modified oestrogen receptor ligand-binding domain as an improved switch for the regulation of heterologous proteins. Nucleic Acids Res 23: 1686–1690.

Liu ML, Mars WM, Zarnegar R, Michalopoulos GK (1994): Collagenase pretreatment and the mitogenic effects of hepatocyte growth factor and transforming growth factor-alpha in adult rat liver. Hepatology 19: 1521–1527.

Loreal O, Levavasseur F, Fromaget C, Gros D, Guillouzo A, Clement B (1993): Cooperation of Ito cells and hepatocytes in the deposition of an extracellular matrix in vitro. Am J Pathol 143: 538–544.

Loyer P, Glaise D, Cariou S, Baffet G, Meijer L, Guguen-Guillouzo C (1994): Expression and activation of cdks (1 and 2) and cyclins in the cell cycle progression during liver regeneration. J Biol Chem 269: 2491–2500.

Loyer P, Cariou S, Glaise D, Bilodeau M, Baffet G, Guguen-Guillouzo C (1996): Growth factor dependence of progression through G1 and S phases of adult rat hepatocytes in vitro. Evidence of a mitogen restriction point in mid-late G1. J Biol Chem 271: 11484–11492.

Maher JJ, Bissell DM, Friedman SL, Roll FJ. (1988): Collagen measured in primary cultures of normal rat hepatocytes derives from lipocytes within the monolayer. J Clin Invest 82: 450–459.

Marion PL, Salazar FH, Alexander JJ, Robinson WS (1979): Polypeptides of hepatitis B virus surface antigen produced by a hepatoma cell line. J Virol 32: 796–802.

Martin DW Jr, Tomkins GM (1970): The appearance and disappearance of the post-transcriptional repressor of tyrosine aminotransferase synthesis during the HTC cell cycle. Proc Natl Acad Sci USA 65: 1064–1068.

McGowan JA, Bucher NL (1983): Pyruvate promotion of DNA synthesis in serum-free primary cultures of adult rat hepatocytes. In Vitro 19: 159–166.

Mesnil M, Fraslin JM, Piccoli C, Yamasaki H, Guguen-Guillouzo C (1987): Cell contact but not junctional communication (dye coupling) with biliary epithelial cells is required for hepatocytes to maintain differentiated functions. Exp Cell Res 173: 524–533.

Michalopoulos GK, Bowen WC, Zajac VF, Beer-Stolz D, Watkins S, Kostrubsky V, Strom SC (1999): Morphogenetic events in mixed cultures of rat hepatocytes and nonparenchymal cells maintained in biological matrices in the presence of hepatocyte growth factor and epidermal growth factor. Hepatology 29: 90–100.

Mitaka T, Mikami M, Sattler GL, Pitot HC, Mochizuki Y (1992): Small cell colonies appear in the primary culture of adult rat hepatocytes in the presence of nicotinamide and epidermal growth factor. Hepatology 16: 440–447.

Mitaka T, Norioka K, Mochizuki Y (1993): Redifferentiation of proliferated rat hepatocytes cultured in L15 medium supplemented with EGF and DMSO. In Vitro Cell Dev Biol Anim 29A: 714–722.

Mitaka T, Kojima T, Mizuguchi T, Mochizuki Y (1996): Subculture of proliferating adult rat hepatocytes in medium supplemented with nicotinamide and EGF. In Vitro Cell Dev Biol Anim 32: 469–477.

Mitaka T, Sato F, Mizuguchi T, Yokono T, Mochizuki Y (1999): Reconstruction of hepatic organoid by rat small hepatocytes and hepatic nonparenchymal cells. Hepatology 29: 111–125.

Miyazaki M, Mars WM, Runge D, Kim TH, Bowen WC, Michalopoulos GK (1998): Phenobarbital suppresses growth and accelerates restoration of differentiation markers of primary culture rat hepatocytes in the chemically defined hepatocyte growth medium containing hepatocyte growth factor and epidermal growth factor. Exp Cell Res 241: 445–457.

Morel F, Beaune PH, Ratanasavanh D, Flinois JP, Yang CS, Guengerich FP, Guillouzo A (1990): Expression of cytochrome P-450 enzymes in cultured human hepatocytes. Eur J Biochem 191: 437–444.

Nakabayashi H, Taketa K, Yamane T, Miyazaki M, Miyano K, Sato J (1984): Phenotypical stability of a human hepatoma cell line, HuH-7, in long-term culture with chemically defined medium. Gann 75: 151–158.

Nakamura T, Tomita Y, Ichihara A (1983): Density-dependent growth control of adult rat hepatocytes in primary culture. J Biochem (Tokyo) 94: 1029–1035.

Nigg EA (1998): Polo-like kinases: Positive regulators of cell division from start to finish. Curr Opin Cell Biol 10: 776–783.

Nishikawa Y, Wang M, Carr BI (1998): Changes in TGF-beta receptors of rat hepatocytes during primary culture and liver regeneration: Increased expression of TGF-beta receptors associated with increased sensitivity to TGF-beta-mediated growth inhibition. J Cell Physiol 176: 612–623.

Orkin RW, Gehron P, McGoodwin EB, Martin GR, Valentine T, Swarm R (1977): A murine tumor producing a matrix of basement membrane. J Exp Med 145: 204–220.

Paine A (2000): Constitutive expression of cytochromes P450 in hepatocyte culture. In Berry MN, Edwards AM (eds.): "The Hepatocyte Review." Dordrecht: Kluwer Academic, pp 411–420.

Paul D, Hohne M, Pinkert C, Piasecki A, Ummelmann E, Brinster RL (1988): Immortalized differentiated hepatocyte lines derived from transgenic mice harboring SV40 T-antigen genes. Exp Cell Res 175: 354–362.

Pfeifer AM, Cole KE, Smoot DT, Weston A, Groopman JD, Shields PG, Vignaud JM, Juillerat M, Lipsky MM, Trump BF, et al. (1993): Simian virus 40 large tumor antigen-immortalized normal human liver epithelial cells express hepatocyte characteristics and metabolize chemical carcinogens. Proc Natl Acad Sci USA 90: 5123–5127.

Pitot JC, Peraino C, Morse PA, Potter VR (1964): Hepatomas in tissue culture compared with adapting liver in vivo. Natl Cancer Inst Monogr 13: 229–242.

Poullain MG, Fautrel A, Guyomard C, Chesne C, Grislain L, Guillouzo A (1992): Viability and primary culture of rat hepatocytes after hypothermic preservation: The superiority of the Leibovitz medium over the University of Wisconsin solution for cold storage. Hepatology 15: 97–106.

Rescan C, Coutant A, Talarmin H, Theret N, Glaise D, Guguen-Guillouzo C, Baffet G (2001): Mechanism in the sequential control of cell morphology and s phase entry by epidermal growth factor involves distinct mek/erk activations. Mol Biol Cell 12: 725–738.

Rialland M, Corlu A, Ilyin G, Cabillic F, Lamy I, Guguen-Guillouzo C (2000): Pattern of cytokine expression by rat liver epithelial cells supporting long-term culture of human CD34(+) umbilical cord blood cells. Cytokine 12: 951–959.

Schrode W, Mecke D, Gebhardt R (1990): Induction of glutamine synthetase in periportal hepatocytes by cocultivation with a liver epithelial cell line. Eur J Cell Biol 53: 35–41.

Seglen PO (1976): Preparation of isolated rat liver cells. Methods Cell Biol 13: 29–83.

Seglen PO (1997): DNA ploidy and autophagic protein degradation as determinants of hepatocellular growth and survival. Cell Biol Toxicol 13: 301–315.

Soriano HE, Kang DC, Finegold MJ, Hicks MJ, Wang ND, Harrison W, Darlington GJ (1998): Lack of C/EBP alpha gene expression results in increased

DNA synthesis and an increased frequency of immortalization of freshly isolated mice [correction of rat] hepatocytes. Hepatology 27: 392–401.

Spray DC, Fujita M, Saez JC, Choi H, Watanabe T, Hertzberg E, Rosenberg LC, Reid LM (1987): Proteoglycans and glycosaminoglycans induce gap junction synthesis and function in primary liver cultures. J Cell Biol 105: 541–551.

Steward AR, Dannan GA, Guzelian PS, Guengerich FP (1985): Changes in the concentration of seven forms of cytochrome P-450 in primary cultures of adult rat hepatocytes. Mol Pharmacol 27: 125–132.

Strom SC, Jirtle RL, Jones RS, Novicki DL, Rosenberg MR, Novotny A, Irons G, McLain JR, Michalopoulos G (1982): Isolation, culture, and transplantation of human hepatocytes. J Natl Cancer Inst 68: 771–778.

Szpirer J, Szpirer C, Wanson JC (1980): Control of serum protein production in hepatocyte hybridomas: Immortalization and expression of normal hepatocyte genes. Proc Natl Acad Sci USA 77: 6616–6620.

Talarmin H, Rescan C, Cariou S, Glaise D, Zanninelli G, Bilodeau M, Loyer P, Guguen-Guillouzo C, Baffet G (1999): The mitogen-activated protein kinase kinase/extracellular signal-regulated kinase cascade activation is a key signalling pathway involved in the regulation of G(1) phase progression in proliferating hepatocytes. Mol Cell Biol 19: 6003–6011.

Tateno C, Yoshizato K (1996): Growth and differentiation in culture of clonogenic hepatocytes that express both phenotypes of hepatocytes and biliary epithelial cells. Am J Pathol 149: 1593–1605.

Tateno C, Yoshizato K (1998): Growth and differentiation of adult rat hepatocytes regulated by the interaction between parenchymal and non-parenchymal liver cells. J Gastroenterol Hepatol 13 Suppl: S83–S92.

Taub R (1998): Blocking NF-kappaB in the liver: The good and bad news. Hepatology 27: 1445–1446.

Theise ND, Badve S, Saxena R, Henegariu O, Sell S, Crawford JM, Krause DS (2000): Derivation of hepatocytes from bone marrow cells in mice after radiation-induced myeloablation. Hepatology 31: 235–240.

Thorgeirsson SS (1996): Hepatic stem cells in liver regeneration. FASEB J 10: 1249–1256.

Tsao MS, Smith JD, Nelson KG, Grisham JW (1984): A diploid epithelial cell line from normal adult rat liver with phenotypic properties of "oval" cells. Exp Cell Res 154: 38–52.

Vandenberghe Y, Morel F, Pemble S, Taylor JB, Rogiers V, Ratanasavanh D, Vercruysse A, Ketterer B, Guillouzo A (1990): Changes in expression of mRNA coding for glutathione S-transferase subunits 1-2 and 7 in cultured rat hepatocytes. Mol Pharmacol 37: 372–376.

Vukicevic S, Kleinman HK, Luyten FP, Roberts AB, Roche NS, Reddi AH (1992): Identification of multiple active growth factors in basement membrane Matrigel suggests caution in interpretation of cellular activity related to extracellular matrix components. Exp Cell Res 202: 1–8.

Webber EM, Godowski PJ, Fausto N (1994): In vivo response of hepatocytes to growth factors requires an initial priming stimulus. Hepatology 19: 489–497.

Webber EM, Bruix J, Pierce RH, Fausto N (1998): Tumor necrosis factor primes hepatocytes for DNA replication in the rat. Hepatology 28: 1226–1234.

Williams GM, Weisburger EK, Weisburger JH (1971): Isolation and long-term cell culture of epithelial-like cells from rat liver. Exp Cell Res 69: 106–112.

Zindy F, Lamas E, Chenivesse X, Sobczak J, Wang J, Fesquet D, Henglein B, Brechot C (1992): Cyclin A is required in S phase in normal epithelial cells. Biochem Biophys Res Commun 182: 1144–1154.

APPENDIX: SOURCES OF MATERIALS

Material	Catalog No.	Supplier
Bovine serum albumin (BSA)	A 8412	Sigma
Cannulae	—	Becton Dickinson
Cell strainer	2360	Becton Dickinson
Gauze	—	Tekto
Growth factors and cytokines	—	Becton Dickinson, ICN, R&D, Sigma
Heparin	H 3149	Sigma
Leibowitz L-15 medium	11415 L 5520	GIBCO Sigma
Matrigel	40234	Becton Dickinson
Medium 199	31150 M 4530	GIBCO Sigma
Nembutal	—	Hospital pharmacy
Scrynel NYHC nylon gauze	Poly Labo 87410.01, 87470.01, 87401.01	Merck
Williams medium E	22551 W 1878	GIBCO Sigma
Winged infusion set	Poly Labo 02183.01 (rat), 02187.01 (mouse)	Merck

12

Culture Of Human Urothelium

Jennifer Southgate,[1] John R. W. Masters,[2] and
Ludwik K. Trejdosiewicz[3]

[1]Jack Birch Unit of Molecular Carcinogenesis, Department of Biology,
University of York,[2] Institute of Urology, University College, London, and
[3]ICRF Cancer Medicine Research Unit, St James's University Hospital,
Leeds, UK. js35@york.ac.uk

Culture of Epithelial Cells, pages 381–399

This chapter is dedicated to the memory of Gisèle M. Hodges.

I. BACKGROUND

Normal urothelium is a transitional epithelium consisting of basal, intermediate, and superficial cell zones (Fig. 12.1a; Plate 2a). The basal cell layer is composed of a single layer of cells in contact with and orientated perpendicular to the plane of the basement membrane (Fig. 12.1b; Plate 2b). The intermediate cell zone contains a variable number of cell layers, which depends on the state of contraction of the tissue. In humans, the luminal or superficial cell layer consists of large, frequently binucleated, "umbrella" cells that are orientated parallel to the basement membrane with their apical edge abutting the lumen. At the ultrastructural level, the umbrella cells are characterized by well-developed tight junctions, the presence of thickened plaques of asymmetric unit membrane (AUM) in the apical membrane, and intracellular fusiform vesicles. The specialized superficial cells display unique morphologic, ultrastructural, antigenic, and gene expression characteristics, which provide unequivocal markers of terminal urothelial cytodifferentiation.

The ability to culture normal epithelial cells derived from different tissues has had an important impact on our understanding of cellular processes such as proliferation and differentiation. A variety of approaches have been taken to study normal human urothelium in vitro, including organ cultures [Knowles et al., 1983; Scriven et al., 1997], primary cultures [de Boer et al., 1996], subcultured cell lines, which are the focus of this chapter, as well as urothelial cell-stroma recombinants [Scriven et al., 1997]. The methods used to initiate urothelial cell lines include outgrowths from explant cultures [Wu et al., 1982; Reznikoff et al., 1983] and the isolation of the urothelium from the stroma. This latter approach has the advantage of eliminating stroma-derived fibroblasts, although fibroblast overgrowth may also be inhibited by

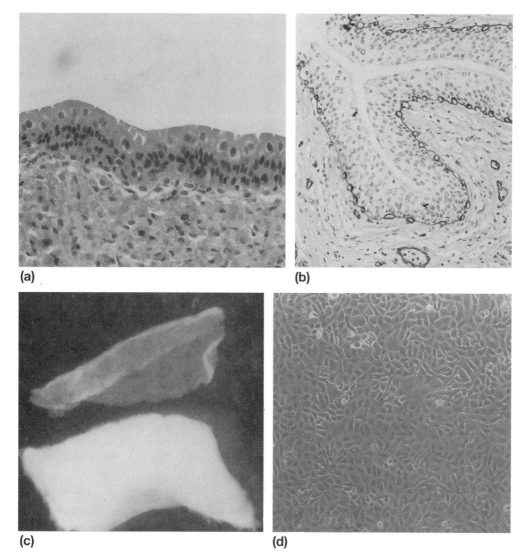

(a)   **(b)**

(c)   **(d)**

Fig 12.1.   Bladder urothelium. (a) Hematoxylin and eosin-stained section of normal human bladder urothelium. A three-layered epithelium is evident, consisting of large, binucleated superficial cells overlying an intermediate and a basal cell layer. Beneath the urothelium is a cellular stroma. (b) Section of human ureter immunolabeled with laminin using an indirect immunoperoxidase technique to show position of basement membrane between urothelium and stroma. Note the "string of beads" effect caused by the prominent capillary bed associated with the epithelial basement membrane. (c) After incubation of urothelial tissue fragments in "stripping solution," the urothelium detaches from the stroma as an intact sheet. (d) When isolated from the stroma, disaggregated, and placed in mon-oculture, normal human urothelial cells appear as an epithelioid cell monolayer.

Culture of Human Urothelium   **383**

the use of serum-free medium formulations (see Section 2). Isolation of the urothelium by scraping with a scalpel blade [Liebert et al., 1990; Cilento et al., 1994] is a simple technique, but it compromises both cell viability and the success rates for establishing primary cultures and cell lines. In contrast, dissociation of the urothelium from the basement membrane using proteolytic enzymes [Hutton et al., 1993] or EDTA [Southgate et al., 1994] results in high yields of cells (typically 2×10^6 cells/cm^2 tissue) that show excellent viability and plating efficiencies.

A number of studies have established epithelial cell cultures from the urine as an accessible source of viable presumptive urothelial cells [Sutherland and Bain, 1972; Felix et al., 1980; Herz et al., 1985]. However, exfoliated cells in the urine may be derived from anywhere in the urogenital tract, including non-urothelial tissues, and therefore, in the absence of other confirmation, the tissue derivation of such cultures must be questioned. Indeed, other groups have used the urine as a source of viable presumptive kidney epithelial cells [Detrisac et al., 1983; Rheinwald and O'Connell, 1985].

The first long-term cultures of human urothelial cells were established from explant cultures, which were maintained in serum-supplemented media and either a 3T3 fibroblast feeder cell layer [Wu et al., 1982] or a collagen type I substratum [Reznikoff et al., 1983]. Subsequent studies aimed to establish more defined systems to limit confounding factors, such as those derived from serum, extracellular matrix, or the stroma. A number of groups have described serum-free culture systems, although most of these include bovine pituitary extract (BPE), which contains an undefined mix of growth factors [Messing et al., 1982; Kirk et al., 1985; Dubeau and Jones, 1987; James et al., 1986; Liebert et al., 1990; Hutton et al., 1993; Cilento et al., 1994; Southgate et al., 1994]. Other factors have also been investigated for their influence on urothelial cell growth. Cholera toxin has been shown to improve the initial plating efficiency of urothelial cells in primary culture [Hutton et al., 1993, Southgate et al., 1994]. In contrast, although known to be mitogenic for keratinocytes and rodent urothelial cells, epidermal growth factor (EGF) has been found to have no effect on survival or proliferation of normal human urothelial (NHU) cells [Reznikoff et al., 1983, Liebert et al., 1990, Southgate et al., 1994], although it is included in most serum-free medium formulations. Using the optimized approaches and conditions developed over the past few decades, NHU cells may now be cultured routinely under relatively defined conditions.

2. PREPARATION OF REAGENTS AND MEDIA

2.1. Media and Supplements

2.1.1. Complete Keratinocyte Serum-Free Medium (KSFMc)

Five hundred-milliliter bottles of KSFM are supplied with frozen aliquots of recombinant EGF and BPE sufficient to give final concentrations of 5 ng/ml and 50 ng/ml, respectively. Add 500 μl of CT working stock (below) and keep at 4°C.

If less than 500 ml KSFMc is used per week, then aliquot KSFM into ten 50-ml sterile containers and store at 4°C until use. Aliquot EGF and BPE supplements into 10 equal portions in sterile vials and store at -20°C. For use, add one aliquot each of BPE and EGF to one 50-ml volume of KFSM and add 50 μl of CT working stock.

2.1.2. Transport Medium

Add 5 ml of 1 M HEPES pH 7.6 and 20 kallikrein inactivating units (KIU) aprotinin to 500 ml of Hanks' balanced salt solution (HBSS) with Ca^{2+} and Mg^{2+} under aseptic conditions. Prepare 15-ml aliquots in sterile plastic universal containers and store at 4°C for up to 3 months.

2.1.3. Freezing Mixture

10% (v/v) fetal bovine serum, 10% (v/v) dimethyl sulfoxide, and 80% (v/v) KSFM. Prepare under aseptic conditions and store at 4°C.

2.1.4. Cholera Toxin (CT)

Reconstitute 1-mg vial of CT in 1 ml of sterile distilled water. Treat as sterile and store at $+4$°C for up to 1 yr. Dilute 150 μl CT to 5 ml in KSFM (below) to make a 30 μg/ml working stock. Use at 1:1000 to give a final concentration of 30 ng/ml.

2.2. Disaggregating Agents

2.2.1. Stripping Solution

Add 5 ml of 1 M HEPES buffer pH 7.6, 20 KIU aprotinin (1 ml of 500,000-KIU stock) and 50 ml of 1% (w/v) EDTA (ethylene diaminetetraacetic acid, disodium salt) to 500 ml of HBSS without Ca^{2+} and Mg^{2+} (HCMF). Prepare under aseptic conditions and store at 4°C for up to 3 months.

2.2.2. Trypsin-EDTA (Containing 0.25% Trypsin and 0.02% EDTA)

Make 20 ml of trypsin, 2.5% (10× solution) and 4 ml of EDTA, 1% (27 mM), up to 200 ml with HBSS without Ca^{2+} or Mg^{2+} (HCMF). Prepare under aseptic conditions, aliquot in 5-ml volumes, and store at $-20°C$. Once thawed, keep at $4°C$ and use within a week.

2.2.3. Collagenase

Dissolve 100 U/ml collagenase type IV in Hanks' balanced salt solution complete with Ca^{2+} and Mg^{2+} (HBSS) and 10 mM sterile HEPES at pH 7.6. Sterilize through a 0.2-μm syringe filter, aliquot in 2-ml volumes, and store at $-20°C$ for up to 1 yr.

2.2.4. Trypsin Inhibitor

Reconstitute 250-mg vial of soybean trypsin inhibitor in 5 ml of PBSA, filter sterilize through 0.2-μm filter, and store in 50-μl aliquots at $-20°C$. For use, thaw one aliquot into 5 ml of KSFM (sufficient to inhibit in excess of 1 ml of trypsin-EDTA solution).

2.3. Fixative

2.3.1. Formalin (10% (v/v) Formalin in PBS)

Make up phosphate-buffered saline (PBSA) from tablets and add, dropwise while stirring, 0.5 ml of 1 M $MgCl_2$ and 0.9 ml of 1 M $CaCl_2$ per liter of PBS. To 450 ml of the complete PBS, add 50 ml of 38% (w/v) formaldehyde. Store at ambient temperature.

3. PROTOCOLS FOR CULTURE OF HUMAN UROTHELIAL CELLS

3.1. Sources of Tissue

Urothelium lines the urinary tract from the renal pelvis through the ureter and bladder to the first part of the urethra. Urothelial cell cultures can be generated readily from each of these regions, and no major differences have been found in cell cultures established from different regions of the urinary tract or from adult or pediatric donors.

Tissue for urothelial cell culture can be obtained from biopsies taken under local anesthetic or tissue removed at surgery. Cadaveric urothelium has been described as a source of viable urothelial cells [Schmidt et al., 1984], but it must be obtained fresh as urothelium deteriorates rapidly when left in contact with urine. Urological tissues can be obtained from children undergoing open urological procedures, such as pyeloplasty for pelvi-ureteric junction obstruction, ureteric reimplantation for vesico-ureteric reflux, bladder diverticulectomy, duplex collecting systems, nephrectomy for nonfunctioning kidney, and bladder augmentation (enterocystoplasty). Useful sources of adult urothelium include pyeloplasty for pelvi-ureteric junction obstruction and renal transplant surgery.

Urothelium from patients with any history of urothelial malignancy should be avoided because of the possibility of field changes in the bladder. Nevertheless, it is possible to use renal pelvis and ureter from patients undergoing nephrectomy for renal cell carcinoma if the renal pelvis is uninvolved. Urothelial cell lines derived from renal cell carcinoma patients are indistinguishable from cell lines derived from other sources of urothelium. Diathermy should be avoided in the area around the tissue to be harvested, as this adversely affects cell viability.

Sterile specimens are collected into plastic Universal containers containing transport medium (see Section 2.1.2, above). Tissue is placed into transport medium either in the operating theater by the surgeon or by the pathologist if there is any diagnostic question (e.g., renal cell carcinoma). Specimens may be processed immediately, although satisfactory recovery of viable cells is possible from specimens stored at 4°C for up to 6 days or kept at ambient temperature for up to 18 h. Thus it is feasible to mail specimens between centers (although a courier service may be preferred).

3.2. Histologic Classification of Tissue

A representative portion of each tissue sample is placed in 10% formalin in complete phosphate-buffered saline (PBS) for routine processing into paraffin wax. Hematoxylin and eosin-stained sections are assessed for morphology. Because of the type of samples used, it would be unexpected to find evidence of urothelial atypia, although benign conditions, such as von Brunn's nests or acute or chronic inflammation, are occasionally found.

3.3. Procedures for Isolation and Culture

Protocol 12.1. Isolation of Human Urothelium

Reagents and Materials

Sterile

- ❑ Transport medium
- ❑ Stripping solution
- ❑ Universal containers
- ❑ Centrifuge tube, 10 ml
- ❑ Petri dishes, 10 cm
- ❑ Pasteur pipettes, wide-tipped plastic (Pastettes)
- ❑ Scalpels, #11
- ❑ Scissors, fine
- ❑ Jeweler's forceps

Nonsterile

- ❑ Dissecting microscope

Protocol

(a) Collect sterile specimens into plastic Universal containers containing transport medium and convey to the laboratory.

(b) Transfer specimen into a 10-cm Petri dish containing 5 ml fresh transport medium.

(c) Trim the specimen to remove any serosa, fat, or debris and dissect into 1- to 2-cm^2 pieces. This can be done under a dissecting microscope.

(d) Transfer pieces to a Universal container containing 15 ml stripping solution.

(e) Leave overnight at 4°C, or for approximately 4 h at 37°C.

(f) Transfer tissue to a Petri dish and, using two pairs of sterile jeweler's forceps, gently separate the urothelium from the underlying stroma. The urothelium should detach easily as intact sheets of cells (Fig. 12.1c).

(g) Pick out the pieces of stroma and, with a wide-tipped sterile plastic Pasteur pipette, transfer the sheets of urothelium into a 10-ml centrifuge tube.

(h) The efficiency of the isolation procedure may be monitored by histologic analysis of the stroma. Immunohistochemical analysis with antibodies against cytokeratins and basement membrane proteins has shown that the urothelium is removed completely, leaving an intact basement membrane [Scriven et al., 1997].

Protocol 12.2. Primary Human Urothelial Cell Culture

Reagents and Materials

Sterile

- ❑ Collagenase, 100 U/ml (see Section 2.2.3, above)
- ❑ Growth medium, KSFMc (see Section 2.1.1, above)
- ❑ Petri dishes or flasks, Primaria®
- ❑ Pastette, fine-tipped

Nonsterile

- ❑ Improved Neubauer hemocytometer and coverslip

Protocol

(a) Collect the urothelial cell sheets by centrifugation at 250 g for 4 min.

(b) Aspirate the supernatant and "flick" the tube to resuspend pellet in the residual volume.

(c) Add 2 ml collagenase and incubate at 37°C for about 20 min.

(d) Add 3 ml KSFMc growth medium and disaggregate the cell sheets by gentle pipetting with a fine-tipped Pastette.

(e) Collect cells by centrifugation, "flick" the tube to resuspend, and add 5 ml KSFMc growth medium.

(f) Use a hemocytometer to estimate the number of urothelial cells in the suspension, which will contain a mixture of single cells and clumps of urothelial cells, erythrocytes, and leukocytes. Plate cells in Primaria® Petri dishes or flasks at a minimum seeding density of 4×10^4 urothelial cells/cm^2 for primary cell culture.

(g) Maintain cultures at 37°C in a humidified atmosphere of 5% (v/v) CO_2 in air.

(h) Replace medium after 24 h and subsequently on alternate days.

Antibiotics should be avoided, as these can mask low-level bacterial contamination. Bacterial contamination of primary urothelial cell cultures is rare, but, if it does occur, it is usually evident within 24 h. Such contaminations may indicate an ongoing urinary tract infection in the patient, and contaminated cell cultures are always discarded. In the absence of contamination, the initiation of primary normal human urothelial cell cultures is very robust and reproducible, permitting the establishment of successful cell lines in virtually all cases.

Δ *Safety note.* Avoid using tissues from patients at high risk for HIV/AIDS or viral hepatitis. Seek immunization for hepatitis B virus before commencing work. Refer to local safety rules for working with primary human tissues and be particularly careful when handling sharp dissection instruments.

Protocol 12.3. Subculture of Human Urothelial Cells

It is important that urothelial cells are not left at confluence before subculture as this increases the subsequent lag phase on replating. Therefore, cells should be passaged when near or just confluent.

Reagents and Materials

Sterile

- ❑ PBSA/EDTA: PBSA containing 0.1% EDTA
- ❑ Trypsin-EDTA (see Section 2.2.2, above)
- ❑ Growth medium, KSFMc (see Section 2.1.1, above)
- ❑ KSFM with trypsin inhibitor (see Section 2.2.4, above)
- ❑ Centrifuge tubes, conical bottom
- ❑ Primaria® flasks
- ❑ Glass slides, 12 well, Teflon coated, Multispot. Ethanol washed and autoclaved

Protocol

(a) Aspirate medium and incubate cell monolayer in 0.2 ml/cm² PBSA-EDTA for 5 min at 37°C, until the cells separate from each other and have visibly begun to "round up" (monitor incubation by periodic inspection under a phase-contrast inverted microscope).

(b) Aspirate PBSA-EDTA solution, add sufficient trypsin-EDTA to cover the monolayer, remove excess, and incubate at 37°C for ~2 min, or until all cells detach when the side of the flask is tapped firmly.

(c) Add 5 ml KSFM with trypsin inhibitor, transfer to 10-ml conical-bottom centrifuge tube, and centrifuge at 250 g for 4 min. Cell counts can be performed at this point; expect to harvest 2 × 10⁶ cells/25-cm² flask.

(d) Resuspend cells and add KSFMc. Seed cells at a ratio of between 1/3 to 1/6 in Primaria® flasks.

(e) For immunofluorescence analysis, seed drops of cell suspension at 4×10^5 cells/ml onto wells of Multispot slides.

(f) The number of passages should be recorded. Cell lines may be serially passaged between 6 and 12 times, before becoming senescent, which is characterized by the appearance of large, nondividing cells.

3.4. Cryopreservation

Urothelial cells may be cryopreserved at any passage, including freshly isolated cells before culture.

Protocol 12.4. Freezing Human Urothelial Cells

Reagents and Materials

Sterile

❑ KSFMc with trypsin inhibitor (see Section 2.2.4, above)
❑ Freezing mixture (see Section 2.1.3, above)
❑ Ampoules: plastic cryotubes

Nonsterile

❑ Programmable freezer or other device to give slow cooling at −1°C/min, e.g., neck-plug cooler, Nalge Nunc cooler, or pack cryotubes in a 12- to 15-mm wall thickness polystyrene foam container or a length of plastic foam pipe insulation.
❑ Cryoprotective gloves
❑ Face mask

Protocol

(a) Harvest cells as described in Protocol 12.3 into KSFMc with trypsin inhibitor and collect by centrifugation.

(b) Aspirate supernatant and "flick" tube to resuspend the cell pellet in the residual volume.

(c) Resuspend the cells at approximately 2×10^6 cells/ml in ice-cold freezing mix and dispense 1-ml volumes into plastic cryotubes kept on ice. In practice, cells harvested from a near-confluent 75-cm^2 flask can be resuspended in 3 ml freezing mix and divided between 3 cryotubes.

(d) Cool cells at a rate of −1°C/min to below the eutectic point

($-18°C$) in a controlled-rate freezer, finally cooling to $-196°C$ in liquid nitrogen. An acceptable, but less satisfactory, method is to pack cryotubes in insulation and leave at $-80°C$ overnight (see *Reagents and Materials*).

(e) Transfer vials to a liquid nitrogen cryogenic refrigerator for long-term storage.

△*Safety note.* A transparent face mask, cryoprotective gloves, and a fastened lab coat must be worn when placing any material into liquid nitrogen.

Protocol 12.5. Thawing

Reagents and Materials

❑ Growth medium, KSFMc
❑ Culture flasks, 25 or 75 cm^2
❑ Dry ice (solid-phase CO_2)

△*Safety note.* Take care in handling solid CO_2. Danger of frostbite; wear gloves.

❑ Bucket with 10 cm warm water at 37°C and lid.
❑ Cryoprotective gloves
❑ Face mask

Protocol

(a) Transfer a cryotube of cells from cryogenic freezer to tissue culture laboratory on dry ice.

△*Safety note.* Wear cryoprotective gloves, a face mask and a fastened lab-coat when removing materials from liquid nitrogen.

(b) Thaw cells rapidly by placing the cryotube in a 500-ml plastic beaker containing about 250 ml water at 37°C. Place a lid over the beaker as soon as the cryotube is inserted.

(c) Transfer the just-thawed contents of the cryotube to a Universal container containing 9 ml KSFMc, prewarmed to 37°C.

(d) Centrifuge at 250 g for 4 min.

(e) Aspirate supernatant, "flick" pellet, and resuspend cells in 3 ml fresh KSFMc.

(f) Seed contents of a single cryotube into one 75-cm^2 or divide among three 25-cm^2 tissue culture flasks.

(g) Maintain as described above (see Protocol 12.3).

4. CELL CHARACTERIZATION

The method used to establish the urothelial cell cultures, which includes the isolation of the urothelium from the underlying tissue and the use of serum-free medium, which discourages growth of nonepithelial cells, ensures that only urothelial cells become established in culture. Urothelial cells grow as nonstratified monolayers in which the urothelial cells can be identified by their epithelioid morphology (Fig. 12.1d) and, more objectively and as discussed below, by the expression of specific antigens. These can be studied using immunochemical techniques [reviewed by Southgate and Trejdosiewicz, 1997].

4.1. Cytokeratins

The cytokeratins are particularly useful markers insofar as their expression is indicative of epithelial derivation and antibodies are available to individual cytokeratin isotypes. CK7, CK8, CK18, and CK19 isotypes are expressed throughout all layers in normal urothelium, and other cytokeratin isotypes show differentiation stage-related expression [reviewed by Southgate et al., 1999b]. Thus CK5 and CK17 are basally expressed (Fig. 12.2a), CK13 is present in all but the superficial cell layer, and CK20 is associated with superficial cells. Cultured urothelial cells largely retain the cytokeratin isotype expression pattern characteristic of the basal cells of normal tissue, with antibodies recognizing CK7, CK8, CK17, CK18, and CK19 reacting with all cells (Fig. 12.2b). However, expression of CK13 tends to be lost in favor of CK14, indicating that urothelial cells in culture tend toward a more squamous phenotype [Southgate et al., 1994]. This squamous differentiation may be reversed by addition of retinoic acid to the culture medium [Southgate et al., 1994].

4.2. Proliferation Markers

A notable phenotypic difference between urothelial cells in situ and in vitro is in the expression of cell cycle-associated antigens. The urothelium is noted as a very slow-turnover epithelium, and immunolabeling of sections for the nuclear Ki67 antigen of dividing cells illustrates that the majority of urothelial cells are not in cell cycle (Fig. 12.2c; Plate 3b). However, urothelium is also noted for its high proliferative potential in response to damage [de Boer et al., 1996; Baskin et al., 1997] and when placed in vitro, urothelial cells appear to adopt this proliferative "wound response" phenotype (discussed in Southgate et al., 1999a; see

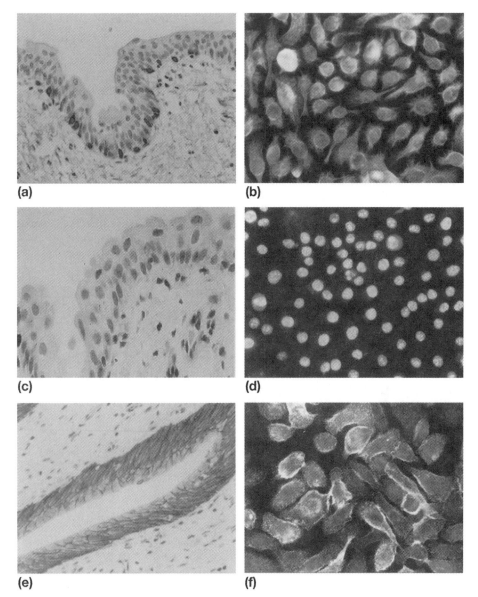

Fig 12.2. Immunophenotypic analysis. (a) Urothelium immunolabeled for CK17, which is expressed predominantly by basal urothelial cells. (b) Cultured normal human urothelial cells immunolabeled for CK17 using an indirect immunofluorescence technique, illustrating expression by essentially all cells in monoculture. (c) Urothelium labeled with the MIB-1 antibody against the Ki67 cell cycle-associated antigen contains very few positive nuclei, suggesting that the majority of cells are out of cell cycle. (d) In culture, normal human urothelial cells adopt a highly proliferative cell phenotype, and the majority express the Ki67 nuclear antigen. (e) E-cadherin is a homotypic cell adhesion molecule that is expressed at intercellular junctions throughout the urothelium. (f) E-cadherin is also expressed at cell-cell junctions in normal human urothelial cell cultures.

also Smith et al., 2001]. Thus cells in vitro typically all express the Ki67 antigen (Fig. 12.2d) and have a very rapid proliferation rate, with an average doubling time of some 15 h [Southgate et al., 1994].

4.3. Cell Adhesion Molecules

In situ, normal urothelium expresses a number of adhesion molecules implicated in cell-cell and cell-matrix interactions, including E-cadherin (Fig. 12.2e), CD44, and several $\beta1$ and $\beta4$ integrins [Southgate et al., 1994; 1995a; 1995b]. In culture, urothelial cells retain a pattern of adhesion molecule expression similar to basal urothelial cells in situ, with intercellular localization of E-cadherin (Fig. 12.2f), $\alpha2\beta1$, $\alpha3\beta1$ integrins, CD44 core and splice exon variants v3, v4/5, v5, and v6, and substrate localization of $\alpha6\beta4$ and $\alpha v\beta4$ integrins [Southgate et al., 1994; 1995a; 1995b]. In addition, normal human urothelial cells express the $\alpha5\beta1$ integrin in vitro [Southgate et al., 1995a].

4.4. Differentiation-Associated Antigens

A number of urothelium-specific proteins have been identified. However, these are expressed only as a consequence of late or terminal cytodifferentiation and hence cannot be used to identify basal or intermediate urothelial cells. The best characterized urothelial differentiation antigens are the four uroplakin (UP) proteins, which constitute the specialized AUM plaques of umbrella cells [Wu et al., 1994; Sun et al., 1999]. A number of antibody reagents have been developed as markers of urothelial cytodifferentiation. Unfortunately, with the exception of a UPIII monoclonal antibody [Moll et al., 1993; Kaufmann et al., 2000], few of these reagents are available commercially.

It appears that normal human urothelial cells in culture do not express terminal differentiation-associated antigens, and expression is neither modulated by retinoic acid nor by increased extracellular calcium concentration. Nevertheless, increasing the extracellular calcium concentration from 0.09 mM to 1 mM does induce cellular stratification and changes in cell phenotype, including desmosome formation, upregulation of E-cadherin and integrin adhesion molecules [Southgate et al., 1994; 1995a], and de novo expression of the Mal-1 gene [Liebert et al., 1997]. Expression of the individual human uroplakin transcripts by normal human urothelial cells has been investigated by ribonuclease protection assay [Lobban et al., 1998]. Such studies confirm that under the culture conditions used, urothelial cytodifferentiation does not proceed. Nevertheless, cultured normal human urothelial cells are able to differentiate, as has been demonstrated by the ability of such cells to form a stratified differentiated urothelium when recombined with an urothelial stroma [Scriven et al., 1997]. This observation shows that the paracrine signals required for urothelial cell maturation to occur have yet to be identified.

5. CONCLUDING REMARKS

In vitro models can provide important insights into the mechanisms regulating normal urothelium and the processes of pathogenesis. The robustness of the normal urothelial cell culture model has made it an ideal subject for investigating how urothelial cells respond to exogenous signaling, for example, using techniques such as differential display RT-PCR [Liebert et al., 1997; Smith et al., 2001]. In addition, it has been shown that normal human urothelial cells may be manipulated by gene transfer, for example, by using recombinant retroviruses. This approach has created immortalized sublines with disabled p53 and/or Rb functions, which are useful for investigating events associated with neoplastic transformation [Reznikoff et al., 1994; Diggle et al., 2000].

In the 1990s, a number of groups became interested in exploiting the high regenerative capacity of urothelium in vitro for bioengineering/tissue reconstructive purposes [Hutton et al., 1993; Cilento et al., 1994]. Notable achievements have included the reconstruction of human urothelial tissues in vitro [Scriven et al, 1997] and the description of a functional and differentiated rabbit urothelium in vitro [Truschel et al., 1999]. The most dramatic development has been the creation of an artificial dog bladder in vitro, which was transplanted and retained urine for up to 11 months [Oberpenning et al, 1999]. Thus advances made in urothelial cell culture are near to achieving genuine benefits for patients requiring bladder augmentation or replacement. In the future, we can expect in vitro studies to lead to a full understanding of the mechanisms involved in the cytodifferentiation and pathogenesis of urothelium.

ACKNOWLEDGMENTS

The authors thank David Russell, Maria Tchetchik, and Wendy Kennedy for their help in preparing the figures.

REFERENCES

Baskin LS, Sutherland RS, Thomson AA, Nguyen HT, Morgan DM, Hayward SW, Hom YK, DiSandro M, Cunha GR (1997): Growth factors in bladder wound healing. J Urol 157: 2388–2395.

Cilento BG, Freeman MR, Schneck FX, Retik AB, Atala A (1994): Phenotypic and cytogenetic characterization of human bladder urothelia expanded in vitro. J Urol 152: 665–670.

De Boer WI, Vermeij M, Diez de Medina SG, Bindels E, Radvanyi F, van der Kwast T, Chopin D (1996): Functions of fibroblast and transforming growth factors in primary organoid-like cultures of normal human urothelium. Lab Invest 75: 147–156.

Detrisac CJ, Mayfield RK, Colwell JA, Garvin AJ, Sens DA (1983): In vitro culture of cells exfoliated in the urine by patients with diabetes mellitus. J Clin Invest 71: 170–173.

Diggle C, Pitt E, Roberts P, Trejdosiewicz LK, Southgate J (2000): n-3 and n-6 polyunsaturated fatty acids induce cytostasis in human urothelial cells independent of p53 function. J Lipid Res 41: 1509–1515.

Dubeau L, Jones PA (1987): Growth of normal and neoplastic urothelium and response to epidermal growth factor in a defined serum-free medium. Cancer Res 47: 2107–2112.

Felix JS, Sun TT, Littlefield JW (1980): Human epithelial cells cultured from urine: Growth properties and keratin staining. In Vitro 16: 866–874.

Herz F, Gazivoda P, Papenhausen PR, Katsuyama J, Koss LG (1985): Normal human urothelial cells in culture. Subculture procedure, flow cytometric and chromosomal analyses. Lab Invest 53: 571–574.

Hutton KA, Trejdosiewicz LK, Thomas DF, Southgate J (1993): Urothelial tissue culture for bladder reconstruction: An experimental study. J Urol 150: 721–725.

James MJ, Nacey JN, Brennan JS, Marshall VR (1986): An improved method for the preparation and culture of urothelial cells. J Urol 136: 1141–1142.

Kaufmann O, Volmerig J, Dietel M (2000): Uroplakin III is a highly specific and moderately sensitive immunohistochemical marker for primary and metastatic urothelial carcinomas. Am J Clin Pathol 113: 683–687.

Kirk D, Kagawa S, Vener G, Narayan KS, Ohnuki Y, Jones LW (1985): Selective growth of normal adult human urothelial cells in serum-free medium. In Vitro Cell Dev Biol 21: 165–171.

Knowles MA, Finesilver A, Harvey AE, Berry RJ, Hicks RM (1983): Long-term organ culture of normal human bladder. Cancer Res 43: 374–385.

Liebert M, Wedemeyer G, Chang JH, Stein JA, McKeever PE, Carey TE, Flint A, Steplewski Z, Buchsbaum DJ, Wahl RL (1990): Comparison of antigen expression on normal urothelial cells in tissue section and tissue culture. J Urol 144: 1288–1292.

Liebert M, Hubbel A, Chung M, Wedemeyer G, Lomax MI, Hegeman A, Yuan TY, Brozovich M, Wheelock MJ, Grossman HB (1997): Expression of *mal* is associated with urothelial differentiation in vitro: Identification by differential display reverse-transcriptase polymerase chain reaction. Differentiation 61: 177–185.

Lobban ED, Smith BA, Hall GD, Harnden P, Roberts P, Selby PJ, Trejdosiewicz LK, Southgate J (1998): Uroplakin gene expression by normal and neoplastic human urothelium. Am J Pathol 153: 1957–1967.

Messing EM, Fahey JL, deKernion JB, Bhuta SM, Bubbers JE (1982): Serum-free medium for the in vitro growth of normal and malignant urinary bladder epithelial cells. Cancer Res. 42: 2392–2397.

Moll R, Laufer J, Wu XR, Sun TT (1993): Uroplakin III, a specific membrane protein of urothelial umbrella cells, as a histological marker for metastatic transitional cell carcinomas. Verhandlungen Deutschen Gesellschaft Pathologie 77: 260–265.

Oberpenning F, Meng J, Yoo JJ, Atala A (1999): De novo reconstitution of a functional mammalian urinary bladder by tissue engineering. Nat Biotechnol 17: 149–155.

Reznikoff CA, Johnson MD, Norback DH, Bryan GT (1983): Growth and characterization of normal human urothelium in vitro. In Vitro 19: 326–343.

Reznikoff CA, Belair C, Savelieva E, Zhai Y, Pfeifer K, Yeager T, Thompson KJ, DeVries S, Bindley C, Newton MA (1994): Long-term genome stability and minimal genotypic and phenotypic alterations in HPV16 E7-, but not E6-, immortalized human uroepithelial cells. Genes Dev 8: 2227–2240.

Rheinwald JG, O'Connell TM (1985): Intermediate filament proteins as distinguishing markers of cell type and differentiated state in cultured human urinary tract epithelia. Ann NY Acad Sci 455: 259–267.

Schmidt WW, Messing EM, Reznikoff CA (1984): Cultures of normal human urothelial cells from ureters of perfused cadaver transplant kidneys. J Urol 132: 1262–1264.

Scriven SD, Booth C, Thomas DF, Trejdosiewicz LK, Southgate J (1997): Reconstitution of human urothelium from monolayer cultures. J Urol 158: 1147–1152.

Smith BA, Kennedy W, Harnden P, Selby PJ, Trejdosiewicz LK, Southgate J (2001): Identification of genes involved in human urothelial cell-matrix interactions: Implications for the progression pathways of malignant urothelium. Cancer Res. 61:1678–85.

Southgate J, Hutton KA, Thomas DF, Trejdosiewicz LK (1994): Normal human urothelial cells in vitro: Proliferation and induction of stratification. Lab Invest 71: 583–594.

Southgate J, Kennedy W, Hutton KA, Trejdosiewicz LK (1995a): Expression and in vitro regulation of integrins by normal human urothelial cells. Cell Adhesion Commun 3: 231–242.

Southgate J, Trejdosiewicz LK, Smith B, Selby PJ (1995b): Patterns of splice variant CD44 expression by normal human urothelium in situ and in vitro and by bladder-carcinoma cell lines. Int J Cancer 62: 449–456.

Southgate J, Harnden P, Selby PJ, Thomas DFM, Trejdosiewicz LK (1999a): Urothelial tissue regulation: Unraveling the role of the stroma. Adv Exp Med Biol 462: 19–30.

Southgate J, Harnden P, Trejdosiewicz LK (1999b): Cytokeratin expression patterns in normal and malignant urothelium: A review of the biological and diagnostic implications. Histol Histopathol 14: 657–664.

Southgate J, Trejdosiewicz LK (1997): Immunolabelling of cells and tissues: approaches and pitfalls. Hum Reprod 12 (Suppl): 65–75.

Sun TT, Liang FX, Wu XR (1999): Uroplakins as markers of urothelial differentiation. Adv Exp Med Biol 462: 7–18.

Sutherland GR, Bain AD (1972): Culture of cells from the urine of newborn children. Nature 239: 231.

Truschel ST, Ruiz WG, Shulman T, Pilewski J, Sun TT, Zeidel ML, Apodaca G (1999): Primary uroepithelial cultures. A model system to analyze umbrella cell barrier function. J Biol Chem 274: 15020–15029.

Wu XR, Lin JH, Walz T, Häner M, Yu J, Aebi U, Sun TT (1994): Mammalian uroplakins. A group of highly conserved urothelial differentiation-related membrane proteins. J Biol Chem 269: 13716–13724.

Wu Y, Parker L, Binder N, Beckett M, Sinard J, Griffiths C, Rheinwald J (1982): The mesothelial keratins: A new family of cytoskeletal proteins identified in cultured mesothelial cells and nonkeratinizing epithelia. Cell 31: 693–703.

APPENDIX: SOURCES OF MATERIALS

Material	Catalog No.	Supplier
Aprotinin (Trasylol®)	—	Bayer
Bovine pituitary extract (BPE)	Included with KSFM 10744	GIBCO
Cholera toxin	C3012	Sigma
Collagenase type IV	C5138	Sigma
Controlled-rate cell freezers: Programmable freezer Neck-plug cooler Cooler tray	— — 5100	Planer Biomed Taylor Wharton Nalge Nunc
Cryoprotective gloves	211-002	Taylor Wharton, Jencons
Cryotubes (ampoules for cell freezing)	123280	Greiner
DMSO, tissue culture grade	D2650	Sigma
EDTA	100935V	BDH (Merck)
EGF	Included with KSFM 10744	GIBCO
Glass slides, 12 well, Teflon coated, Multispot	PH-057	Hendley, Essex
HBSS with Ca^{2+} and Mg^{2+}	24020091	GIBCO
HBSS without Ca^{2+} and Mg^{2+}	14170088	GIBCO
HEPES, 1 M solution	15630	GIBCO
KSFM	10744	GIBCO
Pastette, fine-tipped	LW 4060	Alpha Laboratories
Pastette, wide-tipped	LW 4635	Alpha Laboratories
PBS tablets	P4417	Sigma
Primaria® flasks and dishes	—	Becton Dickinson (Falcon)
Trypsin, 2.5%	T4674	Sigma
Trypsin inhibitor, soya bean	T9003	Sigma

13

Other Epithelial Cells

R. Ian Freshney

CRC Department of Medical Oncology, University of Glasgow, CRC Beatson Laboratories, Garscube Estate, Bearsden, Glasgow G61 1BD, UK. I.Freshney@beatson.gla.ac.uk.

I. INTRODUCTION

In the preceding chapters of this book, we have tried to cover methods and applications for the culture of epithelium from a range of tissues thought to be those most intensively studied. This will be unsatisfactory for some readers whose interest lies in other epithelial cells, not covered in the preceding chapters, but nonetheless important, especially to them. Epithelial tissues have received considerable attention (a) because they are the most frequent site of malignancy, (b) for their importance in transplantation studies, for example, skin and cornea, (c) as regulated transporters of nutrients, ions, gases, and toxins, and (d) as targets for potential cytotoxicity, irritation, and inflammation. It would not have been possible, within the confines of a relatively compact and inexpensive manual, to cover in detail all epithelia of potential interest to the cell culture fraternity. It is to be hoped that the techniques already described for several of the main types of epithelia may be applicable, with some modification, to other epithelial cell types; there is already considerable overlap in technology among those presented, for example, epidermal and vaginal keratinocytes. What will now be attempted is to present some background and literature references for other types of epithelia, not covered in the preceding chapters, in the hope that this will make it easier to apply and extend the protocols presented so far. In addition, some previously published protocols [Freshney and Freshney, 1996; Freshney, 2000] have been incorporated.

Some of the features common to the culture of several different epithelia have been discussed in the first chapter and will be reviewed briefly here. When some of the techniques described in the previous chapters are consulted for their potential application to the culture of a different type of epithelium, a number of common features become apparent:

(i) Disaggregation is often best achieved using collagenase or dispase, or a combination of both, and with perfusion if the tissue is lobular like liver, pancreas, or kidney. Disaggregation can also be achieved in cold trypsin (4°C overnight), and, like collagenase, this procedure does not disaggregate the epithelium completely but leaves it in small clusters, which can be separated by sedimentation velocity and which survive better when plated out (Fig. 13.1).

(ii) Attachment of the disaggregated cells, deprived of matrix by the enzymic digestion, can often be helped by coating the primary culture flask with collagen and/or fibronectin (see Chapters 8 and 11).

(iii)   Selection of epithelial cells will probably require a serum-free medium, such as MCDB 153, designed for epidermal keratinocytes but modified for a number of other cell types, such as mammary epithelium (MCDB 170; see Chapter 4), oral mucosa (see Chapter 7), and lung (see Chapter 8). Common requirements for supplements to serum-free basal media include iron-saturated transferrin, insulin, hydrocortisone, and selenium, with some other epithelia requiring ethanolamine and/or phosphoethanolamine, isoproterenol (isoprenaline) or cholera toxin (to elevate cAMP), EGF, and triiodothyronine. The concentrations of these supplements

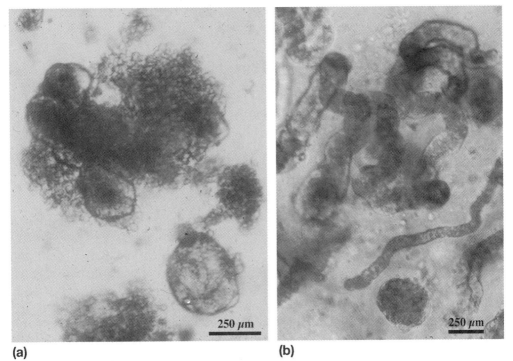

(a)   **(b)**

Fig 13.1.   Partial disaggregation of epithelial tissue (see also Plate 4). (a) Biopsy of human colonic carcinoma after 3 days at 37°C in 200 U/ml crude collagenase in Ham's F12 supplemented with Eagle's MEM amino acids, nonessential amino acids, and 10% FBS. The well-circumscribed aggregates are undisaggregated epithelium, the spongy material is stroma; further pipetting would disperse the stroma but not the epithelial aggregates, if done carefully. (b) Newborn mouse kidney, disaggregated in cold crude trypsin (0.25% in PBSA, 4°C, 18 h, followed by 20 min at 37°C, after removal of trypsin). Again, after gentle pipetting, the stroma has dispersed, leaving whole fragments of tubules and glomeruli. Reproduced from Freshney [1999] (a) and from Freshney [2000] (b) with the permission of the publisher.

may need to be modified for a new type of epithelium and additional supplements added, for example, specific growth factors such as KGF or HGF or trophic hormones such as MSH or hCG.

(iv) Subculture of the primary may also require carefully selected gentle-acting proteases such as collagenase or dispase, but by this stage, the cells may be able to tolerate trypsin, particularly purified trypsin applied at 4°C.

(v) Characterization and identification will usually be achievable with some knowledge of the cytokeratins expressed by that tissue (see Table 1.1). Several specific antibodies are available (see Appendix: Sources of Materials) directed against undifferentiated basal cells or more mature precursor cells, which would be applicable to cultured cells. Coupled with immunocytological or molecular probes for specific products or mRNAs, this should enable confirmation of identity of the cells in the culture.

2. SPECIFIC TYPES OF EPITHELIUM

This section covers a number of epithelial cell types not previously discussed, including cornea, salivary gland, nasal, esophageal, thyroid, gastric, biliary, pancreatic, renal, ovarian surface, and endometrial epithelium. It is not possible to present detailed protocols for all of these, but appropriate references should lead the reader into the literature where, hopefully, such protocols will be found.

2.1. Corneal Epithelium

Culture of corneal epithelium has been stimulated by the opportunity to provide tissue-engineered corneal grafts [Schneider et al., 1999]. In vitro models have also been used in assays for cytotoxicity [Tripathi et al., 1992; Germain et al., 1999] or irritation, for example, from contact lenses [Thakur et al., 1997], during allergic reactions [Trocme et al., 1997], or from infection [Fleiszig et al., 1996], in attempts to cut down on the Draze test, which is both expensive and subject to protest from animal rights groups. Corneal epithelium can be obtained from outdated donated tissue when deterioration in the endothelium makes it unsuitable for grafting. The cells are usually plated onto collagen [Germain et al., 1999] or fibronectin [Kamiyama et al., 1998]. KGF has been found to be mitogenic for corneal epithelium [Liu et al., 1998] and may be beneficial in serum-free media, and

PDGF and EGF stimulate epithelial cell migration [Kamiyama et al., 1998; Maldonado and Furcht, 1995]. KGF and HGF are among the paracrine factors released from the corneal stroma in response to IL-1 and IL-10 from the corneal epithelium [Weng et al., 1997], and they bind only to the epithelium. TGF-α, IL-1β, and PDGF-B are expressed exclusively by epithelial cells, and receptors are found exclusively on stroma [Li et al., 1995]. This suggests that stromal coculture may be important in recreating an accurate model in vitro.

The following protocol, written by Carolyn Cahn, has been reproduced from Freshney [2000].

Protocol 13.1. Corneal Epithelial Cells

Reagents and Materials

Sterile or Aseptically Prepared

❏ Keratinocyte serum-free medium (KGM) containing 0.15 mM calcium, human epidermal growth factor (0.1 ng/ml), insulin (5 μg/ml), hydrocortisone (0.5 μg/ml), and bovine pituitary extract (30 μg/ml)
❏ Eagle's minimal essential medium
❏ PBSA
❏ Fetal bovine serum (FBS)
❏ Trypsin-EDTA: Trypsin, 0.05%, EDTA, 0.5 mM
❏ Fibronectin-Collagen (FNC). This solution consists of fibronectin, 10 μg/ml, collagen, 35 μg/ml, with bovine serum albumin (BSA), 100 μg/ml, added as a stabilizer.
❏ Biocoat six-well plate precoated with rat-tail collagen, type I

Protocol

Primary Cultures

(a) Place donor corneas epithelial-side up on a sterile surface and cut into 12 triangle-shaped wedges, using a single cut of the scalpel and avoiding any sawing motion. Careful handling of the cornea in this manner decreases damage to the collagen matrix of the stroma and minimizes liberation of fibroblasts.

(b) Turn each corneal segment epithelial-side down and place four segments in each well of a six-well tray (precoated with rat-tail collagen, type I).

(c) Press each segment down gently with forceps to ensure

good contact between the tissue and the tissue culture surface and allow tissue to dry for 20 min.

(d) Place one drop of keratinocyte serum-free medium carefully upon each segment and incubate overnight at 37°C in 5% CO_2. Although the donor corneas received from the eye bank are stored in antibiotic-containing medium (either McCarey-Kauffman or Dexsol), all manipulations are performed under antibiotic-free conditions.

(e) The following day, add 1 ml of medium to each well.

(f) During the initial culture period, emigration of cells is observed only from the limbal region of the cornea. No cells are observed to migrate away from the central cornea or the sclera. Fibroblast outgrowth is minimized by utilizing a serum-free medium low in calcium (0.15 mM) and minimizing disruption of the collagen matrix.

(g) Remove the tissue segment with forceps 5 days after the explantation of the donor cornea slice and add 3 ml of medium.

(h) After donor tissue is removed with sterile forceps, adherent cells continue to proliferate and, within 2 wk from the time of establishment of the culture, confluent monolayers form, displaying the typical cobblestone morphology associated with epithelia. The yield is approximately $1-5 \times 10^6$ cells/cornea.

Propagation

(i) After the initial outgrowth period, feed cultures twice per week.

(j) At 70–80% confluence, rinse cells in Dulbecco's phosphate-buffered saline (PBSA) and release with trypsin-EDTA (0.05% trypsin, 0.5 mM EDTA) for 4 min at 37°C.

(k) Stop the reaction with 10% FBS in PBSA.

(l) Wash cells (centrifugation followed by resuspension in KGM), count, and plate at 1×10^4 cells/cm^2 onto tissue culture surfaces coated with FNC.

(m) Incubate at 37°C in 95% air, 5% CO_2.

(n) Exchange culture medium with fresh medium 1 day after trypsinization and reseeding.

Immediately after passage, cells appear more spindle shaped, are refractile, and are highly migratory. Within 7 days, control cultures become 70–80% confluent, continue to display a cobblestone morphology, and if allowed to become postconfluent, the cultures retain the ability to stratify in discrete areas.

Although corneal epithelial cultures can be expanded until P5 (approximately 9–10 population doublings), most of the proliferation occurs between passages 1 and 3. Approximate yields are $1-5 \times 10^6$ cells/cornea. Senescence always ensues by P5.

There are several reports of immortalization of corneal epithelial cells, mostly employing SV40 infection or transfection with the SV40 LT gene [Cahn, 2000; McDermott et al., 1998; Sharif et al., 1998; Araki-Sasaki et al., 1995] with some retention of normal function.

2.2. Salivary Gland

Interest in the salivary gland comes from several directions. It is an excellent model to study morphogenesis [Furue et al., 1999] and cell interaction during organogenesis [Lawson, 1974]. It produces EGF, probably from the mesenchyme [Venkateswaran et al., 1993; Ram et al., 1991], presumed to act in wound repair when a wound is licked, and has provided interesting models for studying IFN-γ- and TNF-α-induced cell death [Wu et al., 1994, 1996].

Human salivary gland epithelial cells from human and macaque have been cultivated using the 3T3 feeder layer system [Sabatini et al., 1991] (see Chapters 3 and 5) and from rat using serum-free selective medium, MCDB 153, with 0.03 mM Ca^{2+} and 1.0 mM pyruvate and an additional 0.76 mM isoleucine, and supplemented with 10 μg/ml bovine insulin, 5 μg/ml human transferrin, 10 μM 2-mercaptoethanol, 10 μM aminoethanol, and 1 ng/ml FGF-1 [Furue et al., 1994, 1999]. These cells show tubular morphogenesis in vitro, induced by HGF in collagen gel cultures and inhibited by activin A [Furue et al., 1999].

2.3. Nasal Mucosa

Two of the predominant differentiated cell types present in nasal epithelium are the ciliated and mucus-secreting cells, and studies with cultures of these cells have examined the harmful effects of toxins and infection on these functions. Subcultured human nasal epithelium can still be shown to express mucin genes MUC4, MUC5A,C, MUC7, and MUC8 when grown at the air-liquid interface [Bernacki et al., 1999; Yoon et al., 2000]. Morphologic evidence of differentiation was also obtained when cells were grown at the air-liquid interface and shown to be induced by high Ca^{2+} (1.8 mM) and coculture with a fibroblast-populated collagen gel [Blank et al., 1997].

Active cilia can be demonstrated in explant culture [Chen et al., 2000] where beating is promoted by TNF-α at low concentrations (0.1–1.0 ng/ml) and inhibited by high concentrations of TNF-α (10 ng/ml) and 1.0 μM dexamethasone. Cell proliferation is also regulated by cytokines where IL-1β and TGF-β have been shown to be inhibitory whereas TNF-α induces proliferation [Min et al., 1998]. Nasal epithelial cultures have also been used in studies on mucin secretion in allergy [Abdelaziz et al., 1998; Mincarini et al., 2000; Yoon et al., 2000] and on chloride, sodium, and fluid transport and transepithelial resistance cystic fibrosis [Denning et al., 1992; Jiang et al., 1993; Blank et al., 1997].

Nasal epithelium, disaggregated in 0.1% pronase, has been cultured in DMEM-F12 supplemented with 4.5 g/l glucose (25 mM), 10 ng/ml cholera toxin, and 2% Ultroser G [Hoefnagels-Schuermans et al., 1999]. A 1-h preincubation on plastic was used to reduce fibroblastic contamination. For analysis of *Staphylococcus aureus* adhesion, cells were plated at 1×10^4 cells/cm^2 on microtitration plates coated with 0.2% rat tail collagen type I (0.1 ml/cm^2). The resultant epithelial population was mainly squamous, but ciliated cells were also retained by this method [Jorrissen et al., 1989]. Further information on the culture of airway cells can be found in Chapter 8, and reference should also be made to culture methods for oral epithelium (Chapter 7).

2.4. Esophagus

The requirements of reconstructive surgery have led to the development of in vitro models suitable for grafting. These have used multilayered cultures grown on collagen sheets with embedded fibroblasts, where 8×10^5 fibroblasts/ml collagen were able to induce multilayering up to 18 cells thick [Miki et al., 1999], which survived for 14 days when xenografted into rats on a polyglycolic acid mesh frame and built up 20 layers of stratified epithelium. Esophageal epithelial cells have been cultured for 11 passages with the use of keratinocyte basal medium with pituitary extract and other supplements and 0.05 mM calcium [Oda et al., 1998]. When cells were grown in organotypic culture, expression of keratins typical of basal cells decreased and stratified keratins increased, including focal expression of K13, implying that these cultures are still capable of at least partial differentiation. Esophageal epithelium has also been grown in LHC8 serum-free medium, a derivative of MCDB 153, for use in carcinogenesis studies [Sasajima et al., 1987].

Methods for culturing human esophagus have been reviewed by Mothersill [1995]. There are also strong similarities with oral epithelium, reviewed in Chapter 7, which would make a good starting point.

2.5. Thyroid

There has been considerable interest in the utilization of thyroid epithelial cells in Ras-induced carcinogenesis [Gire et al., 1999; Gire and Wynford-Thomas, 2000] and its effect on the differentiated phenotype [Portella et al., 1999]. Thyroid epithelium has also been a good model for the demonstration of cellular polarity as a component of the differentiated phenotype, where apical secretion of thyroglobulin and basal secretion of triiodothyronine can be demonstrated on a collagen matrix in a filter well insert [Chambard et al., 1987]. Further evidence of polarization is shown by the basal location of TSH receptors and the apicolateral localization of junctional complexes. These junctional complexes allow the epithelial layer to become "tight," that is, to have a high transepithelial electrical resistance (TEER). TEER can be enhanced by TSH [Nilsson et al., 1996] and reduced by IL-1α [Nilsson et al., 1998]. TSH also elevates cAMP and stimulates the production of thyroglobulin, a marker of the differentiated phenotype [Rasmussen et al., 1996].

A heparin-binding factor from conditioned medium from a subclone of NIH3T3 cells stimulates proliferation in cultured thyroid epithelial cells [Bond et al., 1992]. This factor is probably HGF, as it has subsequently been possible to demonstrate that HGF is a potent mitogen for thyroid epithelium [Eccles et al., 1996], which correlates with the observation that HGF/met signaling is often upregulated in thyroid carcinoma. Thyroid has also been shown to be amenable to the potential for gene therapy by the demonstration that cells from primary culture can be orthotopically transplanted back into the thyroid and become incorporated into the follicles [O'Malley et al., 1993]. Transfection of thyroid epithelial cells is reviewed by Lemoine and Wynford-Thomas [1997].

Culture methods for thyroid epithelium have been reviewed by Williams and Wynford-Thomas [1997]. The following protocol is reproduced from Wynford-Thomas [1996] with the permission of the author and publisher.

The best source of tissue is freshly excised surgical material. Use macroscopically normal regions of thyroid lobectomies performed for nonmalignant disease (ideally, isolated "cold" nodules), sampling as far from the lesion as possible. Take sections for subsequent histologic confirmation of normality. Success can also be achieved with post mortem material, although viability is, of course, less reproducible.

Protocol 13.2. Culture of Human Thyroid Epithelium

Reagents and Materials

Sterile

- ❏ HBSS: ice-cold Hanks' balanced salt solution plus antibiotics (penicillin 100 U/ml, streptomycin 100 μg/ml)
- ❏ RPMI/SF: RPMI 1640 medium, serum-free, ice-cold
- ❏ RPMI/5FB: RPMI 1640 medium containing 5% FBS
- ❏ RPMI/10FB: RPMI 1640 medium containing 10% FBS
- ❏ Enzyme mixture: collagenase, 0.8 mg/ml, dispase, 1 mg/ml, in serum-free RPMI/SF
- ❏ Petri dishes, plastic, 90 mm
- ❏ Centrifuge tubes, 15 ml
- ❏ Universal container or 30- to 50-ml centrifuge tube
- ❏ Scalpel and blades, #22

Nonsterile

- ❏ Ice

Protocol

(a) Transport the sample to the tissue culture laboratory in a universal container containing ice-cold HBSS with antibiotics. Speed is not particularly crucial because viability seems to be unimpaired up to several hours in this state.

(b) Tissue is processed as follows (see summary, Fig. 13.2) in a Class II microbiological cabinet under sterile conditions. Rinse twice in HBSS to reduce blood and surface contamination.

(c) Transfer to 90-mm plastic Petri dish containing a few ml of ice-cold HBSS.

(d) Trim off any connective tissue.

(e) Dice the tissue as finely as possible ($\sim$2-mm^3 pieces) using "crossed" scalpel blades. Ensure that tissue remains moist.

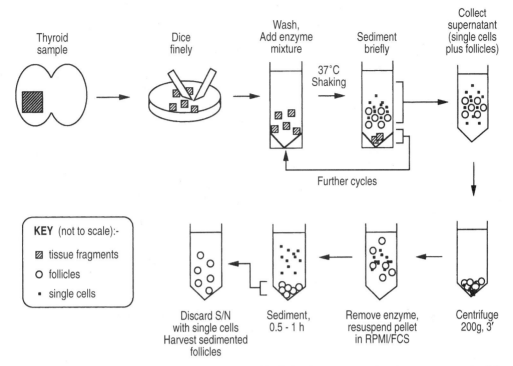

Fig 13.2. Schematic outline of primary thyroid epithelial culture preparation (some steps omitted for clarity). Reproduced from Wynford-Thomas [1996] with the permission of the publisher. S/N, supernatant; FCS, fetal calf serum.

(f) Transfer the fragments in HBSS to a suitable container (e.g., a 25-ml universal container for up to 2 g of tissue) using a 25-ml plastic pipette.

(g) Wash three times by gentle agitation in ~15 ml ice-cold RPMI/SF to remove as much blood as possible, allowing pieces to settle to allow removal of supernatant.

Note: the procedure may be temporarily suspended after this step for up to 18 h, e.g., overnight. Top up the tube with RPMI/SF, seal, and place on ice until restart.

(h) Wash fragments in a minimal volume of enzyme mixture.

(i) Resuspend in 10 volumes of prewarmed enzyme mixture.

(j) Place in 37°C static water-bath.

(k) Remove tube every 15 min and agitate gently for 20 s.

(l) After 1 h, harvest the first "fraction" from the digest as follows:

　　i) Remove tube from water bath, wipe with 70% ethanol,

agitate for 20 s, and then allow undigested tissue fragments to sediment under gravity.

ii) Using a plastic (not glass) 5-ml pipette, carefully remove and save supernatant (containing released single cells and follicles) to a 15-ml centrifuge tube (Falcon).

iii) Store on ice.

Note: Strands of sticky connective tissue, which occasionally contaminate the supernatant, can be conveniently removed by stirring with a glass Pasteur pipette.

(m) Add 10 volumes of fresh, prewarmed enzyme mixture to the remaining tissue fragments and continue the digestion process.

(n) Harvest successive "fractions" at 30-min intervals until disaggregation is complete.

(o) While digestion of the next fraction is proceeding, remove the enzyme solution from the supernatant of step (l) by centrifugation (200 g for 2 min in a swinging-bucket rotor) followed by resuspension in $\sim$1 ml of RPMI/5FB (to reduce clumping).

(p) Remove a small aliquot ($\sim$10 μl) for examination by phase-contrast microscopy. The content of follicles should reach a maximum from fraction 3 onward. Digestion is normally complete within 3–4 h.

(q) Allow the suspended mixtures of single cells and follicles (step (o)) to sediment on ice for at least 45 min.

(r) Carefully remove most of the supernatant containing single cells and erythrocytes and discard.

(s) Progressively pool the remaining pellets as successive fractions are processed.

(t) Make up to 5 ml with cold RPMI/5FB. Rinse tubes with a further 5 ml and add to first.

(u) Centrifuge (200 g, 3 min) and resuspend in required volume of RPMI/10FB. Because the preparation is in the form of follicles, cell number cannot be assessed by the usual methods. We have found the simplest guide is to estimate the volume of the follicle pellet: 1×10^6 cells occupies approximately 8 μl.

(v) Plate out and/or freeze as necessary.

Note: For freezing resuspend at $\sim$4 $\times$ 10^6 cells per ml in ice-cold RPMI/10FB, add an equal volume of 20% DMSO in FBS, and freeze at $\sim$2 $\times$ 10^6 cells per 1-ml vial using standard procedures.

Immortalization of thyroid epithelial cells can be achieved with SV40 LT [Wynford-Thomas, 1996], but immortalized cell lines tend to lose their differentiated properties [Bond et al., 1996]. Overexpression of Ras can also extend the proliferative lifespan of thyrocytes, but this is ultimately limited by a mechanism independent of telomerase [Jones et al., 2000].

2.6. Gastric Mucosa

Culture studies on epithelial cells derived from the stomach have focused mainly on toxic damage, for example, from chloroacetonitrile in drinking water [Abdel-Naim, 1999] and superoxide generation by ethanol [Hiraishi et al., 1999], and on the effect of antiinflammatory drugs on cytokine release [Shimada et al., 1999] and the effect of inflammation on the repair process. Although TGF-α induces repair of wounded monolayer cultures, this is inhibited by macrophage products such as IL-1β [Nakamura et al., 1999]. The production of IL-8 [Ogura et al., 1998; Kassai et al., 1999] and other signs of an inflammatory response, such as neutrophilic infiltration, which can be simulated with filter well inserts [Fujiwara et al., 1997], are induced by *Helicobacter pylori*. This has been shown to be inhibited by rebamipide [Kim et al., 2000], whereas some other nonsteroidal antiinflammatory drugs induce apoptosis in gastric epithelial cells [Watanabe et al., 1999] via the generation of active oxygen species.

In recent years there has also been a lot of interest in the effects of *H. pylori* after its implication in ulceration and, possibly, gastric carcinoma. Cultures have also been used to show that ammonia, hydrogen peroxide, and monochloramine produced by *H. pylori* infection inhibit wound repair [Watanabe et al., 1999]. *H. pylori* also inhibits the production of mucus at the basal level or when stimulated by IL-1β and IL-6 [Takahashi et al., 1998], and this is potentiated by IFN-γ.

Growth of gastric epithelial cells in vitro is stimulated by HGF [Kong et al., 1998], and EGF, insulin, and PDGF-BB accelerate repair of wounded monolayers by increasing proliferation and migration [Watanabe et al., 1996, 1997]. Repair of wounded monolayers is also accelerated by coating the plates with collagen type I and type IV and laminin [Fujiwara et al., 1995], and adhesion is enhanced by Matrigel and collagen IV by a protein synthesis-dependent mechanism [Rhodes et al., 1994].

Cells have been cultured from a number of mammalian species, including rat [Pu et al., 1999], rabbit [Sato et al., 1999], guinea pig [Schwenk et al., 1992; Rokutan et al., 1997], dog [Boland et al., 1990; Chen et al., 1991], and human [Rutten et al., 1996]. Rat mucosa can be detached after overnight trypsinization (0.2% trypsin with 5 mM EDTA) at 4°C, the epithelial cells disaggregated in collagenase (0.01%, type I), and the cells cultured in medium supplemented with 0.18 mM $CaCl_2$, 10 μg/ml insulin, 10 μg/ml transferrin, 1×10^{-6} M dexamethasone, 1×10^{-8} M selenious acid, 10 ng/ml cholera toxin, 1 ng/ml recombinant bovine FGF-2, and 2% FBS [Pu et al., 1999]. An alternative technique for rabbit used scraping of the fundic mucosa, followed by mincing into 2- to 3-mm^2 pieces, which were then incubated in BME containing crude type I collagenase (0.35 mg/ml) and then 1 mM EDTA, followed by two more sequential incubations in collagenase [Takahashi et al., 1995]. Cells from the last incubation were washed in HBSS and plated out in Ham's F12 supplemented with 10% heat-inactivated FBS, 15 mM HEPES buffer, 100 U/ml penicillin, 100 U/ml streptomycin, and 5 μg/ml Fungizone. Culture methods for human gastric mucosa have been reviewed [Rutten et al. 1996; Park et al., 2002] Dispase and collagenase have been used to disaggregate human gastric epithelium, giving cultures that originated primarily from small epithelial clusters grown in Ham's F12 with 10% FBS. The release of epithelial cells from mouse mucosa by chelating agents is mentioned briefly in Chapter 10, so the application of this and other techniques described in this chapter, particularly the use of collagenase/dispase and 3T3 feeder layers, should be considered. Modified MCDB 153, originally devised for selective culture of keratinocytes, has also been used successfully for oral (see Chapter 7) and bronchial (see Chapter 8) epithelia, and might be considered for this application.

2.7. Biliary Epithelium

The isolation and culture of hepatocytes are covered in detail in Chapter 11, and the establishment of a human biliary epithelial cell line has been reported by the same group [Rumin et al., 1997], based on similar methodology. Although many groups use collagenase/hyaluronidase perfusion to disaggregate liver, bile duct segments can also be recovered from liver disaggregated by treatment with trypsin at 4°C overnight in Ca^{2+}-free HBSS [Yamada et al., 1992]. Cells growing out from these disaggregated segments were positive for biliary epithelial markers γ-glutamyl transpeptidase and cytokeratin 19. Rats with bile ductular hyperplasia induced by ligation and furan yield high numbers of bile duct epithelial cells that can differentiate, when grown on collagen type I in medium with 25 ng/ml EGF and 10% FBS, into polarized epithelial cells similar to those in the ductules in vivo [Sirica and Gainey, 1997].

Biliary epithelial cells have also been isolated from disaggregated human liver and purified by immunomagnetic sorting [Leon et al., 1996]. Alternatively, biliary epithelium may be separated from hepatocytes by density centrifugation on Percoll following collagenase digestion. After a preliminary separation by differential centrifugation at 50 g without density medium, the supernatant cells were washed by centrifugation in PBS and sedimented through 10, 20, and 30% layered Percoll. Cells collected from the 20–30% interface and cultured in Williams E medium with 1 $\times$ 10^{-6} M insulin, 15 mM HEPES, 10% low-endotoxin calf serum, and 25 mg/ml human recombinant EGF showed biliary epithelial characteristics, such as cytokeratin 19 and γ-glutamyl transpeptidase, but also showed some hepatocyte markers, such as α1-antitrypsin, cytokeratins 8 and 18, and glycogen but not albumin or tyrosine aminotransferase [Nussler et al., 1999].

Biliary epithelium and hepatocytes may share a common origin as cultures have been observed in which cells in cloned colonies express markers of both phenotypes [Tateno and Yoshizato, 1996] when the cells are cultured in vitamin C, EGF, nicotinamide, and dimethyl sulfoxide. Isolated hepatocytes, grown in collagen gels in the presence of EGF, HGF, and insulin undergo morphologic differentiation similar to bile canaliculi (microvilli) and express cytokeratin 19 [Nishikawa et al., 1996]. HGF (1–50 ng/ml) and IL-6 (1–1000 U/ml) are mitogenic for biliary epithelial cells in serum-free medium [Matsumoto et al., 1994]. Immortalized lines have been established from mouse biliary epithelium [Hreha et al., 1999] and shown to be positive for cytokeratin 19 and cystic fibrosis transmembrane conductance regulator (CFTR). CFTR chloride channel function has been the subject of studies by several groups [e.g., McGill et al., 1999].

2.8. Pancreatic Epithelium

Although much of the interest in culture of cells from pancreas revolves around the β-islet cells and their role in insulin deficiency in diabetes, there has also been considerable interest in pancreatic acinar and ductal epithelium. Because of the demand for islet tissue for transplantation, the residual ductal and acinar tissue is often available. Ductal epithelial cells have been cultured satisfactorily by sieving the disaggregated pancreas, allowing ductal cysts to form, and inhibiting fibroblast growth with cholera toxin [Kolar et al., 1997]. These cells expressed the ductal markers cytokeratin 19 and CFTR. Partial digestion in collagenase followed by Ficoll density gradient centrifugation and culture on matrix-coated filter well inserts produces cultures that are predominantly ductal in phenotype, expressing the ductal markers carbonic anhydrase and CFTR but not the acinar markers amylase or chymotrypsin [Githens et al., 1994]. Acinar cells have been cultured from rat and shown to secrete zymogen granules [Anderson and McNiven, 1995] under the influence of the hormone agonist cholecystokinin octapeptide (CCK-8) at 2×10^{-9} M or $2-5$ μM 12-O-tetradecanoylphorbol-13-acetate (TPA), and other workers have shown that exclusively exocrine cell cultures, isolated with collagenase and dispase, rapidly transdifferentiate into ductal cells within 4 days of culture [Hall and Lemoine, 1992].

Both acinar [Bosco et al., 1994] and islet [Vonen et al., 1992; Cao et al., 1997] cells have been grown from pancreas, and lines have been established from the "immortomouse" [Blouin et al., 1997]. The conversion of adenoma to carcinoma has generated particular interest [Perl et al., 1998]. The following protocol for the culture of pancreatic acinar cells was contributed by Robert J. Hay and Maria das Gracas Miranda (American Type Culture Collection, 10801 University Boulevard, Manassas, VA 20110–2209) to Freshney [2000] and is reproduced here with the permission of the author and the publisher.

Protocol 13.3. Culture of Pancreatic Epithelium

Reagents and Materials

Sterile

- ❏ Conical flask, 25 ml siliconized
- ❏ Pipettes, 5 or 10 ml wide bore
- ❏ Büchner funnel
- ❏ Dialysis tubing
- ❏ Sidearm flask, 250 ml
- ❏ Polypropylene centrifuge tubes, 50 ml
- ❏ Cheesecloth
- ❏ F12K tissue culture medium with 20% bovine calf serum (F12K-CS20)
- ❏ Collagenase
- ❏ Trypsin 1:250 (Difco)
- ❏ Dextrose (Difco, No. 0155-174)
- ❏ HBSS

- HBSS without Ca^{2+} and Mg^{2+} (HCMF)
- Bovine serum albumin, fraction V
- Collagen-coated culture dishes (Biocoat, Becton Dickinson)
- Collagenase solution: Dissolve collagenase in 1× HCMF (pH 7.2) to give 1800 U/ml. Adjust to pH 7.2 and dialyze using a 12-kDa exclusion membrane for 4 h at 4°C, against 1× HCMF containing 0.2% glucose. The HBSS is discarded and this step is repeated for 16–18 h with fresh HCMF. Filter, sterilize, and store in 10- to 20-ml aliquots at −70°C or below.
- Trypsin solution: Trypsin 1:250, 0.25% in citrate buffer; 3 g/l trisodium citrate; 6 g/l NaCl, 5 g/l dextrose; 0.02 g/l phenol red; pH 7.6.

Nonsterile

- Agitating water bath
- Centrifuge

Protocol

(a) Make up the dissociation fluid fresh before use by mixing 1 part of collagenase with 2 parts of trypsin solution.

(b) Aseptically remove the entire pancreas (0.5–1.0 g) and place in F12K-CS20. Trim away mesenteric membranes and other extraneous matter and mince into 1- to 3-mm^3 fragments.

(c) Transfer to a siliconized 25-ml conical flask in 5 ml of pre-warmed dissociation fluid. Agitate at about 120 rpm for 15 min at 37°C in a shaker bath. Repeat this dissociation step two or three times with fresh fluid until most of the tissue has been dispersed.

(d) After each dissociation, allow large fragments to settle and transfer the supernate to a 50-ml polypropylene centrifuge tube with approximately 12 ml of cold F12K-CS20 to neutralize the dissociation fluid. Spin down at 600 rpm for 5 min and resuspend pellet in 5–10 ml of cold F12K-CS20. Keep cell suspension in ice.

(e) Pool the cell suspensions and pass through several layers of sterile cheesecloth in a Büchner funnel. Apply light suction by inserting the funnel stem into a vacuum flask during filtration. Take an aliquot for cell quantitation.

(f) Generally, 1–2 × 10^5 cells/mg of tissue are obtained at this step with 90–95% viability.

(g) Layer 5×10^7 to 5×10^8 cells from the resulting fluid on to the surface of 2–4 columns consisting of 35 ml of 4% cold BSA in HCMF (pH 7.2) in polypropylene 50-ml centrifuge tubes. Centrifuge at 600 rpm for 5 min. This step is critical to achieve good separation of acinar cells from islet, ductal, and stromal cells of the pancreas. Discard the supernate and repeat this fractionation step twice more, pooling and resuspending the pellets in cold F12K-CS20 after each step.

(h) Collect the cell pellets in 5–10 ml cold F12K-CS20. Take an aliquot for counting. Yields of $2–5 \times 10^4$ cells/mg of tissue are obtained, with 80–95% of the total being acinar cells. Inoculation densities can be $3 \times 10^5/cm^2$. Cells adhere as aggregate colonies within 72 h.

After cells have adhered, F12K-CS20 can be replaced by serum-free MEM with insulin (10 ng/ml), transferrin (5 ng/ml), selenium (9 ng/ml), and EGF (21 ng/ml). This medium supports pancreatic cell growth for at least 15 days without altering cell morphology. This method has been applied for studies with guinea pig and human (transplant donor) tissues. Addition of human lung irradiated feeder-fibroblasts produces a marked stimulation (up to 500%) in [^{3}H]thymidine incorporation and prolongs survival at least by a factor of two.

2.9. Kidney Epithelium

Kidney tubular epithelium has been selected using a positive immunomagnetic sort for epithelial membrane antigen (EMA) [Carr et al., 1999]. These cells were enriched for kallikrein activity, indicating their origin in the distal tubules. When grown in filter well inserts, tubular epithelial cells establish polarity as evidenced by apical secretion of IL-8, induced by IL-1 [Kruger et al., 2000] and basolateral secretion of PDGF and monocyte chemoattractant protein-1 (MCP-1) [Burton et al., 1999]. In a further increase in histotypic complexity, kidney tubular epithelial cells have been grown in hollow fiber bioreactors and show polarized transport of bicarbonate and glucose [Humes et al., 1999].

Given the kidney's role in regulating plasma concentrations of inorganic ions, it is not surprising that many studies on kidney have focused on this. A 1,25-dihydroxyvitamin D_3-dependent Ca^{2+} channel has been identified in distal tubular epithelium [Hoenderop et al., 1999], and insulin, EGF, and carbachol have been shown to regulate the Na^+–HCO_3^- cotransporter in proximal tubule epithelial cells [Ruiz et al., 1998]. Ascorbic acid has been shown to have a beneficial effect on the culture of renal proximal tubule cells (RPTC) by increasing cell density at the end of the growth phase, stimulating in vivo-like respiration and inducing differentiated properties such as Na^+-K^+-ATPase and brush-border enzyme activity [Nowak and Schnellmann, 1996].

The role of the cytotoxicity of drugs and bacterial toxins in renal failure is also amenable to in vitro analysis. Both glomerular and cortical tubular cells have been shown to be sensitive to vero-cytotoxin from *E. coli* [Williams et al., 1999], and the release of TGF-β and PDGF by proximal tubular epithelial cells has been implicated in cyclosporin-induced fibrosis [Johnson et al., 1999] and in fibronectin deposition [Burger et al., 1998]. The toxicity of drug solvents such as propylene glycol has been investigated by measuring inhibition of DNA synthesis and mitochondrial metabolic activity and increased uptake of neutral red [Morshed et al., 1998], and it has been shown that HIV-1 replicates in proximal tubule epithelial cells and induces apoptosis [Conaldi et al., 1998].

Although many workers prefer to use primary cultures of tubular or glomerular epithelium, continuous cell lines have also been used. LLC-PK1 cells, from porcine kidney, have been used to study the potential role of growth factors in kidney repair [Anderson and Ray, 1998] and renal tubulogenesis [Anderson et al., 1998] and the role of P-glycoprotein in efflux-induced resistance to antivirals after HIV infection [Leung and Bendayan, 1999]. MDCK cells, from canine kidney, have been used for studies on junctional communication [Noguchi et al., 1998] and to show that propafenone inhibits P-glycoprotein activity [Woodland et al., 1997]. A procedure for the primary culture of monkey kidney epithelium and subsequent immortalization with SV40LT has been described by Clarke [1996].

The following text and protocol for the culture of human kidney epithelium are reproduced from McAteer et al. [2000].

The kidney is a structurally complex organ in which the system of nephrons and collecting ducts is made up of numerous functionally and phenotypically distinct segments. This segmental heterogeneity is compounded by cellular diversity that has yet to be fully characterized. Some tubular segments possess several morphologically distinct cell types. In addition, evidence points to rapid adaptive changes in cell ultrastructure that may correlate with changes in cell function [Stanton et al., 1981]. This structural and cellular heterogeneity presents a challenge to the cell culturist interested in isolating pure or highly enriched cell populations. The difficulty of the problem is further compounded for studies of the human kidney, where form and access to the specimen may make some manipulations such as vascular perfusion difficult or impossible.

Several approaches have been used successfully to culture the cells of specific tubular segments. Density gradient methods are now commonly used to isolate enriched populations of enzyme-digested tubule segments and are particularly effective in establishing proximal tubule cell cultures from experimental animals [Taub et al., 1989]. Specific nephron or collecting duct segments can also be isolated by microdissection, then explanted to the culture substrate. This method, developed using experimental animals [Horster, 1979], has been applied to culture of human kidney [Wilson et al., 1985] and the cyst wall epithelium of polycystic kidneys [Wilson et al., 1986]. Immunodissection [Smith and Garcia-Perez, 1985] and immunomagnetic separation [Pizzonia et al., 1991] methods have also been developed to isolate specific nephron cell types on the basis of expression of cell type-specific ectoantigens. These elegant methods hold considerable promise for the study of specific kidney cell types in health and disease but as yet have been applied almost exclusively to studies on experimental animals. The limited (and unscheduled) availability and inconsistent form (e.g., excised pieces, damaged vasculature, lengthy postnephrectomy period) of human donor kidneys make progressive enzymatic dissociation a more practical means to isolate human kidney cells for culture.

A number of methods for primary culture of human kidney have been reported [Detrisac et al., 1984; States et al., 1986; McAteer et al., 1991]. Primary culture of tissue fragments excised from the outer cortex of human kidney provides a means to isolate cells that express many of the functional characteristics of the proximal tubule [Kempson et al., 1989]. Progressive enzymatic dissociation and crude filtration yields single cells and small aggregates of cells that when seeded at high density give rise to a heterogeneous epithelium-enriched population. Large numbers of cells can be harvested, making it practical to establish multiple replicate primary cultures or to propagate cells for frozen storage. Experience with the method shows that the functional characteristics of such primary and subcultured cells are reproducible for kidneys from different donors, and that with proper handling of specimens good cultures can be derived from kidneys following even a lengthy postnephrectomy period.

Protocol 13.4. Culture of Renal Proximal Tubule Epithelial Cells (RPTCs)

Reagents and Materials

Sterile

- ❏ Basal medium: DMEM-F12, 50:50
- ❏ Fetal bovine serum
- ❏ Complete medium: DMEM-F12 with 10% FBS
- ❏ Collagenase (type IV), 0.1%, trypsin (1:250), 0.1% solution in 0.15 M NaCl
- ❏ DNase, 0.5 mg/ml in saline
- ❏ Trypsin-EDTA solution: trypsin (1:250), 0.1%, EDTA, 1 mM
- ❏ Scalpels, tissue forceps
- ❏ Nitex screen (160 μm) (Tetko)
- ❏ Culture dishes, flasks
- ❏ Tubes, sterile 50 ml

Nonsterile

- ❏ Orbital shaker
- ❏ Centrifuge, e.g., Centra 4-B

Protocol

(a) Cut 5- to 10-mm-thick coronal slices of kidney and wash fragments in chilled basal medium.

(b) Excise fragments from outer cortex and use crossed blades to mince the tissue into 1- to 2-mm^3 pieces.

(c) Transfer approximately 5 ml of tissue fragments to a 50-ml tube containing 20 ml warm collagenase-trypsin solution. Secure the tube to the platform of an orbital shaker within a 37°C incubator.

(d) Incubate with gentle agitation for 1 h.

(e) Discard and replenish the enzyme solution.

(f) Subsequently, collect the supernatant at 20-min intervals after addition of 20 ml basal medium containing 0.05 mg/ml DNase and gentle trituration through a 10-ml pipette (10 cycles).

(g) Dilute collected supernatant with an equal volume of complete culture medium and hold on ice.

(h) Repeat (5 or more times) this cell collection procedure until fragments are spent.

(i) Pool the harvested supernatants and aliquot to 50-ml tubes.

(j) Sediment by centrifugation (1200 rpm, 15 min) and resuspend each pellet with 45 ml complete medium containing DNase.

(k) Filter the suspension through Nitex cloth (160 μm).

(l) The isolation protocol yields cell aggregates as well as single cells. Therefore, cell counting is unreliable, so use 15 ml of the filtrate to seed each 75-cm^2 flask.

(m) When approaching confluence, subculture with trypsin-EDTA, which produces a monodisperse suspension suitable for hemocytometer counting.

(n) Seed dishes or flasks at approximately 1 × 10^5 cells per cm^2.

(o) Cryopreservation is performed by routine methods using complete medium containing 10% dimethyl sulfoxide [Freshney, 2000].

A prominent variable in this method is the quality of the kidney specimen itself. Procedures for tissue procurement are impossible to standardize. Donor tissue commonly includes segments of kidney collected at surgical nephrectomy (e.g., for renal cell carcinoma) and intact kidney that is judged unsuitable (e.g., anomalous vasculature) for transplantation. These specimens are collected under different conditions (e.g., with or without perfusion, varying periods of warm ischemia, different duration of the postnephrectomy period). In addition, differences in the age and health of the donor ensure that no two specimens are equivalent. Although not all kidneys yield satisfactory cultures, this protocol has been effective for a wide variety of specimens, including fresh surgical specimens and intact, perfused kidney held on wet ice for nearly 100 h.

Cells cultured by this protocol exhibit predominantly the functional characteristics of the renal proximal tubule, including a parathyroid hormone (PTH)-inhibitable Na$^+$-dependent inorganic phosphate transport system [Kempson et al., 1989]. They also show phlorizin-sensitive Na$^+$-dependent hexose transport, exhibit a proximal tubulelike pattern of hormonal stimulation of cAMP (PTH responsive, vasopressin insensitive), and express several proximal tubule brush-border enzymes (maltase, leucine aminopeptidase, γ-glutamyl transpeptidase). These cells have also been used to demonstrate the specificity of phosphonoformic acid, an inhibitor of Na$^+$-Pi cotransport [Yusufi et al., 1986], and they serve as a model of oxidant injury in the renal tubule [Andreoli and McAteer, 1990].

2.10. Ovarian Surface Epithelial (OSE) Cells

The surface epithelium of the ovary is mesothelial in origin, and cultures can exhibit a dual epithelial-mesenchymal phenotype [Kruk et al., 1994]. It is the major site of ovarian carcinogenesis, and many studies with the normal epithelium have attempted to define events associated with malignant transformation. Gap junctional proteins (connexins) are often downregulated in transformed cells, and a comparison of normal human surface epithelial cells and various transformed cell lines showed reduced gap junctional communication and an associated reduction in the expression of Cx43 [Hanna et al., 1999]. Aberrant expression of E-cadherin in cultures of OSE cells has also been associated with genetic predisposition to ovarian cancer [Wong et al., 1999]. Cellular changes associated with metaplasia have been described in cultures of OSE cells [Wong et al., 1998].

Human OSE (HOSE) cells have been cultured from tissue scraped from the surface of the ovary of women undergoing laparotomy for benign gynecological conditions [Hillier et al., 1998] and shown to express both the α- and β-subunits of the estrogen receptor. HOSE cells show an increase in [^{3}H]thymidine incorporation in response to PDGF in vitro [Dabrow et al., 1998], and retention of the receptor PDGFR-β correlates with a prolonged relapse-free interval in ovarian cancer patients who have received chemotherapy. IL-1 and TNF also increase cell proliferation in OSE cells [Marth et al., 1996]. OSE cells in filter well inserts cultured over ovarian stromal cells showed a 50% increase in cell proliferation in response to the stromal cells [Giacomini et al., 1995]. OSE cells, as well as ovarian carcinoma cells, produce M-CSF and IL-6 in vitro [Lidor et al., 1993].

OSE cells have been cultured from rabbits by scraping off the epithelium after a 1-h incubation in 300 U/ml collagenase I. After 1 g sedimentation of organoids (equivalent to ~1 $\times$ 10^6 cells/animal) through 5% BSA, they were cultured serum-free in HL-1 medium supplemented with 4 μg/ml fibronectin [Giacomini et al., 1995]. HOSE cells have been cultured by scraping the surface of ovaries after 40-min exposure to 300 U/ml collagenase I, sedimentation of the cell clusters through 5% BSA (as for rabbit, above) and culture in medium 199 (M199) with 15% FBS. HOSE can also be propagated in a low-serum medium, OSEM-1, which is a 1:1 mixture of M199 and MCDB 105 supplemented with insulin, transferrin, ethanolamine, lipoic acid, phosphatidylcholine and Pedersen's fetuin. The further addition of highly purified (>99%) fetuin, α2-macroglobulin, and hydrocortisone resulted in a serum-free medium (OSEM-2) capable of supporting 1–2 doublings per week [Elliott and Auersperg, 1993].

HOSE cells can be immortalized with human papillomavirus E6 and E7 genes [Tsao et al., 1995] and still express cytokeratins, 7, 8, 18, and 19, although they have an increased growth rate, plating efficiency, and saturation density. Immortalization is associated with a decrease in senescence-associated β-galactosidase SA-βGal and an increased expression of telomerase [Litaker et al., 1998]. This has given rise to a continuous cell line, HOSE 6-3.

2.11. Endometrial Epithelial Cells

Much of the work reported with endometrial epithelial cell culture relates to the effects of cytokines on proliferation and on secondary cytokine or prostaglandin release. Human chorionic gonadotrophin (hCG) and luteinizing hormone (LH) increase cyclooxygenase-2 (COX-2) mRNA and protein and the secretion of PGE$_2$ via cAMP and protein kinase A signaling [Zhou et al., 1999]. Although oxytocin stimulates the production of prostaglandin PGF$_{2\alpha}$ by bovine endometrial epithelial cells, stromal cells seem to be the target for TNF-α-induced release of PGF$_{2\alpha}$ [Skarzynski et al., 2000]. Protease inhibitors, secretory leukocyte protease inhibitor (SLPI) and uterine plasmin/trypsin inhibitor (UPTI), increase DNA synthesis in endometrial epithelial cells [Badinga et al., 1999], and IGF-II stimulates epithelial cell proliferation via the type II receptor and IGFBP-2 [Badinga et al., 1999].

Primary cultures initiated from various stages of the menstrual cycle exhibit different types of differentiation that can be manipulated in vitro [Fleming, 1999] making this a valuable model for understanding hormonally regulated epithelial phenotypic changes during the menstrual cycle [Classen-Linke et al., 1998]. Insulin can be shown to induce Na$^+$ transport via the α-1 and α-2 isoforms of Na$^+$-K$^+$-ATPase [Deachapunya et al., 1999], and diethylstilbestrol increases the production of KGF by endometrial stroma, which in turn, increase proliferation in endometrial epithelial cells [Li and Rinehart, 1998]. Evidence for other paracrine effects is demonstrated by the expression of c-met (HGF receptor) in endometrial epithelium and the response of the epithelium to HGF, which stimulates cell migration, proliferation, and morphogenesis [Sugawara et al., 1997]. Enhanced epithelial proliferation is linked to increased telomerase expression [Tanaka et al., 1998; Yokoyama et al., 1998].

Filter well cultures of endometrial epithelial cells show polarized localization of VEGF at the apical surface, implying secretion into the lumen [Hornung et al., 1998] that may have significance in blastocyst implantation. Blastocysts, in turn, may influence the endometrial epithelial phenotype locally by down-regulating Muc1 otherwise up-regulated by progesterone [Hoffman et al., 1998]. Filter well inserts have also been used to demonstrate polarization of endometrial epithelial cells by electron microscopy [Classen-Linke et al., 1997] and by secretagogue-dependent ion flux [Liu et al., 1997].

REFERENCES

Abdelaziz MM, Devalia JL, Khair OA, Bayram H, Prior AJ, Davies RJ (1998): Effect of fexofenadine on eosinophil-induced changes in epithelial permeability and cytokine release from nasal epithelial cells of patients with seasonal allergic rhinitis. J Allergy Clin Immunol 101: 410–420.

Abdel-Naim AB (1999): Chloroacetonitrile-induced toxicity and oxidative stress in rat gastric epithelial cells. Pharmacol Res 40: 377–383.

Anderson KL, McNiven MA. (1995): Vesicle dynamics during regulated secretion in a novel pancreatic acinar cell in vitro model. Eur J Cell Biol 66: 25–38.

Anderson RJ, Ray CJ, Hattler BG (1998): Retinoic acid regulation of renal tubular epithelial and vascular smooth muscle cell function. J Am Soc Nephrol 9: 773–781.

Anderson RJ, Ray CJ (1998): Potential autocrine and paracrine mechanisms of recovery from mechanical injury of renal tubular epithelial cells. Am J Physiol 274: F463–F472.

Andreoli SP, McAteer JA (1990): Reactive oxygen molecule-mediated injury in endothelial and renal tubular epithelial cells in vitro. Kidney Int 38: 785–794.

Araki-Sasaki K, Ohashi Y, Sasabe T, Hayashi K, Watanabe H, Tano Y. Handa H (1995): An SV40-immortalized human corneal epithelial cell line and its characterization. Invest. Ophthalmol Vis Sci 36: 614–21.

Badinga L, Michel FJ, Simmen RC (1999): Uterine-associated serine protease inhibitors stimulate deoxyribonucleic acid synthesis in porcine endometrial glandular epithelial cells of pregnancy. Biol Reprod 61: 380–387.

Badinga L, Song S, Simmen RC, Clarke JB, Clemmons DR, Simmen FA (1999): Complex mediation of uterine endometrial epithelial cell growth by insulin-like growth factor-II (IGF-II) and IGF-binding protein-2. J Mol Endocrinol 23: 277–285.

Bernacki SH, Nelson AL, Abdullah L, Sheehan JK, Harris A, William Davis C, Randell SH (1999): Mucin gene expression during differentiation of human airway epithelia in vitro. Muc4 and muc5b are strongly induced. Am J Respir Cell Mol Biol 20: 595–604.

Blank U, Ruckes C, Clauss W, Hofmann T, Lindemann H, Munker G, Weber W (1997): Cystic fibrosis and non-cystic-fibrosis human nasal epithelium show analogous Na^+ absorption and reversible block by phenamil. Pflügers Arch 434: 19–24.

Blouin R, Grondin G, Beaudoin J, Arita Y, Daigle N, Talbot BG, Lebel D, Morisset J (1997): Establishment and immunocharacterization of an immortalized pancreatic cell line derived from the H-2Kb-tsA58 transgenic mouse. In Vitro Cell Dev Biol Anim 33: 717–726.

Boland CR, Kraus ER, Scheiman JM, Black C, Deshmukh GD, Dobbins WO 3d (1990): Characterization of mucous cell synthetic functions in a new primary canine gastric mucous cell culture system. Am J Physiol 258: G774–G787.

Bond JA, Graham GJ, Freshney M, Dawson T, Sawhney N, Williams ED, Wynford-Thomas D (1992): Detection and partial purification of a potent mitogenic factor for human thyroid follicular cells. Mol Cell Endocrinol 84(1–2): R15–R21.

Bond JA, Oddweig Ness G, Rowson J, Ivan M, White D, Wynford-Thomas D (1996): Spontaneous de-differentiation correlates with extended lifespan in transformed thyroid epithelial cells: An epigenetic mechanism of tumour progression? Int J Cancer 67: 563–572.

Bosco D, Soriano JV, Chanson M, Meda P (1994): Heterogeneity and contact-dependent regulation of amylase release by individual acinar cells. J Cell Physiol 160: 378–388.

Burger A, Wagner C, Viedt C, Reis B, Hug F, Hansch GM (1998): Fibronectin synthesis by human tubular epithelial cells in culture: Effects of PDGF and TGF-beta on synthesis and splicing. Kidney Int 54: 407–415.

Burton CJ, Combe C, Walls J, Harris KP (1999): Secretion of chemokines and cytokines by human tubular epithelial cells in response to proteins. Nephrol Dial Transplant 14: 2628–2633.

Cahn C (2000): Cornea. In Freshney RI (ed): "Culture of Animal Cells" (4th ed). New York: Wiley, pp 349–350.

Cao D, Lin G, Westphale EM, Beyer EC, Steinberg TH (1997): Mechanisms for the coordination of intercellular calcium signaling in insulin-secreting cells. J Cell Sci 110: 497–504.

Carr T, Evans P, Campbell S, Bass P, Albano J (1999): Culture of human renal tubular cells: Positive selection of kallikrein-containing cells. Immunopharmacology 44: 161–167.

Chambard M, Mauchamp J, Chaband O (1987): Synthesis and apical and basolateral secretion of thyroglobulin by thyroid cell monolayers on permeable substrate: Modulation by thyrotropin. J Cell Physiol 133: 37–45.

Chen JH, Takeno S, Osada R, Ueda T, Yajin K (2000): Modulation of ciliary activity by tumor necrosis factor-alpha in cultured sinus epithelial cells. Possible roles of nitric oxide. Hirosh J Med Sci 49: 49–55.

Chen MC, Lee AT, Soll AH (1991): Mitogenic response of canine fundic epithelial cells in short-term culture to transforming growth factor alpha and insulinlike growth factor I. J Clin Invest 87: 1716–1723.

Clarke JB (1996): Monkey kidney epithelium. In Freshney RI, Freshney MG (eds): "Culture of Immortalized Cells." New York: Wiley-Liss, pp 145–160.

Classen-Linke I, Alfer J, Hey S, Krusche CA, Kusche M, Beier HM (1998): Marker molecules of human endometrial differentiation can be hormonally regulated under in-vitro conditions as in-vivo. Human Reprod Update 4: 539–549.

Classen-Linke I, Kusche M, Knauthe R, Beier HM (1997): Establishment of a human endometrial cell culture system and characterization of its polarized hormone responsive epithelial cells. Cell Tissue Res 287: 171–185.

Conaldi PG, Biancone L, Bottelli A, Wade-Evans A, Racusen LC, Boccellino M, Orlandi V, Serra C, Camussi G, Toniolo A (1998): HIV-1 kills renal tubular epithelial cells in vitro by triggering an apoptotic pathway involving caspase activation and Fas upregulation. J Clin Invest 102: 2041–2049.

Dabrow MB, Francesco MR, McBrearty FX, Caradonna S (1998): The effects of platelet-derived growth factor and receptor on normal and neoplastic human ovarian surface epithelium. Gynecol Oncol 71: 29–37.

Deachapunya C, Palmer-Densmore M, O'Grady SM (1999): Insulin stimulates transepithelial sodium transport by activation of a protein phosphatase that increases Na-K ATPase activity in endometrial epithelial cells. J Gen Physiol 114: 561–574.

Denning GM, Ostedgaard LS, Welsh MJ (1992): Abnormal localization of cystic fibrosis transmembrane conductance regulator in primary cultures of cystic fibrosis airway epithelia. J Cell Biol 118(3): 551–559.

Detrisac CJ, Sens MA, Garvin AJ, Spicer SS, Sens DA (1984): Tissue culture of human kidney epithelial cells of proximal tubule origin. Kidney Int 25: 383–390.

Eccles N, Ivan M, Wynford-Thomas D (1996): Mitogenic stimulation of normal and oncogene-transformed human thyroid epithelial cells by hepatocyte growth factor. Endocrinology 117: 247–251.

Elliott WM, Auersperg N (1993): Growth of normal human ovarian surface epithelial cells in reduced-serum and serum-free media. In Vitro Cell Dev Biol 29A: 9–18.

Fleiszig SM, Zaidi TS, Preston MJ, Grout M, Evans DJ, Pier GB (1996): Relationship between cytotoxicity and corneal epithelial cell invasion by clinical isolates of *Pseudomonas aeruginosa*. Infect Immun 64: 2288–2294.

Fleming H (1999): Structure and function of cultured endometrial epithelial cells. Reprod Endocrinol 17: 93–106.

Freshney RI (1999): "Freshney's Culture of Animal Cells—a Multimedia Guide." New York: Wiley-Liss.

Freshney RI (2000): "Culture of Animal Cells, a Manual of Basic Technique" (4th ed). New York: Wiley.

Freshney RI, Freshney MG (1996): "Culture of Immortalized Cells." New York: Wiley.

Fujiwara Y, Arakawa T, Fukuda T, Higuchi K, Kobayashi K, Tarnawski A (1995): Role of extracellular matrix in attachment, migration, and repair of wounded rabbit cultured gastric cells. J Clin Gastroenterol 21 Suppl 1: S125–S130.

Fujiwara Y, Arakawa T, Fukuda T, Sasaki E, Nakagawa K, Fujiwara K, Higuchi K, Kobayashi K, Tarnawski A (1997): Interleukin-8 stimulates leukocyte migration across a monolayer of cultured rabbit gastric epithelial cells. Effect associated with the impairment of gastric epithelial barrier function. Dig Dis Sci 42:1210–1215.

Furue M, Okamoto T, Hayashi H, Sato JD, Asashima M, Saito S (1999): Effects of hepatocyte growth factor (HGF) and activin on the morphogenesis of rat submandibular gland-derived epithelial cells in serum-free collagen gel culture. In Vitro Cell Dev Biol Anim 35: 131–135.

Furue M, Okamoto T, Ikeda M, et al. (1994): Primitive neuroectodermal tumor cell lines derived from a metastatic pediatric tumor. In Vitro Cell Dev Biol Anim 30A: 813–816.

Germain L, Auger FA, Grandbois E, Guignard R, Giasson M, Boisjoly H Guerin SL (1999): Reconstructed human cornea produced in vitro by tissue engineering. Pathobiology. 67:140–7.

Giacomini G, Nicosia SV, Saunders BO, Fultz C, Sun X, Jasonni VM (1995): Ovarian mesothelial and extramesothelial cells in interactive culture. In Vitro Cell Dev Biol Anim 31: 300–309.

Gire V, Marshall CJ, Wynford-Thomas D (1999): Activation of mitogen-activated protein kinase is necessary but not sufficient for proliferation of human thyroid epithelial cells induced by mutant Ras. Oncogene 18: 4819–4832.

Gire V, Wynford-Thomas D (2000): RAS oncogene activation induces proliferation in normal human thyroid epithelial cells without loss of differentiation. Oncogene 19: 737–744.

Githens S, Schexnayder JA, Moses RL, Denning GM, Smith JJ, Frazier ML (1994): Mouse pancreatic acinar/ductular tissue gives rise to epithelial cultures that are morphologically, biochemically, and functionally indistinguishable from interlobular duct cell cultures. In Vitro Cell Dev Biol Anim 30A: 622–635.

Guerin SL (1999): Reconstructed human cornea produced in vitro by tissue engineering. Pathobiology 67:140–147.

Hall PA, Lemoine NR (1992): Rapid acinar to ductal transdifferentiation in cultured human exocrine pancreas. J Pathol 166: 97–103.

Handa H. (1995): An SV40-immortalized human corneal epithelial cell line and its characterization. Invest Ophthalmol Vis Sci 36: 614–621.

Hanna EA, Umhauer S, Roshong SL, Piechocki MP, Fernstrom MJ, Fanning JD, Ruch RJ (1999): Gap junctional intercellular communication and connexin43 expression in human ovarian surface epithelial cells and ovarian carcinomas in vivo and in vitro. Carcinogenesis 20: 1369–1373.

Hillier SG, Anderson RA, Williams AR, Tetsuka M (1998): Expression of oestrogen receptor alpha and beta in cultured human ovarian surface epithelial cells. Mol Human Reprod 4: 811–815.

Hiraishi H, Shimada T, Ivey KJ, Terano A (1999): Role of antioxidant defenses against ethanol-induced damage in cultured rat gastric epithelial cells. J Pharmacol Exp Ther 289: 103–109.

Hoefnagels-Schuermans A, Peetermans M, Jorissen M, Van Lierde S, Van Den Orde J, De Vos R, Van Eldere J (1999): *Staphylococcus aureus* adherence to nasal epithelial cells in a physiological in vitro model. In Vitro Cell Dev Biol Anim 35: 472–480.

Hoenderop JG, van der Kemp AW, Hartog A, van de Graaf SF, van Os CH, Willems PH, Bindels RJ (1999): Molecular identification of the apical Ca^{2+} channel in 1, 25-dihydroxyvitamin D_3-responsive epithelia. J Biol Chem 274: 8375–8378.

Hoffman LH, Olson GE, Carson DD, Chilton BS (1998): Progesterone and implanting blastocysts regulate Muc1 expression in rabbit uterine epithelium. Endocrinology 139: 266–271.

Hornung D, Lebovic DI, Shifren JL, Vigne JL, Taylor RN (1998): Vectorial secretion of vascular endothelial growth factor by polarized human endometrial epithelial cells. Fertil Steril 69: 909–915.

Horster M. (1979): Primary culture of mammalian nephron epithelia: Requirements for cell outgrowth and proliferation from defined explanted nephron segments. Pflügers Arch 382: 209–215.

Hreha G, Jefferson DM, Yu CH, Grubman SA, Alsabeh R, Geller SA, Vierling JM (1999): Immortalized intrahepatic mouse biliary epithelial cells: Immunologic characterization and immunogenicity. Hepatology 30: 358–371.

Humes HD, MacKay SM, Funke AJ, Buffington DA (1999): Tissue engineering of a bioartificial renal tubule assist device: In vitro transport and metabolic characteristics. Kidney Int 55: 2502–2514.

Jiang C, Finkbeiner WE, Widdicombe JH, McCray PB Jr, Miller SS (1993): Altered fluid transport across airway epithelium in cystic fibrosis. Science 262: 424–427.

Johnson DW, Saunders HJ, Johnson FJ, Huq SO, Field MJ, Pollock CA (1999): Cyclosporin exerts a direct fibrogenic effect on human tubulointerstitial cells: Roles of insulin-like growth factor I, transforming growth factor beta1, and platelet-derived growth factor. J Pharmacol Exp Ther 289: 535–542.

Jones CJ, Kipling D, Morris M, Hepburn P, Skinner J, Bounacer A, Wyllie FS, Ivan M, Bartek J, Wynford-Thomas D, Bond JA (2000): Evidence for a telomere-independent "clock" limiting RAS oncogene-driven proliferation of human thyroid epithelial cells. Mol Cell Biol 20: 5690–5699.

Jorissen M, Van Der Schueren B, Van Der Berghe H, Cassiman JJ (1989): The preservation and regeneration of cilia on human nasal epithelial cells cultured in vitro. Arch Otorhinolaryngol 246: 308–314.

Kamiyama K, Iguchi I, Wang X, Imanishi J (1998): Effects of PDGF on the migration of rabbit corneal fibroblasts and epithelial cells. Cornea 17: 315–325.

Kassai K, Yoshikawa T, Yoshida N, Hashiramoto A, Kondo M, Murase H (1999): *Helicobacter pylori* water extract induces interleukin-8 production by gastric epithelial cells. Dig Dis Sci 44: 237–242.

Kempson SA, McAteer JA, Al-Mahrouq HA, Dousa TP, Dougherty GS, Evan AP (1989): Proximal tubule characteristics of cultured human renal cortex epithelium. J Lab Clin Med 113: 285–296.

Kim H, Seo JY, Kim KH (2000): Inhibition of lipid peroxidation, NF-kappaB activation and IL-8 production by rebamipide in *Helicobacter pylori*-stimulated gastric epithelial cells. Dig Dis Sci 45: 621–628.

Kolar C, Caffrey T, Hollingsworth M, Scheetz M, Sutherlin M, Weide L, Lawson T (1997): Duct epithelial cells cultured from human pancreas processed for transplantation retain differentiated ductal characteristics. Pancreas 15: 265–271.

Kong W, Yee LF, Mulvihill SJ (1998): Hepatocyte growth factor stimulates fetal gastric epithelial cell growth in vitro. J Surg Res 78: 161–168.

Kruger S, Brandt E, Klinger M, Kreft B (2000): Interleukin-8 secretion of cortical tubular epithelial cells is directed to the basolateral environment and is not enhanced by apical exposure to *Escherichia coli*. Infect Immun 68: 328–334.

Kruk PA, Uitto VJ, Firth JD, Dedhar S, Auersperg N (1994): Reciprocal interactions between human ovarian surface epithelial cells and adjacent extracellular matrix. Exp Cell Res 215: 97–108.

Lawson KA (1974): Mesenchyme specificity in rodent salivary gland development: the response of salivary epithelium to lung mesenchyme in vitro. J Embryol Exp Morphol 32: 469–493.

Lemoine NR, Wynford-Thomas D (1997): Transfection and transformation of human thyroid epithelial cells. Methods Mol Biol 75: 441–447.

Leon MP, Bassendine MF, Gibbs P, Burt AD, Thick M, Kirby JA (1996): Hepatic allograft rejection: Regulation of the immunogenicity of human intrahepatic biliary epithelial cells. Liver Transpl Surg 2: 37–45.

Leung S, Bendayan R (1999): Role of P-glycoprotein in the renal transport of dideoxynucleoside analog drugs. Can J Physiol Pharmacol 77: 625–630.

Li DQ, Tseng SC (1995): Three patterns of cytokine expression potentially involved in epithelial-fibroblast interactions of human ocular surface. J Cell Physiol 163: 61–79.

Li Y, Rinehart CA (1998): Regulation of keratinocyte growth factor expression in human endometrium: Implications for hormonal carcinogenesis. Mol Carcinog 23: 217–225.

Lidor YJ, Xu FJ, Martinez-Maza O, Olt GJ, Marks JR, Berchuck A, Ramakrishnan S, Berek JS, Bast RC Jr. (1993): Constitutive production of macrophage colony-stimulating factor and interleukin-6 by human ovarian surface epithelial cells. Exp Cell Res 207: 332–339.

Litaker JR, Pan J, Cheung Y, Zhang DK, Liu Y, Wong SC, Wan TS, Tsao SW (1998): Expression profile of senescence-associated beta-galactosidase and activation of telomerase in human ovarian surface epithelial cells undergoing immortalization. Int J Oncol 13: 951–956.

Liu CQ, Fong SK, Law SH, Leung PS, Leung PY, Fu WO, Cheng Chew SB, Wong PY (1997): Electrogenic ion transport in the mouse endometrium: Functional aspects of the cultured epithelium. Biochim Biophys Acta 1356: 140–148.

Liu JJ, Shay JW, Wilson SE (1998): Characterization of a soluble KGF receptor cDNA from human corneal and breast epithelial cells. Invest Ophthalmol Vis Sci 39: 2584–2593.

Maldonado BA, Furcht LT (1995): Epidermal growth factor stimulates integrin-mediated cell migration of cultured human corneal epithelial cells on fibro-nectin and arginine-glycine-aspartic acid peptide. Invest Ophthalmol Vis Sci 36: 2120–2126.

Marth C, Zeimet AG, Herold M, Brumm C, Windbichler G, Muller-Holzner E, Offner F, Feichtinger H, Zwierzina H, Daxenbichler G (1996): Different effects of interferons, interleukin-1beta and tumor necrosis factor-alpha in normal (OSE) and malignant human ovarian epithelial cells. Int J Cancer 67: 826–830.

Matsumoto K, Fujii H, Michalopoulos G, Fung JJ, Demetris AJ (1994): Human biliary epithelial cells secrete and respond to cytokines and hepatocyte growth factors in vitro: Interleukin-6, hepatocyte growth factor and epidermal growth factor promote DNA synthesis in vitro. Hepatology 20: 376–382.

McAteer J, Kempson S, Evan A (2000): Kidney. In Freshney RI (ed): "Culture of Animal Cells, a Manual of Basic Technique" (4th ed). New York: Wiley, pp 359–361.

McAteer JA, Kempson SA, Evan AP (1991): Culture of human renal cortex epithelial cells. J Tissue Cult Methods 13: 143–148.

McDermott AM, Kern TS, Murphy CJ (1998): The effect of elevated extracellular glucose on migration, adhesion and proliferation of SV40 transformed human corneal epithelial cells. Curr Eye Res 17: 924–932.

McGill JM, Yen MS, Basavappa S, Mangel AW, Kwiatkowski AP (1995): ATP-activated chloride permeability in biliary epithelial cells is regulated by calmodulin-dependent protein kinase II. Biochem Biophys Res Commun 208: 457–462.

Miki H, Ando N, Ozawa S, Sato M, Hayashi K, Kitajima M (1999): An artificial esophagus constructed of cultured human esophageal epithelial cells, fibroblasts, polyglycolic acid mesh, and collagen. ASAIO J 45: 502–508.

Min YG, Rhee CS, Kwon SH, Lee KS, Yun JB (1998): Effects of IL-1 beta, TNF-alpha, and TGF-beta on proliferation of human nasal epithelial cells in vitro. Am J Rhinol 12: 279–282.

Mincarini M, Cagnoni F, Canonica GW, Cordone G, Sismondini A, Semino C, Pietra G, Melioli G (2000): Quantitative flow cytometric analysis of the effects of cetirizine on the expression of ICAM-1/CD54 on primary cultured nasal cells. Allergy 55: 226–231.

Morshed KM, Jain SK, McMartin KE (1998): Propylene glycol-mediated cell injury in a primary culture of human proximal tubule cells. Toxicol Sci 46: 410–417.

Mothersill C (1995): Human esophageal culture. Methods Mol Biol 43: 75–79.

Nakamura E, Takahashi S, Ishikawa M, Okabe S (1999): Inhibitory effect of macrophage-derived factors on the recovery of wounds induced in rat gastric epithelial monolayers. Biochem Pharmacol 58: 1221–1227.

Nilsson M, Husmark J, Bjorkman U, Ericson LE (1998): Cytokines and thyroid epithelial integrity: Interleukin-1alpha induces dissociation of the junctional complex and paracellular leakage in filter-cultured human thyrocytes. J Clin Endocrinol Metab 83: 945–952.

Nilsson M, Husmark J, Nilsson B, Tisell LE, Ericson LE (1996): Primary culture of human thyrocytes in Transwell bicameral chamber: thyrotropin promotes polarization and epithelial barrier function. Eur J Endocrinol 135: 469–480.

Nishikawa Y, Tokusashi Y, Kadohama T, Nishimori H, Ogawa K (1996): Hepatocytic cells form bile duct-like structures within a three-dimensional collagen gel matrix. Exp Cell Res 223: 357–371.

Noguchi M, Nomata K, Watanabe J, Kanetake H, Saito Y (1998): Changes in the gap junctional intercellular communication in renal tubular epithelial cells in vitro treated with renal carcinogens. Cancer Lett 122: 77–84.

Nowak G, Schnellmann RG (1996): L-Ascorbic acid regulates growth and metabolism of renal cells: Improvements in cell culture. Am J Physiol 271: C2072–C2080.

Nussler AK, Vergani G, Gollin SM, Dorko K, Gansauge S, Morris SM, Demetris AJ, Nomoto M, Beger HG, Strom SC (1999): Isolation and characterization of a human hepatic epithelial-like cell line (AKN-1) from a normal liver. In Vitro Cell Dev Biol Anim 35: 190–197.

Oda D, Savard CE, Eng L, Sekijima J, Haigh G, Lee SP (1998): Reconstituted human oral and esophageal mucosa in culture. In Vitro Cell Dev Biol Anim 34: 46–52.

Ogura K, Takahashi M, Maeda S, Ikenoue T, Kanai F, Yoshida H, Shiratori Y, Mori K, Mafune KI, Omata M (1998): Interleukin-8 production in primary cultures of human gastric epithelial cells induced by *Helicobacter pylori*. Dig Dis Sci 43: 2738–2743.

O'Malley BW Jr, Finegold MJ, Ledley FD (1993): Autologous, orthotopic thyroid follicular cell transplantation: a surgical component of ex vivo somatic gene therapy. Otolaryngol Head Neck Surg 108(1): 51–62.

Park J-G, Ku J-L, Kim H-S, Park S-Y, Rutten MJ (2002): Culture of Normal and Malignant Gastric Epithelium. In Culture of Human Tumor Cells, R Pfragner & RI Freshney, eds. John Wiley & Sons, New York (in press).

Perl A-K, Wilgenbus P, Dahl U, Semb H, Christofori G (1998): A causal role for E-cadherin in the transition from adenoma to carcinoma. Nature 392: 190–193.

Pizzonia JH, Gesek FA, Kennedy SM, Coutermarach BA, Bacskal BJ, Friedman PA (1991): Immunomagnetic separation, primary culture, and characterisation of cortical thick ascending limb plus distal convoluted tubule cells from mouse kidney. In Vitro Cell Dev Biol 27A: 409–416.

Portella G, Vitagliano D, Borselli C, Melillo RM, Salvatore D, Rothstein JL, Vecchio G, Fusco A, Santoro M (1999): Human N-ras, TRK-T1, and RET/PTC3 oncogenes, driven by a thyroglobulin promoter, differently affect the expression of differentiation markers and the proliferation of thyroid epithelial cells. Oncol Res 11: 421–427.

Pu H, Gao C, Yuasa T, Namba M, Kondo A, Inada K-I, Sakaguchi M (1999): Establishment and characterisation of a rat pepsin-producing gastric cell line (OUMS-37). In Vitro Cell Dev Biol Anim 35: 488–490.

Ram TG, Venkateswaran V, Oliver SA, Hosick HL (1991): Title A transforming growth factor related to epidermal growth factor is expressed by fetal mouse salivary mesenchyme cells in culture. Biochem Biophys Res Commun 175: 37–43.

Rasmussen AK, Kayser L, Perrild H, Brandt M, Bech K, Feldt-Rasmussen U (1996): Human thyroid epithelial cells cultured in monolayers. II. Influence of serum on thyroglobulin and cAMP production. Mol Cell Endocrinol 116: 173–179.

Rhodes D, Revis D, Lacy ER (1994): Extracellular matrix constituents affect superficial gastric epithelial cell adhesion. Gastroenterol Hepatol 9 Suppl 1: S72–S77.

Rokutan K, Teshima S, Miyoshi M, Nikawa T, Kishi K (1997): Oxidant-induced activation of nuclear factor-kappa B in cultured guinea pig gastric epithelial cells. Dig Dis Sci 42: 1880–1889.

Ruiz OS, Qiu YY, Cardoso LR, Arruda JA (1998): Regulation of the renal Na-HCO$_3$ cotransporter: IX. Modulation by insulin, epidermal growth factor and carbachol. Regul Pept 77: 155–161.

Rumin S, Loreal O, Drenou B, Turlin B, Rissel M, Campion JP, Gripon P, Strain AJ, Clement B, Guguen-Guillouzo C (1997): Patterns of intermediate filaments, VLA integrins and HLA antigens in a new human biliary epithelial cell line sensitive to interferon-gamma. J Hepatol 26: 1287–1299.

Rutten MJ, Campbell DR, Luttropp CA, Fowleer WM, Hawkey MA, Boland RC, Kraus ER, Sheppard BC, Crass RA, Deeveney KE, Deveney CW (1996): A method for the isolation of human gastric mucous epithelial cells for primary cell culture: A comparison of biopsy vs. surgical tissue. Methods Cell Sci 18: 269–281.

Sabatini LM, Allen-Hoffmann BL, Warner TF, Azen EA (1991): Serial cultivation of epithelial cells from human and macaque salivary glands. In Vitro Cell Dev Biol 27A: 939–948.

Sasajima K, Willey JC, Banks-Schlegel SP, Harris CC (1987): Effects of tumor promoters and cocarcinogens on growth and differentiation of cultured human esophageal epithelial cells. J Natl Cancer Inst 78: 419–423.

Sato K, Watanabe S, Yoshizawa T, Hirose M, Murai T, Sato N (1999): Ammonia, hydrogen peroxide, and monochloramine retard gastric epithelial restoration in rabbit cultured cell model. Dig Dis Sci 44: 2429–2434.

Schneider AI, Maier-Reif K, Graeve T (1999): Constructing an in vitro cornea from cultures of the three specific corneal cell types. In Vitro Cell Dev Biol Anim 35: 515–526.

Schwenk M, Linz C, Rechkemmer G (1992): First pass effect of 1-naphthol in the gastric mucosa. Studies with isolated epithelium and cultured mucous cells of guinea pig. Biochem Pharmacol 43: 771–774.

Sharif NA, Wiernas TK, Griffin BW, Davis TL (1998): Pharmacology of [^{3}H]-pyrilamine binding and of the histamine-induced inositol phosphates generation, intracellular Ca^{2+}-mobilization and cytokine release from human corneal epithelial cells. Br J Pharmacol 125: 1336–1344.

Shimada T, Watanabe N, Ohtsuka Y, Endoh M, Kojima K, Hiraishi H, Terano A (1999): Polaprezinc down-regulates proinflammatory cytokine-induced nuclear factor-kappaB activation and interleukin-8 expression in gastric epithelial cells. J Pharmacol Exp Ther 291: 345–352.

Sirica AE, Gainey TW (1997): A new rat bile ductular epithelial cell culture model characterized by the appearance of polarized bile ducts in vitro. Hepatology 26: 537–549.

Skarzynski DJ, Miyamoto Y, Okuda K (2000): Production of prostaglandin f(2alpha) by cultured bovine endometrial cells in response to tumor necrosis factor alpha: Cell type specificity and intracellular mechanisms. Biol Reprod 62: 1116–1120.

Smith WL, Garcia-Perez A (1985): Immunodissection: Use of monoclonal antibodies to isolate specific types of renal cells. Am J Physiol 248: F1–F7.

Smoot DT, Sewchand J, Young K, Desbordes BC, Allen CR, Naab T (2000): A method for establishing primary cultures of human gastric epithelial cells. Methods Cell Sci 22: 89–99.

Stanton BA, Biemesderfer D, Wade JB, Giebisch G (1981): Structural and functional study of the rat distal nephron: Effects of potassium adaptation and depletion. Kidney Int 19: 36–48.

States B, Foreman J, Lee J, Segal S (1986): Characteristics of cultured human renal cortical epithelia. Biochem Med Metab Biol 36: 151–161.

Sugawara J, Fukaya T, Murakami T, Yoshida H, Yajima A (1997): Hepatocyte growth factor stimulated proliferation, migration, and lumen formation of human endometrial epithelial cells in vitro. Biol Reprod 57: 936–942.

Takahashi M, Ota S, Shimada T, Hamada E, Kawabe T, Okudaira T, Matsumura M, Kaneko N, Terano A, Nakamura T (1995): Hepatocyte growth factor is the most potent endogenous stimulant of rabbit gastric epithelial cell proliferation and migration in primary culture. J Clin Invest 95: 1994–2003.

Takahashi S, Nakamura E, Okabe S (1998): Effects of cytokines, without and with *Helicobacter pylori* components, on mucus secretion by cultured gastric epithelial cells. Dig Dis Sci 43: 2301–2308.

Tanaka M, Kyo S, Takakura M, Kanaya T, Sagawa T, Yamashita K, Okada Y, Hiyama E, Inoue M (1998): Expression of telomerase activity in human endometrium is localized to epithelial glandular cells and regulated in a menstrual phase-dependent manner correlated with cell proliferation. Am J Pathol 153: 1985–1991.

Tateno C, Yoshizato K (1996): Growth and differentiation in culture of clonogenic hepatocytes that express both phenotypes of hepatocytes and biliary epithelial cells. Am J Pathol 149: 1593–1605.

Taub ML, Yang SI, Wang Y. (1989): Primary rabbit proximal tubule cell cultures maintain differentiated functions when cultured in a hormonally defined serum-free medium. In Vitro Cell Dev Biol 25: 770–775.

Thakur A, Clegg A, Chauhan A, Willcox MD. (1997): Modulation of cytokine production from an EpiOcular corneal cell culture model in response to *Staphylococcus aureus* superantigen. Aust NZ J Ophthalmol 25 Suppl 1: S43–S45.

Tripathi BJ, Tripathi RC, Kolli SP (1992): Cytotoxicity of ophthalmic preservatives on human corneal epithelium. Lens Eye Toxicol Res 9: 361–375.

Trocme SD, Hallberg CK, Gill KS, Gleich GJ, Tyring SK, Brysk MM (1997): Effects of eosinophil granule proteins on human corneal epithelial cell viability and morphology. Invest Ophthalmol Vis Sci 38: 593–599.

Tsao SW, Mok SC, Fey EG, Fletcher JA, Wan TS, Chew EC, Muto MG, Knapp RC, Berkowitz RS (1995): Characterization of human ovarian surface epithelial cells immortalized by human papilloma viral oncogenes (HPV-E6E7 ORFs). Exp Cell Res 218: 499–507.

Venkateswaran V, Oliver SA, Ram TG, Hosick HL (1993): Salivary mesenchyme cells that induce mammary epithelial hyperplasia up-regulate EGF receptors in primary cultures of mammary epithelium within collagen gels. Growth Regul 3(2): 138–145.

Vonen B, Bertheussen K, Giaever AK, Florholmen J, Burhol PG (1992): Effect of a new synthetic serum replacement on insulin and somatostatin secretion from isolated rat pancreatic islets in long term culture. J Tissue Cult Methods 14: 45–50.

Watanabe S, Hirose M, Iwazaki R, Miwa H, Sato N (1997): Effects of epidermal growth factor and insulin on migration and proliferation of primary cultured rabbit gastric epithelial cells. J Gastroenterol 32: 573–578.

Watanabe S, Wang XE, Hirose M, Oide H, Kitamura T, Miwa H, Miyazaki A, Sato N (1996): Platelet-derived growth factor accelerates gastric epithelial restoration in a rabbit cultured cell model. Gastroenterology 110(3): 775–779.

Watanabe S, Yoshizawa T, Hirose M, Murai T, Sato N (1999): Ammonia, hydrogen peroxide, and monochloramine retard gastric epithelial restoration in rabbit cultured cell model. Dig Dis Sci 44: 2429–2434.

Weng J, Mohan RR, Li Q, Wilson SE (1997): IL-1 upregulates keratinocyte growth factor and hepatocyte growth factor mRNA and protein production by cultured stromal fibroblast cells: interleukin-1 beta expression in the cornea. Cornea 16: 465–471.

Williams JM, Boyd B, Nutikka A, Lingwood CA, Barnett Foster DE, Milford DV, Taylor CM (1999): A comparison of the effects of verocytotoxin-1 on primary human renal cell cultures. Toxicol Lett 105: 47–57.

Williams DW, Wynford-Thomas D (1997): Human thyroid epithelial cells. Methods Mol Biol 75: 163–172.

Wilson PD, Dillingham MA, Breckon R, Anderson RJ (1985): Defined human renal tubular epithelia in culture: Growth, characterization, and hormonal response. Am J Physiol 248: F436–F443.

Wilson PD, Schrier RW, Breckon RD, Gabow PA (1986): A new method for studying human polycystic kidney disease epithelia in culture. Kidney Int 30: 371–378.

Wong AS, Leung PC, Maines-Bandiera SL, Auersperg N (1998): Metaplastic changes in cultured human ovarian surface epithelium. In Vitro Cell Dev Biol Anim 34: 668–670.

Wong AS, Maines-Bandiera SL, Rosen B, Wheelock MJ, Johnson KR, Leung PC, Roskelley CD, Auersperg N (1999): Constitutive and conditional cadherin expression in cultured human ovarian surface epithelium: Influence of family history of ovarian cancer. Int J Cancer 81: 180–188.

Woodland C, Verjee Z, Giesbrecht E, Koren G, Ito S (1997): The digoxin-propafenone interaction: Characterization of a mechanism using renal tubular cell monolayers. J Pharmacol Exp Ther 283: 39–45.

Wu AJ, Chen ZJ, Tsokos M, O'Connell B, Ambudkar IS, Baum BJ (1996): Interferon-gamma induced cell death in a cultured human salivary gland cell line. J Cell Physiol 167: 297–304.

Wu AJ, Kurrasch RH, Katz J, Fox PC, Baum BJ, Atkinson JC (1994): Effect of tumour necrosis factor-alpha and interferon-gamma on the growth of a human salivary gland cell line. J Cell Physiol 16: 217–226.

Wynford-Thomas D (1996): In Freshney RI, Freshney MG (eds): "Culture of Immortalized Cells." New York: John Wiley & Sons, pp 183–201.

Yamada G, Sawada N, Mori M (1992): Evidence for fluid-phase pinocytosis of extrahepatic bile duct cells isolated from normal rats in culture. Cell Struct Funct 17: 67–75.

Yokoyama Y, Takahashi Y, Shinohara A, Lian Z, Xiaoyun W, Niwa K, Tamaya T (1998): Telomerase activity is found in the epithelial cells but not in the stromal cells in human endometrial cell culture. Mol Hum Reprod 4: 985–989.

Yoon JH, Kim KS, Kim SS, Lee JG, Park IY (2000): Secretory differentiation of serially passaged normal human nasal epithelial cells by retinoic acid: expression of mucin and lysozyme. Ann Otol Rhinol Laryngol 109: 594–601.

Yusufi ANK, Szczepanska-Konkel M, Kempson SA, McAteer JA, Dousa TP (1986): Inhibition of human renal epithelial Na^+/Pi cotransport by phosphonoformic acid. Biochem Biophys Res Commun 139: 679.S–686.S

Zhou XL, Lei ZM, Rao CV (1999): Treatment of human endometrial gland epithelial cells with chorionic gonadotropin/luteinizing hormone increases the expression of the cyclooxygenase-2 gene. J Clin Endocrinol Metab 84: 3364–3377.

APPENDIX: SOURCES OF MATERIALS

Material	Catalog no.[1]	Supplier
Aminoethanol (see ethanolamine)		
Agitating water bath	M5B#11-22-1	Baker
Bovine serum albumin (BSA)	A 3156	Sigma
Centrifuge	Centra 4-B	IEC (see ThermoQuest or ThermoLife)
Collagen Bovine type I Human type I Rat tail type I	 40231 12166-013 C 7661	 Becton Dickinson GIBCO BRL Sigma
Collagenase I[2] Collagenase IV	17100-017 C 2674 CLS —	GIBCO Sigma Boehringer Mannheim (see Roche) Worthington Worthington
Cytokeratin antibodies		Santa Cruz Biotechnology; Zymed Laboratories; Lab Vision; Dako
DNase I	D4263	Sigma
EDTA	E 6758	Sigma
EGF, human, recombinant		Pepro Tech Inc, Rocky Hill, NJ
Ethanolamine	E 0135	Sigma
FGF, human recombinant		Upstate Biotechnology
Fibronectin	40008 F 2518	Becton Dickinson Biofluids Sigma
Insulin, bovine	I 6634	Sigma
Keratinocyte growth medium KGM-2 K-SFM	 BW 3107 17005-022	 BioWhittaker GIBCO
2-Mercaptoethanol	M 7522	Sigma
MCDB 153	M 7403	Sigma
Nitex screen	160 μm	Tekto
Orbital shaker		Bellco

Appendix continues

Material	Catalog no.[1]	Supplier
Pipettes, wide bore		Bellco
Pronase	P 8811	Sigma
Transferrin, human	T 2158	Sigma
Trypsin, 1:250	T4799	Sigma
Ultroser G	15950-017	GIBCO

[1]These catalog numbers are suggestions only. In some cases, it may be necessary to try alternative types or suppliers.

[2]Batches of collagenase vary considerably in purity and activity. When attempting a new procedure it is often advisable to try several batches of differing purity and from different suppliers. The purest collagenase is not always the best, as other proteases may contribute.

Suppliers

Abbott Diagnostics Div: 100 Abbott Park Rd., Abbott Park, IL 60064-3500 USA; 5440 Patrick Henry Dr., Santa Clara, CA 95054, USA.

Alpha: Alpha Laboratories, 40 Parham Drive, Eastleigh, Hampshire SO50 4NU, UK. *alphalabs@ukbusiness.com*, *www.ukbusiness.com/alphalabs*.

Alfa Inorganics: See Fisher Corporation.

ATCC (American Type Culture Collection): 10801 University Boulevard, Manassas, VA 20110-2209, USA. *www.atcc.org*.

Austral Biologicals: 125 Ryan Industrial Ct., Suite 207, San Ramon, CA 94583, USA *sales@australbio.com*; *www.australbiologicals.com*.

Baker Co., Inc: Old Sandford Airport Rd., P.O. Drawer E, Sanford, ME 04073, USA.

Baker Chem. Co: See J.T. Baker.

Bayer Vital, Bayer AG Geschaftsbereich Pflansenschutz: Zentrum Landwirtschaft Monheim Div., Alfred-NobelStrasse 50, D-509 Leverkusen-Bayerwerk, Germany.

Bayer: Bayer PLC, Bayer House, Strawberry Hill, Newbury RG14 1JA, UK; Diagnostics Division, 511 Benedict Ave, Tarrytown, NY 10591, USA. *www.bayermhc.com/*.

Beckman Coulter Corporation: P.O. Box 169015, Miami, FL 33116-9015, USA. *www.BeckmanCoulter.com*.

Becton Dickinson, Collaborative Biomedical Products Division: Labware Div., 2 Oak Park, Bedford, MA 01730, USA. *www.bd.com/labware*.

Becton Dickinson: 1 Becton Drive, Franklin Lakes, NJ 07417-1886, USA. *mail@bdl.com*; *www.bd.com/labware*.

Bellco Glass Inc: 340 Edrudo Rd., Vineland, NJ 08360-3493, USA. *sales@bellcoglass.com*; *www.bellcoglass.com*.

Bibby Sterilin Ltd: Tilling Drive, Stone, Staffordshire ST15 0SA, UK. *sterilin@bibby-sterilin.com*; *www.bibby-sterilin.com*.

Biochrom: Leonorenstr. 2-6, D-12247 Berlin, Germany; *www.biochrom.de/*; *info@biochrom.de*.

Biofluids Inc: 1146 Taft St., Rockville, MD 20850, USA; *biofluids@erols.com*.

BioWhittaker: 8830 Biggs Ford Road, P.O. Box 127, Walkersville, MD 21793-0127, USA. *sales@biowhittaker.com*; *www.biowhittaker.com*.

Britannia Pharmaceuticals: 41-51 Brighton Road, Redhill, Surrey RH1 6YS, UK. *enquiries@britannia-pharm.co.uk*; *www.britannia-pharm.co.uk*.

Boehringer Mannheim: Sandhofer Str 116, P.O. Box 310120, D-68298 Mannheim 31, Germany; Bell Lane Lewes West Sussex BN7 1LG, UK; 9115 Hague Rd., P.O. Box 50414, Indianapolis, IN 46250, USA. *biochemts_us@bmc.boehringer-mannheim.com*. *www.biochem.boehringer-mannheim.com*. (see also Roche Diagnostics).

Celtrix Laboratories: 3055 Patrick Henry Drive, Santa Clara CA-95054-1815, USA. *www.informagen.com/Resource_Informagen/Full/3024.html*; *info@NHBiotech.com*.

Clonetics: See BioWhittaker.

Cohesion Technologies: 2500 Faber Place, Palo Alto, CA 94303, USA; Fax: (650) 320-5522.

Collaborative Biomedical Products: See Becton Dickinson

Collagen Corp.: 2500 Faber Place, Palo Alto, CA 94303, USA. *www.collagen.com/*.

Coriell Institute for Medical Research: 401 Haddon Avenue, Camden, NJ 08103, USA. http://arginine.umdnj.edu/; *www.locus.umdnj.edu/*.

Corning: One Riverfront Plaza, Corning, NY 14831-0001, USA. *labware@corning.com*. *www.scienceproducts.corning.com*.

Corning Separations: 45 Nagog Park, Acton, MA 01720, USA. *separations@corning.com*; *www.corningcostar.com*.

CP Pharmaceuticals Ltd: Ash Road North, Wrexham Industrial, Estate, Wrexham LL13 9UF, Wales, UK; *www.cppharma.co.uk/home.htm*.

Dako Corp: 6392 Via Real, Carpinteria, CA 93013, USA; *www.dakousa.com/*.

Dako Ltd: Marketing Dept., Denmark House, Angel Drove, Ely, Cambridge, CB2 4ET, UK; *www.dako.co.uk*.

Dako A/S: Produktionsvej 42, DK-2600 Glostrup, Denmark.

ECACC (European Collection of Cell Cultures): CAMR Div., Porton Down, Wilts., Salisbury SP4 0JG, UK; *ecacc@camr.org.uk*; *www.camr.org.uk*.

Elkins-Sinn: Cherry Hill, NJ 08003-4099, USA.

Fa. Greiner and Söhne: P.O. Box 1320, D-72622 Nürtingen, Germany.

Falcon: Becton Dickinson, Between Towns Road, Cowley, Oxford OX4 3LY, UK; 1 Becton Drive, Franklin Lakes, NJ 07417-1886, USA. *mail@bdl.com*; *www.bd.com/labware*.

Fisher: 2000 Park Ln, Pittsburgh, PA 15275, USA. *www.fisher1.com*.

Funakoshi Pharmaceutical Company: 2-3 Surugadai, Tokyo, Japan.

Gelman Sciences: See Pall Gelman.

Gemini Bio-Products: 5115-M Douglas Fir Rd. Calabasas, CA 91302, USA.

GIBCO: See Invitrogen.

GlaxoSmithKline: SmithKline Beecham Consumer Healthcare, Great West Road, Greenford, Middlesex TW8 9BD, UK. *ukpharma.customer@sb.com*; http://uk.gsk.com/.

GlaxoSmithKline: Five Moore Dr., P.O. Box 13398, Research Triangle Park, NC, 27709, USA. http://us.gsk.com/.

Glen Research Corp: 22825 Davis Drive, Sterling, VA 20164, USA. *support@glenres.com*; *www.glenres.com/*.

GMI: 3874 Bridgewater Drive, St. Paul, MN, 55123, USA. *rpowell@gmi-inc.com*; *www.gmi-inc.com/Products.*

Greiner Labortechnik Ltd: Brunel Way, Stonehouse, Gloucestershire, UK. Tel 01453 825255; Fax 01453 826266; *sales@greiner-lab.de*; *http://www.greiner-lab.com.*

Hammond Cell Technology: P.O. Box 147, Alameda, CA 94501, USA *hctculture@aol.com*; *www.hammondcelltech.com.*

Hendley: CA Hendley, Oakwood Hill Industrial Estate, Loughton, Essex IG10 3TZ, UK.

HyClone Laboratories, Inc: 1725 South HyClone Road, Logan, UT 84321-6212, USA. *www.hyclone.com.*

IBFB (Institut für Biomedizinische Forschung und Beratung): Leipzig, Germany.

Invitrogen (GIBCO BRL): 3 Fountains Drive, Inchinnan Business Park, Paisley PA4 9RF, Scotland, UK.; 1600 Faraday Avenue, Carlsbad, CA 92008, USA; *tech_service@invitrogen.com*; *www.invitrogen.com*

Johnson Matthey Co: See Fisher Scientific Co.

JRH Biosciences: 13804 West 107th Street, Lenexa, KS 66215, USA. *www.jrhbio.com/.*

J.T.Baker: Mallinckrodt Baker, Inc., 222 Red School Lane, Phillipsburg NJ 08865, USA. *infombi@mkg.com*; *www.jtbaker.com*

Kebo Care–Niko: Jernholmen 41, 2650 Hvidovre, Denmark.

KeLab: KeLab, Karl-Erik Ljung AB, Knipplagatan 10, 414 74 Göteborg, Sweden. *www.kelab-biochem.com/kontakt.html*; *goteborg@kelab-biochem.com.*

Lab Vision Corporation: 47770 Westinghouse Drive, Fremont, CA 94539, USA; *neomark@ix.netcom.com*; *www.labvision.com.*

LGC (Laboratory of the Government Chemist): Queens Road, Teddington, Middlesex TW11 0LY, UK. *info@lgc.co.uk*; *www.lgc.co.uk.*

Life Technologies: see Invitrogen.

List Biological Laboratories: 501-B Vandell Way, Campbell, CA 95008, USA. *info@listlabs.com*; *www.listlabs.com.*

Merck Eurolab Ltd: Merck House, Poole, Dorset BH15 1TD, UK. *www.merckeurolab.ltd.uk.*

Merck Inc: P.O. Box 2000, RY7-220, Rahway, NJ 07065, USA. *www.merck.com/.*

Merck KGaA: Frankfurter Strasse 250, Postfach 4119, D-64293 Darmstadt, Germany.

Miles Scientific: See Bayer.

Millipore: 80 Ashby Rd., Bedford, MA 01730, USA. *www.millipore.com/.*

Millipore (U.K.), Ltd: The Boulevard, Blackmoor Lane, Watford, Herts., WD1 8YW, UK. *www.millipore.com/.*

Miltenyi Biotec GmbH: Friedrich-Ebert-Strasse 68, 51429 Bergisch Gladbach, Germany. *macs@miltenyibiotec.de. www.MiltenyiBiotec.com.*

Miltenyi Biotech Inc: 12740 Earhart Avenue, Auburn, CA 95602, USA. *macs@miltenyibiotec.com. www.MiltenyiBiotec.com.*

Miltenyi Biotec Ltd: Almac House, Church Lane, Bisley, Surrey GU24 9DR, UK. *macs@miltenyibiotec.co.uk. www.MiltenyiBiotec.com.*

Nalge Nunc International: P.O. Box 20365, Rochester, NY 14602-0365, USA. *intlmktg@nalgenunc.com. www.nalgenunc.com.*

NEN Life Sciences: 549 Albany St., Boston, MA 02118, USA. *techsupport@nen.com; www.nen.com.*

NEN Life Science Products: P.O. Box 66, Hounslow TW5 9RT, UK. *www.nen.com.*

Nuclepore Co: Falkenweg 47, Tübingen, Germany; Victoria House, 28-38 Desborough Street, High Wycombe, Bucks., HP11 2NF, UK (*see also Corning Separations*).

Nunc: see Nalge Nunc.

Pall Gelman, Laboratory Products Div: 600 S. Wagner Rd., Ann Arbor, MI 48103, USA. *gelmanlab@pall.com. www.pall.com/gelman.*

Parke-Davis: D-10562 Berlin, Germany; Fax: (++)49 [0]761 5183070.

Pel-Freez Clinical Systems Inc: 9099 N. Deerbrook Tr., Brown Deer, WI 53223, USA. *www.pel-freez.com.*

Pepro Tech, Inc: Princeton Business Park, 5 Crescent Ave., Rocky Hill, NJ 08553-0275, USA. *info@peprotech.com; www.peprotech.com.*

Promega Biotech: 2800 Woods Hollow Rd., Madison, WI 53711, USA. *custserv@promega.com; www.promega.com.* Delta House, Chilworth Research Centre, Southampton SO16 7NS, UK. *ukmarketing@uk.promega.com; www.euro.promega.com/uk.*

R & D Systems: 614 McKinley Place, NE, Minneapolis, MN 55413, USA. *info@rndsystems.com.*

Raymond A. Lamb: 7304 Vanclaybon Drive, Apex, NC 27502, USA. *sales.na@ralamb.com; www.ralamb.net/information.html.*

Raymond A. Lamb Ltd: Units 4 & 5 Parkview Industrial Estate, Lottbridge Grove, Eastbourne, East Sussex BN23 6QE, UK. *sales@ralamb.com; www.ralamb.co.uk/.*

Renner KG: Riedstr. 6, D-67125 Darmstadt, Germany.

Research Organics Inc: 4353 E. 49th St., Cleveland, OH 44125-1083, USA. *www.resorg.com; info@resorg.com.*

ROBOZ Surgical Instruments: 9210 Corporate Blvd., Ste. 220, Rockville, MD 20850, USA. *maryfrances@starpower.net; www.roboz.com.*

Roche Laboratories: 340 Kingsland St., Nutley, NJ 07110, USA.

Sakura: See Raymond A. Lamb.

Santa Cruz Biotechnology: 2161 Delaware Ave., Santa Cruz, CA 95060-5706, USA. *scbt@netcom.com; www.scbt.com.*

Schärfe System: Krammerstrasse 22, D-72764 Reutlingen, Germany. *mail@CASY-Technology.com. www.CASY-Technology.com.*

Scientific Laboratory Supplies Ltd: Unit 27, Nottingham South & Wilford Industrial Estate, Ruddington Lane, Wilford, Nottingham NG11 7EP, UK.

Sefar America: 333 S. Highland Ave., Briarcliff Manor, NY 10510, USA. *www.sefaramerica.com.*

Seikagaku America Inc.: 704 Main St., Falmouth, MA 02540, USA. . *dnaman@seikagaku.com; www.seikagaku.com.*

Serva Feinbiochemica GmBH: P.O. Box 105260, D-69042 Heidelberg, Germany.

Sigma-Aldrich: P.O. Box 14508, St. Louis, MO 63178. *sigma-techserv@sial.com*; *www.sigma.sial.com.*

Sigma-Aldrich Company Ltd: Fancy Road, Poole, Dorset BH12 4QH, UK. *ukcustsv@vns.sial.com.*

Spectrum Europe B.V: P.O. Box 3262, 4800 Breda, The Netherlands.

Spectrum Laboratories Inc: 18617 Broadwick St., Rancho Domingas, CA 90220, USA. *webmaster@spectrapore.com*; *dkamps@spectrumlabs.com*; *www.spectrapore.com*; *www.spectrumlabs.com.*

Sorvall: See GMI.

Taylor-Wharton RDF Cryogenics: P.O. Box 568, Theodore, AL 36590-0568, USA. *twsales@taylor-wharton.com*; *www.taylor-wharton.com/cryohom.htm.*

TCS Biologicals: Botolph Claydon, Buckingham MK18 2LR, UK. *office@tcsgroup.co.uk.*

Techno Plastic Products AG: Zollstrasse 155, CH-8219 Trasadingen, Switzerland. *info@tpp.ch*; *sales@tpp.ch*; *customservice@tpp.ch*; *www.tpp.ch.*

Tekto Inc: See Sefar America.

Thermo Life Sciences: Unit 5, The Ringway Centre, Edison Road, Basingstoke, Hampshire RG21 6YH, UK. *ukservice@tmquest.com*; *www.thermo-lifesciences.co.uk*

ThermoQuest Scientific Equipment: 71 Bradley Road, Suite 10B, Madison, CT 06443, USA. *www.thermoquest.com.*

UCSF Cell Culture Facility: (415) 476-1450.

Unipath, Oxoid Division: 800 Proctor Avenue, Ogdensburg, NY 13669-2205, USA.

Upstate Biotechnology: 1100 Winter Street, Suite 2300, Waltham, MA 02451, USA. *info@upstatebiotech.com*; *www.upstatebiotech.com.*

Vector Laboratories: 30 Ingold Road, Burlingame, CA 94010, USA. *www.vectorlabs.com.* 3 Accent Park, Blakewell Road, Orton Southgate, Peterborough PE2 6XS, UK.

VWR Scientific Products: 1310 Goshen Pkwy, West Chester, PA 19380, USA; *www.vwrsp.com.*

Whatman Inc: 9 Bridewell Place, Clifton, NJ 07014, USA. *info@whatman.com*; *www.whatman.com.*

Whatman International Ltd: Whatman House, St Leonard's Road, 20/20 Maidstone, Kent, ME16 0LS, UK. *information@whatman.co.uk*; *www.whatman.plc.uk.*

Worthington Biochemical Corp: 730 Vassar Avenue, Lakewood, NJ 08701, USA. *www.worthington-biochem.com.* U.K. Agents: Lorne Biochemicals, Reading, Berks., UK.

Zymed Laboratories Inc: 458 Carlton Court, South San Francisco, CA 94080, USA. *tech@zymed.com*; *www.zymed.com.*

Index